THE NEW REPRODUCTIVE ORDER

The New Reproductive Order

Technology, Fertility, and Social Change around the Globe

Edited by

Sarah Franklin *and* Marcia C. Inhorn

NEW YORK UNIVERSITY PRESS

New York

NEW YORK UNIVERSITY PRESS
New York
www.nyupress.org

© 2025 by New York University

Please contact the Library of Congress for Cataloging-in-Publication data.

ISBN: 9781479832620 (hardback)
ISBN: 9781479832644 (paperback)
ISBN: 9781479832668 (library ebook)
ISBN: 9781479832651 (consumer ebook)

This book is printed on acid-free paper, and its binding materials are chosen for strength and durability. We strive to use environmentally responsible suppliers and materials to the greatest extent possible in publishing our books.

Manufactured in the United States of America

10 9 8 7 6 5 4 3 2 1

Also available as an ebook

CONTENTS

List of Figures and Tables   ix

Introduction: Why Do Changing In-Fertilities Matter to Us All?   1
Sarah Franklin and Marcia C. Inhorn

PART I: IN-FERTILE FAMILIES   27

1: Technological Convergence: Creating the New Arab Family
through Contraception, Assisted Reproduction, Selective
Abortion, and Son Selection   29
Marcia C. Inhorn

2: Pursuit of Pregnancy: Assisted Reproduction and Women's
Repro-Activity in Japan   47
Nana Okura Gagné

3: Reproductive Heterosexism: Assisted Reproduction and
Family Making in the "Best Interests of the Child" in Greece   67
Venetia Kantsa

4: Reproductive Imaginations: Process versus Outcome in
Queer Family Making in Britain   86
Robert Pralat

5: Queer Calculations: Spreadsheet Fertility and British
Gay Men's Reproductive Projects   103
Marcin Smietana

PART II: IN-FERTILE NATIONS   123

6: Fertility Figures: The Reconfiguring of "One-Child" China   125
Ayo Wahlberg

7: Resilient Pronatalism: Reproductive Politics among
Jews in Israel   142
Daphna Birenbaum-Carmeli

8: Fertility Paradoxes: Mexico's Shifting Reproductive Agendas   163
Sandra P. González-Santos

9: Reproductive Rebellion: Challenging Authority and
Seeking Autonomy in Iran's Fertility Regime   182
Soraya Tremayne

10: Rethinking Demography: Assisted Reproduction and the
"Proximate Determinants of Fertility" Reexamined   199
Nitzan Peri-Rotem

PART III: IN-FERTILE ECONOMIES   219

11: Fertility Efficiency: Rationalizing Reproductive Extensions
in Financialized IVF   221
Lucy van de Wiel

12: Mobile Reproductive Labor: Fly-in Fly-out Clinicians,
Batched Patients, and Extraction in African
Assisted Reproduction   238
Andrea Whittaker and Trudie Gerrits

13: Motherworkers of Tbilisi: The Housewifization of
Commercial Surrogates in Post-Soviet Georgia   254
Sigrid Vertommen

14: Haunted Data "Goldmine": Repropolitical Anxieties and
Injustice in Finland   273
Mwenza Blell and Riikka Homanen

PART IV: IN-FERTILE ENVIRONMENTS   291

15: Reproductive Extractivism: Mining and the Reproductive
Grammar of Multispecies Destruction in Peru   293
Julieta Chaparro-Buitrago

16: Maternity amid Disaster: Childbearing and Moral
Vulnerabilities in Tectonic Japan   309
Tsipy Ivry

17: Landscapes of Infertility: The Afterlives of Colonialism
in Indian Plantation Economies   327
Sharmila Rudrappa

18: Heterotopian Ecologies of Abundance: Saving Seeds and
   (Bio)Diversity in London   348
      Katharine Dow

19: Fruitility Activism: Restoring Roots, Branches, and
   Rot Holes in the English Orchard Revival   364
      Sarah Franklin

   Afterword: In-Fertilities in the New Reproductive Order   383
      Aditya Bharadwaj

   Acknowledgments   387

   About the Contributors   389

   About the Editors   395

   Index   397

LIST OF FIGURES AND TABLES

FIGURES

Figure 2.1. Total Fertility Rate of Japan (1947–2021)   51

Figure 2.2. Numbers of Neonate Births by Assisted Reproductive Technology in Japan (1985–2020)   51

Figure 2.3. Various *Ninkatsu*-Related Books   53

Figure 2.4. Riko Higashio's Best-Selling Book, *Not Infertility, but TGP (Trying to Get Pregnant)*   55

Figure 5.1. Harvey and Oliver's Surrogacy Expense Spreadsheet, Arrangement 1   108

Figure 5.2. Harvey and Oliver's IVF Expense Spreadsheet, Arrangement 2   110

Figure 5.3. Harvey and Oliver's Surrogacy Expense Spreadsheet, Arrangement 2   111

Figure 5.4. Paul and Federico's Expense Spreadsheet   115

Figure 6.1. "Let People Dare to Give Birth to 'Two Children'"   127

Figure 6.2. Still Image from *The Marriage Market Takeover*   133

Figure 6.3. Characters in Jie Hao's *Single Man* Watch as the Sun Sets   135

Figure 6.4. Screenshot of Blog Post "Is a New DINK Family Form Emerging?"   137

Figure 7.1. Total Fertility Rate by Religious Group, 2002–2022   144

Figure 7.2. An Orthodox City Street in Israel   149

Figure 7.3. Women's Educational Attainment vs. Fertility, 2020   150

Figure 7.4. Cover Page Featuring Geula Even at the End of Her Fifth Pregnancy   154

Figure 7.5. Photo from the Delivery Room of "Little Michal"   156

Figure 7.6. Total Fertility Rate of Jewish Women in Israel by
Religiosity, 1990–2021   158

Figure 10.1. Path Diagram Modeling Hypothesized
Relationships between Education and Fertility   212

Figure 13.1. Kartlis Deda (Mother Georgia)   255

Figure 13.2. Hotline—Know Our Rights Facebook Page   269

Figure 17.1. Robusta Coffee under Thinned Silver Oak   330

Figure 17.2. Woman Worker in Field of Robusta Coffee   332

Figure 17.3. Tiny Coffee Berry Borer   333

Figure 17.4. *Aedes aegypti*   337

Figure 17.5. Jenu Kurubas, Kodagu Region (1859–1861)   339

Figure 17.6. Shoal Creek, Austin, Texas   342

Figure 17.7. Chucklee the Cat Investigates
Unidentified Mushrooms   343

Figure 17.8. Unidentified Mushrooms   344

Figure 19.1. Image of Author's Home Orchard   366

Figure 19.2. The "Orchard Habitat" Page on Website of People's
Trust for Endangered Species   370

Figures 19.3 and 19.4. Two Best-Selling Books That Helped
to Catalyze the Countryside Protection Movement in
the United Kingdom   372

Figure 19.5. 1972 Magazine Ad for Robertson's Food Products   375

Figures 19.6 and 19.7. Screenshot of Hawkes London Website   378

TABLES

Table 1.1. Arab Countries in the Top Fifteen for Fertility Decline   31

Table 1.2. Decline in Arab Fertility Levels over Forty-Five Years   32

Table 1.3. Arab Countries Performing the Most ART Cycles
per Capita   36

Table 7.1. Fertility among FSU Immigrants and Jewish Women
in Israel   148

Table 7.2. Fertility Rates in Jewish Communities in the United
States and Israel by Religiosity   151

Table 9.1. Iran's Population according to Successive Censuses   188

Introduction

Why Do Changing In-Fertilities Matter to Us All?

SARAH FRANKLIN AND MARCIA C. INHORN

Ever since the inception of in vitro fertilization (IVF) in 1978, feminist research on new forms of assisted conception has emphasized the far-reaching implications of these technologies in terms of the way reproductive futures are imagined, desired, and pursued. Despite varying theoretical frameworks and methodologies, scholars in this field have continually emphasized the importance of fertility technologies as both indexical and symptomatic of fundamental changes to society, economy, culture, and politics (Franklin 2013a). Notably, too, techniques such as IVF were seen from the outset by feminist researchers both as objects of inquiry and as reading devices—or optics—for feminist analysis, so much so that the term "reprolens" has been coined to describe the use of assisted reproductive technologies (ARTs) and IVF as a "looking glass" or hermeneutic device (Franklin 2013b; Inhorn 2020). IVF has been interpreted not only as "the perfect feminist text," as Charis Thompson notes (2002, 2005), but also as a mapping device for what we have called "repronationalisms" across the globe (Franklin and Inhorn 2016). It has taken many decades for the feminist analysis of ARTs to become recognized as more than a "specialist" topic, but increasingly feminist perspectives on reproduction, technology, and society are being mainstreamed in many disciplines. For all of these reasons, this field of feminist reproductive studies has come to play an ever more important role in "dragging reproduction to the center" of both social theory and social life (Ginsburg and Rapp 1991, 1995).

This book represents an effort to document the effects of half a century of new reproductive technologies on ideas and practices surrounding fertility, infertility, fertility control, and fertility decline—that is, on reproduction itself. It brings together research from across the globe and seeks to understand the ways in which technologies such as IVF have changed perceptions, expectations, and experiences of fertility and infertility. Using a combination of anthropological, sociological, and feminist intersectional approaches, we argue that *in-fertilities*—or the complicated and dialectical relationship between fertility and infertility (Inhorn 1994), and ongoing concerns over both (Franklin 2013a, 2022)—are increasingly central to social life and social thought. Their newly explicit prominence calls for bold new models in the social sciences to chart what we characterize as a *new reproductive order*. By this we refer to substantial shifts in what we are calling *reproductive cause and effect*, or the ways in which changing perceptions of in-fertility are altering how people imagine, pursue, and experience reproductivity, both individually and collectively.

These changing perceptions of in-fertility not only are changing individual attitudes and orientations toward reproduction but are generating cumulative and consequential effects at an aggregate level. These effects include falling birth rates, delayed parenting, greater reliance on fertility-enhancement products and services, higher numbers of children born from IVF and related technologies, and greater anxiety about fertility precarity (Franklin 2022). Furthermore, new forms of fertility extension through technologies such as egg freezing (Inhorn 2023; Van de Wiel 2020) are now complemented by a new commercial emphasis on fertility efficiencies (Van de Wiel, chapter 11), which seek to reduce the cost, labor, and time required to achieve the goal of a "take-home baby" by introducing new technologies and business models in IVF. These not only are changing the actual mechanics of reproductive biology but are also altering the way reproductivity itself is conceived, understood, navigated, and controlled.

The transformed fertility logics of this new reproductive order include new knowledges, aspirations, rationales, and calculations that shape and guide the way babies and families are imagined and made. Young, presumed-to-be-fertile women can freeze, sell, or donate their eggs to research or to other women or couples. Fertility brokers run agencies that create "Google Babies" for wealthy clients—often involving transnational arrangements with paid surrogates and the purchase of donor eggs. These twenty-first-century fertility workers participate in a new reproductive order that is highly stratified, commercialized, globalized, and precarious.

The intensive marketization of fertility has also changed the way people imagine creating families. Increasingly, individuals and couples struggling to create their own families are invited to join online support groups, buy fertility apps, consult fertility services, and attend fertility fairs in order to prepare for a complex baby-making journey, which involves a host of products and services, as well as the investment of substantial time and resources. And while the pursuit of ever more assistance to the achievement of pregnancy has become an increasingly widely shared experience for many people across the globe, fertility precarity has become headline news. The rapid expansion of ARTs has consequently gained increasing social, political, and economic prominence in the twenty-first century, altering perceptions and representations of in-fertility on both the individual and aggregate levels. These trends are evident from social media sites dedicated to IVF users, egg donors, and gay dads to the promotion of ART services by governments in many countries facing "ultra-low fertility," such as Japan, Singapore, South Korea, and Taiwan. The idea that fertility can no longer be taken for granted, and is instead in dire need of help, is one of the reversals that most defines the new reproductive order and its accompanying fertility logics, orientations, and industries.

Anxiety related to fertility decline, as well as the growth of fertility markets and the accompanying expansion of what Vertommen, Pavone, and Nahman (2022) refer to as "global fertility chains," are all contributing to the emergence of new political economies of reproduction, and to what Pavone (2017) has characterized as the "reproductive bioeconomy." In the context of the new reproductive order, we can even more precisely refer to the emergence of a distinctive "fertinomics," encompassing the explicit marketization of both fertility products and fertility services but also emphasizing the rising importance of "fertility value" in geopolitical economic calculations more generally. The argument that reproductive politics are fundamental to the formation of the social order at every level has become increasingly cogent amid the rise of twenty-first-century populist alt-right and theocratic ethnonationalisms, often linked to neo-patriarchal heads of state (Briggs 2018; Franklin and Ginsburg 2019). For example, in September 2023, at a European fertility summit hosted by the "Great Replacement" theory advocate Viktor Orban, far-right leaders from across Europe met in Budapest to compare strategies to jump-start flagging EU birthrates.

Government promotion of increased domestic fertility as a means to rescue declining national economies has become an increasingly explicit worldwide trend. Indeed, Laura Briggs's (2018) argument that "all politics have become reproductive politics" in the United States is equally evident across the globe. Ethnonationalist claims to sovereignty based on racialized equations of people, nation, and security are increasingly used not only to justify territorial expansion by governments such as Russia, China, and Israel but also to pour money into fertility technologies such as IVF to increase some populations at the expense of others. Such "political arithmetic" has been explicit in the case of Israel and Palestine (Kanaaneh 2002). In its efforts to "reproduce Jews" (Kahn 2000), Israel continues to be the world's most generous subsidizer of IVF services for its citizens, leading to the "resilient pronatalism" described in chapter 7 of this volume. Yet, it is important to emphasize that Israel's state-sponsored pronatalism and settler-colonial expansion have come at the expense of the Palestinian population (Shalhoub-Kevorkian 2022; Vertommen et al. 2023), which has experienced, among other things, refugee flight, ethnic cleansing, humanitarian crises, war crimes, and genocide in Gaza. Sadly, these forms of ethnocratic domination and violence have been experienced by many populations in the twenty-first century—including the Rohingyas of Myanmar (Ware and Laoutides 2018), the residents of Darfur in Sudan (Hastrup 2012; Kohnert 2023), the Uyghurs in western China (Byler 2022; Roberts 2022), and Ukrainians, particularly in the Donbas region (Channell-Justice 2022; Uehling 2023; Wanner 2023). In general, ethnic and civil strife leading to violent population disruptions and dispossession represents a truly deleterious "reproductive effect" in the twenty-first-century new world order—one in which political conflict has led to massive forms of reproductive suffering and injustice (Inhorn 2018).

Yet, the twenty-first century has also witnessed the growth of a dynamic reproductive justice (RJ) movement, forwarded by women of color. The right *not* to have children, the right *to* have children, and the right to *parent* children in safe and healthy environments have been held up by RJ activists as basic human rights (Luna 2020), serving to empower women of color through RJ social activism (Davis 2019; Luna 2020; Zavella 2020). RJ activism has also facilitated an important international movement to return abortion politics to the front line of political struggle, not only in the United States (Munson 2018) but in societies around the globe (Maffi 2020; Singer 2022; Suh 2021). The importance of this struggle has unfolded most dramatically in the United States, where the 2022 *Dobbs v. Jackson Women's Health Organization* case heard by the US Supreme Court effectively reversed *Roe v. Wade*, the 1973 US Supreme Court decision upholding abortion prior to the viability of the fetus as a fundamental right. With the 2022 *Dobbs* reversal, many US states moved quickly to curtail abortion services. The Alabama Supreme Court went even further in 2024, asserting that frozen embryos in the state's IVF clinics should be considered "extrauterine children," and their destruction seen as equivalent to "wrongful death."

The importance of the RJ movement for women's health and reproductive rights could not be clearer. However, other recent influences have fueled a renewed global emphasis on changing in-fertilities. For example, the effort to decarbonize the economy has highlighted the high costs of extractive economies and invited a reevaluation of the interconnected fertilities of people, plants, microorganisms, and the soil (Hoover 2018; Kimmerer 2013; Murphy 2017)—the key theme of part 4 of this volume. Similarly, recent reevaluations of the legacies of colonial-imperialism, slavery, and neoliberal capitalism have demonstrated in detail how economic logics of reproduction and fertility have been at the core of these projects (Davis 2019; Morgan 2004, 2021; Weinbaum 2019). Most recently, a radical rethinking of both political economy and reproductivity has occurred in the context of COVID-19 (Rao 2021) and the serial credit crises punctuating the first quarter of the twenty-first century (Sultana 2021). The refugee flows produced by several major wars since 2000 (Inhorn 2018; Inhorn and Volk 2021), as well as the accelerating rate of climate change (Crate and Nuttall 2016), have confirmed that we are living through a period of dramatic social disruption and political change, in which many of the core axioms guiding previous phases of modern development and post-Enlightenment global planning are revealed as fundamentally misguided and myopic. Like eugenics and colonialism, the Green Revolution and many Western aid programs have worsened rather than improved the life conditions for many of the world's most impoverished peoples (Mezzadri, Newman, and Stevano 2022). Rather than signs of progress, they are now implicated in global extractive decline. These forces demonstrate how changes in reproductive cause and effect are perceived not only in the present but also historically, and how the new reproductive order implicates fundamental political, economic, and environmental concerns.

Remodeling Fertility

The study of fertility thus continues to be a source of radically revisionist remodelings, not only of political economy and reproductive cause and effect but also of the very idea of modernity and its associated values—such as the equation of industrial economic growth with modern progress and of modern progress with the improvement of the human condition. As Susan Greenhalgh (1990, 1996) has so convincingly shown, demography is one of the most illuminating case studies of classic modernization theory and its misapprehensions. Serial models of fertility transition for over half a century have relied on a standard model of population change according to which decreasing fertility follows decreasing morbidity and mortality and leads to increasing wealth and better, more prosperous lives. Even after the Princeton European Fertility Project convincingly disproved the causal and empirical basis of transition models in the 1980s (Coale and Watkins 1986), the modernization-of-fertility paradigm has continued to play a dominant role in research on both population and reproduction, as well as in economic development programs. This is the case because the foundational assumptions of demographic transition modeling are ideological rather than scientific, and because the science of demography remains so deeply entrenched in the logics, calculations, and policies it has helped to create (Greenhalgh 2013; Szreter 1993).

Today, the challenges for both demographers and governments attempting to identify the causal drivers of fertility change are even greater. One of our key arguments is that many contemporary logics of fertility care, planning, and awareness—be they at the global, national, medical, marital, or individual levels—do not add up in any simple way, and indeed in many cases do not add up at all. The new reproductive order is characterized by the topsy-turvy, often contradictory logics that have come to characterize contemporary fertility decision making—be it in the context of the clinic, the board room, or the bedroom. As this volume shows through numerous and detailed case studies, the zig-zagging logics of fertility planning reveal the often-overlooked complexity of reproductive causality. This is a familiar feminist argument, as well as a hallmark of ethnographic empiricism. For example, as Inhorn's (2023) recent research on egg freezing in the United States has shown, the rationale that fertility delay helps women to maximize their career potential—although much hyped by the media—turns out to be the wrong causal factor in women's turn to egg freezing. Rather, a shortage of potential partners is the primary cause of their reproductive delay—a sometimes insurmountable problem that egg-freezing technology itself cannot fix. As Inhorn notes, a significant demographic factor at work is the rapid decline in men's educational attainment levels, a disparity exacerbated by the opposite trend among women in more than half the world's nations.

It is of course not news for demographers or feminists—or governments or fertility professionals—that the causal factors driving a significant worldwide fertility decline are social as well as biological, structural as well as individual, and complex as well as often tacit. These factors also overlap. For example, environmental factors such as pesticide use, which manifests biologically as diminished fertility, have their roots in social life—in historically specific approaches to agricultural productivity, scientific progress, and economic growth. This means that at a basic causal level, fertility has never been easy to determine or predict. The much-debated question of how birth rates are reshaped over time is, if anything, even more obscure today than in the past.

Our reference to a new reproductive order is deliberately intended to foreground this uncertainty about reproductive cause and effect, as is our use of "in-fertilities" as a hyphenated conjunction. As noted earlier, this latter term derives from the increasing overlap—and proximity—between fertility and infertility in popular consciousness, as well as in terms of the marketing of in-fertility services (and the two are not unconnected). Although it is often noted, for example, that egg freezing is one of the first major fertility technologies to be primarily marketed to young, single, presumed-to-be-fertile women (Gürtin and Tiemann 2021), this trend is now beginning to characterize IVF marketing as well. The "straight to IVF" route for the mid-thirty-something presumed-to-be-fertile couple that has either the funds to afford it or subsidized access to high-tech fertility care is increasingly being promoted as the safest way to guarantee a take-home baby, for two main reasons. First, since time is tight, couples can avoid the potential risk of trying IVF later when it is already too late to succeed. Second, doing IVF now will be a faster way to find a fertility problem if there is one, thus leading to a crucial head start in achieving a family, especially for those who would like more than one child.

In such a formulation—which is increasingly recommended by IVF professionals as the safest bet for thirty-somethings who do not achieve a pregnancy within three to six months of trying—we see the melding together of fertility and infertility as copresent conditions rather than as a pair of linear opposites. Rather than presumed fertility gradually (and painfully) fading into the limbo and anxiety of possible infertility, it is precisely the increased taken-for-grantedness of IVF that has established it as a new fact of life for those who can afford it (and indeed for many who cannot)—creating a new social norm that is coupled with the other new fact of increased fertility precarity, thus conjoining fertility and infertility within a single spectrum.

The blending together of fertility and infertility is not only evident at an individual or clinical level, and it is not only a product of in-fertility marketing. Importantly, the hyphenated conundrum of in-fertility is now fundamentally embedded in the very core of contemporary demographic research—and at the highest levels. For example, despite their critical location at the heart of global planning, long-standing stalwarts of fertility statistics and prediction, such as the specialist demography units informing the United Nations, World Health Organization, International Monetary Fund, and World Bank, increasingly struggle to offer reliable and reproducible methodologies or models to predict fertility change—even in specific regions or communities. Indeed, amid accelerating fertility decline and increasing uncertainty about the factors that determine either fertility intentions or their outcomes, it appears increasingly hard for demographers to provide even roughly accurate baseline data about actual fertility change (Billari 2022). Thus, forecasting has become increasingly unreliable.

As a case in point, the UN Population Division Report from May 2021 about the impact of the COVID-19 epidemic on fertility shows the widespread demographic uncertainty concerning both short- and long-term fertility predictors, measures, and models, even at the very highest levels of policymaking. The Population Division is one of the oldest, most prestigious, and best-resourced agencies within the United Nations, best known for its benchmark annual publication, *World Population Prospects*. This report is the main source of baseline data about fertility and birth rates for national governments worldwide, providing the most authoritative population forecasts available.

To assess population change and offer policy advice, Population Division staff use the same three standard demographic indices that have defined the field since its inception: fertility, mortality, and migration. At their May 2021 meeting in New York, the focus was on how fertility had been affected by the global pandemic (United Nations 2021). Although the experts predicted that the shocks to fertility caused by COVID-19 would lead in the first year to diminishing cycles and a drop in fertility rates, followed by a rebound in the second year and subsequent stabilization in years three and four, they agreed on little else due to how many other fertility-influencing factors, in addition to COVID-19, had come into play. Indeed, participants reclassified the pandemic as a "syndemic," due to how many synergistic economic, biological, and environmental "shocks" were occurring simultaneously. This made it difficult to disentangle the lingering effects of the global economic downturn of 2008 from those of ongoing climate change and the COVID-19 pandemic of 2020–2021. In such a context, demographers assumed that biological, social, and behavioral factors would combine to influence sexual activity, partnering, marriage rates, and reproductive intentions, thus shaping fertility decisions and other proximate determinants of conception and birth rates, such as marriage rates. However, by 2021, it had become almost impossible for even leading world experts to disaggregate the discrete causal drivers of these trends.

These difficulties were reinforced by highly divergent fertility patterns from well-researched individual geographic regions. For example, fertility rates in both the sub-Saharan and wider African context remained relatively unchanged by the COVID-19 pandemic and other syndemic effects that so heavily affected Anglo-European, Scandinavian, and Australian fertility and natality rates in the same period. In sub-Saharan Africa, contraceptive uptake did not appear to be significantly impaired, and women's "fertility desires" and "fertility intentions" appeared to be stable or increasing in Kenya and Nigeria, as well as in other parts of Africa. In contrast, the steep fertility decline appeared to be largely independent of COVID-19 across all of mainland China, where, according to demographers, the three most significant "proximate" fertility factors driving down birth rates were the increasing number of never-married women, the declining number of children desired by both married and cohabiting couples, and the rising age of both first marriage and first birth. Similarly, for high- and middle-income countries in the southeast Asian region, such as Singapore and Thailand, experts claimed that below-replacement fertility rates were already "baked in" to such an extent that the 2020 pandemic's impact was undetectable (United Nations 2021).

Tomas Sobotka, representing the prestigious Vienna Institute of Demography at the UN meeting, described the COVID-19 effect on fertility in terms of "cycles of busts and recoveries" roughly corresponding to lockdowns, and he attributed the "significant differences" between European countries to "more long-lasting scars in the economy" of southern Europe (United Nations 2021). Adding further texture to this picture, one of the world's leading demographers, Francesco Billari, questioned whether "internetization" might be having an increasing effect on fertility, citing research demonstrating a link between mobile phone use and higher contraceptive uptake in low-income countries and other examples of "digital fertility," such as "broadband diffusion linked to higher fertility for highly educated women in Germany" (United Nations 2021; see also Billari 2022).

At the close of the meeting, participants were directly asked whether they believed it would be possible for a post-COVID fertility recovery phase to "rebound to above pre-pandemic levels." Rather than reply with a simple "yes" or "no," however, a majority of experts instead voiced their increasing skepticism about the accuracy or reliability of even rudimentary predictions about future fertility fluctuations, other than "short-term trends" based on close analysis of specific regional factors such as birth registrations. The uncertainty is so great at so many levels, they claimed, that even the core concept of a "fertility rate" is no longer a viable basis for extrapolating future population prospects. This is due in part to the increasing role of "both quantum and tempo" effects on fertility, otherwise known as the effects of unpredictable or highly varied birth "cycles," "seasonality," and "timing" on birth totals, or "rates." These complex variations are in turn the consequence of a wide variety of global trends: concerns about the economy, declines in women's paid employment, lack of accessible childcare, declining adolescent fertility, increases in sexual abstinence, the depressive effect of COVID-19 on fertility, delayed first marriage, delayed first birth, and poorly characterized factors such as "internetization" (Billari, Rotondi, and Trinitapoli 2020), the latter of which, through dating apps, may be altering patterns of sexual behavior. At the close of the meeting, the director of the division confessed that he was "struck by the overarching message of uncertainty" and the "repeated mentions of fear as a driver of fertility behavior," noting that this suggested increasingly "unpredictable outcomes" (United Nations 2021: 14).

Such doubts have increasingly become the demographic norm. Like linear, causal explanations of conception, birth rates can only be either calculated or confirmed retrospectively. From any other point of view, they are merely hypothetical. In the aggregate, changes to population can be calculated as a rate, or predicted in terms of rises and falls. However, the manner in which such changes develop—their causal determinants, either individually or collectively—remains far more elusive. As the overarching message of uncertainty emerging from the world's leading demographic experts in the wake of COVID-19 suggests, calculating fertility change has become increasingly less feasible, even using the most mathematically advanced methods of statistical demographic analysis (Vanella, Greil, and Deschermeier 2023).

Beyond Demography through Anthropology

As this book argues, the new in-fertility uncertainty is a defining condition of the new reproductive order, making it vital to revisit basic questions of reproductive cause and effect. The value of more qualitative approaches to in-fertility has never been greater, especially in terms of identifying the more recent, twenty-first-century factors influencing fertility, many of them technological, such as mobile phone–based dating apps, emergency contraception, new forms of fertility tracking, IVF "add-ons," and a variety of "selective" reproductive technologies used to eliminate certain embryos and fetuses (Wahlberg and Gammeltoft 2017).

Since the 1980s, in-depth qualitative analysis of in-fertility, IVF, and other ARTs has been particularly well developed within the burgeoning anthropology of reproduction, but also in the sociology of reproductive biomedicine. For more than forty years, anthropologists and sociologists have been producing a rich literature on "where the quest for conception has taken us" (Inhorn 2020), leading to many lessons learned about the masculine, moral, selective, stratified, technological, and transnational dimensions of in-fertility and the rapidly proliferating movement of ARTs across the globe.

Three anthropological anthologies were particularly field defining. The first was *Conceiving the New World Order: The Global Politics of Reproduction*, coedited by Faye Ginsburg and Rayna Rapp (1995). This volume demonstrated the powerfully transformative effects of placing reproduction at the heart of social theory, while also introducing a framework through which reproduction could be analyzed as a site of intersecting social structures. Drawing upon Shellee Colen's (1995) concept of "stratified reproduction," *Conceiving the New World Order* theorized the ways in which transnational inequalities structure reproductive practices, policies, and politics in ways that are both intersectional and interconnected. As Ginsburg and Rapp (1995: 3) made clear, "The concept of stratified reproduction helps us see the arrangements by which some reproductive futures are valued while others are despised."

A similarly broad and ambitious agenda for the anthropology of reproduction was articulated in Susan Greenhalgh's anthology, *Situating Fertility: Anthropology and Demographic Inquiry*, published in the same year (1995). Calling for a "broad, synthetic agenda" (Greenhalgh 1995: 4), this volume aimed to "situate fertility" by identifying four of the reproductive dynamics most often omitted from conventional demographic theory and analysis—namely, culture and agency, history, gender, and power and politics. The larger aim of the volume was to draw anthropological attention to reproduction as an "arena of social life in the hope of making reproductive research more central to the anthropological project" (Greenhalgh 1995: 4).

This aim was clearly manifest in the third volume, *Infertility around the Globe: New Thinking on Childlessness, Gender, and Reproductive Technologies*, coedited by Marcia C. Inhorn and Frank van Balen (2002). *Infertility around the Globe* homed in on "reproductive disruptions," or the many ways in which reproduction "goes badly and sadly awry" (Inhorn and van Balen 2002: 4). Such disruptions have major implications for individuals' identities and couples' family making, but particularly in cultural contexts where parenthood is socially mandatory and globalizing ARTs have yet to reach. Focusing on "non-normative reproductive scenarios and experiences" (Inhorn and van Balen 2002: 4) in societies around the globe, the volume placed special emphasis on gender and body politics, particularly the ways in which women suffer the social onus and physical burden of fertility failures and involuntary childlessness, thus bringing into sharper focus both the suffering caused by infertility and its highly stratified distribution.

These pathbreaking anthologies dedicated to the retheorization of reproduction and in-fertility—as both *situated* and *stratified*—were published amid the burgeoning feminist literature on what were then called the "new reproductive technologies" (NRTs, later recast as ARTs). Feminist anthropologists working in this area provided extensive theoretical analyses of the ways in which nature, culture, and gender, as well as kinship, religion, property, and political institutions, were being reconfigured with the advent of these new technologies. Marilyn Strathern (1992a, 1992b) was among the first anthropologists to link the emergence of the new market in fertility services such as IVF to the economic and political changes initiated in the 1980s under Reagan and Thatcher, as well as to emerging ideologies of neoliberal choice among "stakeholder citizens." Early ethnographic studies of consumers of IVF similarly located its importance not only in relation to the gendered experiences of infertility (Inhorn 1996), and within the wider context of poverty (Inhorn 1994, 2003), but also in relation to changing meanings of the biological "facts of life" (Edwards et al. 1993; Franklin 1997) and emergent media narratives about overcoming infertility using new technological options (Franklin 1990, 1995). These studies were followed by similarly expansive feminist accounts of IVF in relation to agency, identity, and personhood in IVF clinics (Cussins 1996, 1998; Sandelowski 1993), new kinship and conception models (Franklin and Ragoné 1998), consumer culture (Becker 2000) and "enterprise culture" (Franklin 1997), ideas about intergenerational identities and transmission (Edwards 2000; Franklin 2013a), and the "ontological choreography" and "strategic naturalization" needed to "make parents" through IVF (Thompson 2005). (See Franklin 2013a, 2022; Franklin and Inhorn 2016; and Inhorn 2020 for overviews of this scholarship.)

This volume draws its primary inspiration from this rich feminist anthropological corpus, in which the study of changing in-fertilities and fertility technologies has been used to provide a hermeneutic "repro-lens" on wider social, political, economic, and cultural changes. Across nineteen chapters, it both reflects and extends the legacy of feminist anthropological research analyzing in-fertility, technology, and social change—thus amplifying the consistent finding and refrain that this area of research is pivotal to contemporary social theory. Indeed, today, in a context in which not only people and populations but the planet itself are perceived to be in a state of increasing reproductive precarity, the study of in-fertility has arguably never had more important or more global implications. Like epidemics, in-fertilities raise fundamental issues of economic justice, social equality, and human rights. The suffering caused by in-fertility is inextricable from histories of colonialism, armed conflict, and ethnonationalism, as well as climate change, migration, and industrial capitalism. As Ginsburg and Rapp (1995) rightly insisted, the stratification of reproduction is a map of intersecting local/global forces that offers unique insights into the current world order. Three decades on, the title of our volume reflects this vital insight, and seeks to extend it precisely by identifying what Greenhalgh (1995) described as the "dynamic" nature of reproductivity.

Today, amid what some commentators describe as the "infertility trap" (Aitken 2022), these questions take on a new set of structural implications. Fertility precarity has risen dramatically in the public consciousness as well as in corporate board rooms, confirming that infertility is not only an increasingly pressing issue in and of itself but also a medium through which other concerns are both amplified and symbolized. In other words, in-fertility has become, among other things, a zeitgeist. Echoing, but reversing, twentieth-century concerns about overpopulation, in-fertility has become both a general and a generalizable condition. In addition, both in-fertility and IVF have become indexical signs not only of imperiled future generations but of the future *of* generation—in all its forms. The links among soil depletion, carbon emission, the food chain, and parenting are today the stuff of both everyday social media messaging and a new ethical calculus shaping decisions about both personal and industrial consumption. In such a context, the feminist axiom that reproductive justice cannot be separated from other justice struggles is becoming more widely legible and playing a more explicit role in shaping national, economic, and social policies. It offers a timely reminder that no political economy can be either credible or accountable if it fails to take account of reproductive cause and effect—in all its complex forms.

The Changing In-Fertilities Project

Inspired by these many concerns, we launched the Changing In-Fertilities Project (CIFP), carried out from 2018 to 2022 and funded by the Wellcome Trust. In designing the CIFP, we built on several of the key findings from the aforementioned decades of feminist work on in-fertilities and ARTs to shape a new agenda for scholarship in this space and to widen it. Our goal was both to confirm how the findings of the ambitious research projects conducted by earlier scholars have been realized, and to demonstrate how many key concepts from this field have indeed helped to reshape social theory. However, additional goals of the CIFP were to launch a global network of scholars to explore the question of how IVF and newer fertility technologies are changing perceptions of in-fertility, and how in turn these changed perceptions are affecting reproductive decision making.

Given the extensive research demonstrating that IVF and related ARTs are reproducing not only babies but also kinship relations, values, institutions, norms, identities, and ideals, it is clearly insufficient to depict these technologies primarily in terms of "responding" to infertility. Moreover, since fertility technologies such as IVF so often fail to deliver what their users hope to achieve by undergoing such costly and demanding procedures, it is more important than ever to understand how these technologies not only "respond" to fertility concerns but actively transform the experience of reproductive failure, and generate new kinds of reproductive affect, identity, consciousness, and agency—as well as markets, services, and products. Again, there are basic reproductive cause-and-effect questions at issue here. As was evident in the very first studies of IVF (Crowe 1985; Sandelowski 1993), the technique itself plays a significant role in shaping future reproductive imaginaries, aspirations, intentions, and, above all, hopes. As a "hope technology" (Franklin 1997, 2022), the very existence of IVF substantially changes the moral, emotional, and practical realities of everyday life for individuals and couples facing unwanted childlessness, and their local networks of support or judgment. For some, it introduces not only a new possibility but a new reproductive imperative or obligation.

This "IVF effect" has become increasingly apparent and powerful over the past four decades, especially as the technology has expanded so rapidly, including to resource-poor settings (Inhorn and Patrizio 2015). Indeed, it is no exaggeration to describe IVF as one of the most influential translational technologies of the twentieth century, one that has transformed understandings not only of human fertility but of developmental biology and, for that matter, of the fundamental mechanisms of cellular differentiation. The IVF technique introduced in the 1950s as an experimental method in mammals has become the "IVF platform" (Franklin 2013a), scaled up since the 1960s to become not only a means of interconnected procedures to deliver clinical IVF and the standardization of this process but also a means to link IVF back to basic research as an experimental technique. In turn, the IVF platform has become a key element in translational biotechnology more widely, leading not only to the cloning of mammals and stem cell research in the 1990s (Franklin 2007, 2013a) and to a host of postmillennial bio-industrial projects but more recently to the introduction of new embryo models. As a result of its expansion and normalization, IVF is now both a confirmation and a symbol of increased biological control and the remaking of life, while at the same time it is a technology of human conception and family creation. For all of these reasons, IVF offers a critical reprolens for understanding contemporary biological and social life, as well as social change.

The CIFP asked thirty ethnographic researchers in sixteen different countries to focus their own reprolenses on changing perceptions of in-fertility in culturally specific settings worldwide. The project had four basic components. First, we posed a main research question, which borrowed an elementary premise from demographic transition theory, namely, How do fertility perceptions play a fundamental role in shaping fertility behaviors? Second, we asked, How have perceptions of in-fertility changed in the post-ART context, and how are these altered perceptions changing in-fertility behaviors? Third, we drew on Greenhalgh's (1995) model of "situating fertility" to focus on "situating *in*-fertility" in a variety of global sites. Finally, we proposed a methodology that would be both qualitative and comparative.

Five years later, we have arrived at both predictable and somewhat surprising findings that together helped us develop the concepts of the new reproductive order and in-fertilities. For example, our research greatly strengthens the arguments made in earlier landmark volumes by Greenhalgh (1995) and Ginsburg and Rapp (1995) that understanding both the intersectional and stratified character of fertility and reproduction both matters in and of itself and can be used as a hermeneutic lens to map other social forces. Our research also confirmed the enormous value of using a detailed, situated approach to individual case studies, which were then put into comparative perspective to forge a more broadly conclusive methodology. A key contribution of this volume that extends these earlier findings is the focus on in-fertility as an increasingly salient feature of reproductive politics, as well as a source of increased suffering in many parts of the world. For example, we have confirmed a significant rise in the way in-fertility is being used as a condensed signifier—or code—for other issues and topics, and similarly how both fertility and infertility have become mediating idioms through which a wide range of nationalist aspirations and anxieties are expressed.

Our work has consequently extended key themes from reproductive politics and increasingly important reproductive justice efforts by offering new perspectives on economy, policy, and governance, as well as health, citizenship, and welfare. We have been able to turn our attention to the "fertility-industrial complex" and to how "fertinomics," "fertility labor," "fertility efficiency," and "fertility value" are linked to new political economies of reproduction. We also show how the new emphasis on fertility benefits by corporate employers, FemTech start-ups, and philanthropy are linked to broader efforts by governments and corporate titans to shape the fertility profiles of national and even global economies. Our case studies document how "fertility consciousness," "fertility planning," and "fertility awareness" take on new meanings and significance in the context of increasing fertility stratification, harmful environmental exposures and concerns, and increasing economic precarity. Building on Franklin's concepts of "iVF" (2013a) and "iFertility" (2022), we describe the ways in which in-fertilities are increasingly technologically mediated—and indeed have become mainstream media tropes themselves through newly iconic visual images, such as those of microinjection (Franklin 2013c).

Through the global range of case studies presented in this volume, we now know how to track, compare, and analyze specific articulations of in-fertility in a range of situated contexts, and therefore how these can be generalized and used to map and characterize wider patterns of social change. We can also document how fertility and infertility have become the focus of various activisms—from campaigns for greater fertility awareness and protests against racially stratified infertility to movements advocating "making kin not babies" and LGBTQI+ parenting networks. Revealingly, many of these campaigns have an explicitly intersectional approach to in-fertility and draw on social justice movements such as abolitionism and environmentalism.

As a result, despite its specific focus, the framework offered here is enormous and expansive. Innumerable additional case studies could be added to the limited number collected here, meaning that our volume is not representative, nor could it be. The global picture of changing in-fertilities is far too complex for any single volume to unravel. Nonetheless, the strength of our findings—both individually and collectively—lies in their confirmation of how pivotal the politics of in-fertilities have become to geopolitical trends and of how important it is for scholars to develop new models and approaches that undertake the challenge of analyzing in-fertilities and their significance in the new reproductive order. If there is one lesson, then, that stands out from our collective effort to document and analyze the significance of changing in-fertilities across the globe—using the core concept of the *new reproductive order*—it is that this area requires research on a much larger scale. To the extent that the new reproductive order is defined by an altered logic of cause and effect, it is vital to understand this relation more fully.

Conclusion

One of the benefits of putting changing in-fertilities center stage is the range of somewhat unexpected topics and questions such an analytic strategy engenders. This volume clearly indicates how much uncertainty and confusion still surround the apparent obviousness of reproduction and its causality. As this volume also demonstrates, "fertility" not only describes a natural condition or biological potential. It is a concept, and its use articulates values, which organize not only activities but also aspirations, and not only families and communities but the social order. Even biologically, "fertility" is a composite condition as well as a basket denomination for everything from individual capacity to aggregate quantity. Demographically, fertility exists simultaneously in several tenses—past, present, and future (and perhaps especially conditionally). A consequent paradox of fertility—especially as an empirical number—is its hidden nature. For all of these reasons, a key objective of this volume is to challenge the narrowness of the way in which both fertility and reproduction are conventionally understood.

Importantly, this effort to interrogate the narrow associations among biology, fertility, and reproduction is neither a new nor a recent effort, but instead one that has been part of many well-established critical traditions of intellectual and academic writing, including both feminist theory and science studies, as well as histories of colonialism and imperialism. Susan Greenhalgh's (1995) pathbreaking effort to both debiologize and decolonize the study of demography, for example, recentered the larger reproductive dynamics underlying population change—which she broadly described in terms of culture, history, gender, and power. As this volume argues, Greenhalgh's call to situate fertility within a more complex set of dynamic social, cultural, and political forces clarifies why the traditional list of fertility "drivers"—such as the ideal number of children couples would like to have and their access to the means to achieve this goal—is far too limited. Similarly, as Nitzan Peri-Rotem's chapter 10 of this volume shows, even the definition of "proximate determinants" of fertility remains too narrow. Social life is far more complex than these demographic constructs and variables can hope to measure.

Understanding fertility and fertility change requires shifting the focus away from such narrow definitions of reproductive causality, and their circular empirical metrics, and toward more complex and inclusive methodologies that encompass the effects of how fertility is perceived, experienced, and imagined, as well as deliberately and consciously planned. But if we are to achieve this goal, what we need to understand better are not only the causal dynamics shaping changing in-fertilities, or patterns of in-fertility change, but the increasing politicization of these perceptions and the ways that "in-fertility" has become an indexical idiom, not only for issues such as climate change and cost-of-living increases but for many other forms of cultural, social, and economic precarity.

Further still, as several chapters in this volume show, this in-fertility idiom registers discontent—with governments, businesses, and even entire industries, such as agriculture, mining, and petroleum. This is what we mean by the new reproductive order, in which awareness of in-fertility is not only a measure of understanding or knowledge but a powerful source of social, economic, and political consciousness and activism. By proposing this argument, we are introducing an altered model of reproductive cause and effect based on the hypothesis that a key influence on in-fertility change is not only how perceptions of in-fertility are transforming but how people feel about these changes, and interpret and react to them. These reactions are highly intersectional, linking the infertilities of seeds and soil to migrant belongings and the history of colonialism. To use Sara Ahmed's (2004) term, in-fertilities have become affectively "sticky"—linking together ideas and objects from disparate domains and morphing into existential idioms about the histories and future of humanity, the environment, parenting, and life itself.

This is why we argue for the importance of understanding in-fertility as an intersectional and indexical site of meaning that offers a unique reprolens on changing social conditions, cultural practices, and political economy. Crucially, we suggest that the new logics and grammars of in-fertility reflect changing value systems in which the causal relationships among the economy, health, food, polity, governance, kinship, and parenting are being perceived and evaluated differently. We need also to note that in-fertilities are subsequently not only political and politicized but fought over and increasingly a source of geopolitical conflict. None of the contemporary militarized conflicts occurring throughout the first quarter of the twenty-first century can be interpreted either accurately or credibly without our understanding of the fundamental importance of a repro-political interpretive lens. Conflicts over borders, land, sovereignty, and territory are never disconnected from reproductive histories, aspirations, and identities—be they of families, races, nations, or religions. And neither can such conflicts be understood without appreciating the politics of in-fertilities in their widest and most existential sense.

In sum, what this volume is intended to demonstrate across a wide range of contexts and communities is how in-fertility has become a prominent medium, idiom, and imaginary through which contemporary concerns are not only articulated and expressed but understood to be interconnected. In all of these ways, and for all of these reasons, we can therefore also track how fertility and infertility have come to be seen as indexical of more widely shared, general, and global conditions.

While the chapters in this volume are inherently valuable based on the findings of their in-depth ethnographic research across the globe, the real impact of this volume is to be found through the extended comparative range and scale it will acquire as its core analytics are further developed and refined. By adding many layers of inquiry to the invitation this book offers to other scholars, we can begin to grasp both the wider global implications of situated in-fertilities in specific settings and the more nuanced aspects of reproductive cause and effect, changing patterns of in-fertility consciousness and behavior, and the ways in which constantly evolving ARTs are changing our world for better and for worse. Ultimately, we hope that this volume opens up new horizons of scholarship on in-fertility and social change, as well as new thinking on policy, practice, and activism in the twenty-first century's new reproductive order.

REFERENCES

Ahmed, Sara. 2004. *The Cultural Politics of Emotion*. Edinburgh: Edinburgh University Press.

Aitken, John. 2022. *The Infertility Trap: Why Life Choices Impact Your Fertility and Why We Must Act Now*. Cambridge: Cambridge University Press.

Becker, Gaylene. 2000. *The Elusive Embryo: How Women and Men Approach New Reproductive Technologies*. Berkeley: University of California Press.

Billari, Francesco C. 2022. "Internet Use and the Postponement of Age Deadlines for Childbearing." Paper presented at the Annual Meeting of the Population Association of America, Atlanta, GA, April 7. https://paa.confex.com/.

Billari, Francesco C., Valentina Rotondi, and Jenny Trinitapoli. 2020. "Mobile Phones, Digital Inequality, and Fertility." *Demographic Research* 42: 1057–96.

Briggs, Laura. 2018. *How All Politics Became Reproductive Politics: From Welfare Reform to Foreclosure to Trump.* Berkeley: University of California Press.

———. 2002. *Reproducing Empire: Race, Sex, Science, and U.S. Imperialism in Puerto Rico.* Berkeley: University of California Press.

Byler, Darren. 2022. *Terror Capitalism: Uyghur Dispossession and Masculinity in a Chinese City.* Durham, NC: Duke University Press.

Channell-Justice, Emily. 2022. *Without the State: Self-Organization and Political Activism in Ukraine.* Toronto: University of Toronto Press.

Coale, Ansley Johnson, and Susan Cotts Watkins. 1986. *The Decline of Fertility in Europe.* Princeton, NJ: Princeton University Press.

Colen, Shellee. 1995. "'Like a Mother to Them': Stratified Reproduction and West Indian Childcare Workers and Employers in New York." In *Conceiving the New World Order: The Global Politics of Reproduction*, ed. Faye D. Ginsburg and Rayna Rapp, 78–102. Berkeley: University of California Press.

Crate, Susan A., and Mark Nuttall, eds. 2016. *Anthropology and Climate Change: From Actions to Transformations.* New York: Routledge.

Crowe, Christine. 1985. "Women Want It: In-vitro Fertilization and Women's Motivations for Participation." *Women's Studies International Forum* 8(6): 547–52.

Cussins, Charis. 1996. *Technologies of Personhood: Human Reproductive Technologies.* PhD dissertation. University of California, San Diego.

———. 1998. "Ontological Choreography: Agency for Women Patients in an Infertility Clinic. In *Differences in Medicine: Unraveling Practices, Techniques, and Bodies*, ed. Marc Berg and Annemarie Mol, 166–201. Durham, NC: Duke University Press.

Davis, Dána-Ain. 2019. *Reproductive Injustice: Racism, Pregnancy, and Premature Birth.* New York: New York University Press.

Edwards, Jeanette. 2000. *Born and Bred: Idioms of Kinship and New Reproductive Technologies in England.* Oxford: Oxford University Press.

Edwards, Jeanette, Sarah Franklin, Eric Hirsch, Frances Price, and Marilyn Strathern. 1993. "Making Representations: The Parliamentary Debate on the Human Fertilisation and Embryology Act." In *Technologies of Procreation*, 96–132. Manchester: Manchester University Press.

Franklin, Sarah. 1990. "Deconstructing 'Desperateness': The Social Construction of Infertility in Popular Media Representations." In *The New Reproductive Technologies*, ed. Maureen McNeil, Ian Varcoe, and Steven Yearley, 200–229. London: Macmillan.

———. 1995. "Postmodern Procreation: A Cultural Account of Assisted Conception." In *Conceiving the New World Order: The Global Politics of Reproduction*, ed. Faye Ginsburg and Rayna Rapp, 323–45. Berkeley: University of California Press.

———. 1997. *Embodied Progress: A Cultural Account of Assisted Conception*. New York: Routledge.

———. 2007. *Dolly Mixtures: The Remaking of Genealogy*. Durham, NC: Duke University Press.

———. 2013a. *Biological Relatives: IVF, Stem Cells, and the Future of Kinship*. Durham, NC: Duke University Press.

———. 2013b. "Conception through a Looking Glass: The Paradox of IVF." *Reproductive BioMedicine Online* 27: 747–55.

———. 2013c. "Embryo Watching: How IVF Has Remade Biology." *TECNOSCIENZA: Italian Journal of Science & Technology Studies* 4(1): 23–44.

———. 2022. *Embodied Progress: A Cultural Account of Assisted Conception*, 2nd ed. London: Routledge.

Franklin, Sarah, and Faye Ginsburg. 2019. "Reproductive Politics in the Age of Trump and Brexit." *Cultural Anthropology* 34: 3–9.

Franklin, Sarah, and Marcia C. Inhorn. 2016. "Introduction: IVF—Global Histories." *Reproductive BioMedicine and Society Online* 2: 1–7.

Franklin, Sarah, and Helena Ragoné, eds. 1998. *Reproducing Reproduction: Kinship, Power, and Technological Innovation*. Philadelphia: University of Pennsylvania Press.

Ginsburg, Faye D., and Rayna Rapp. 1991. "The Politics of Reproduction." *Annual Review of Anthropology* 20: 311–43.

———, eds. 1995. *Conceiving the New World Order: The Global Politics of Reproduction*. Berkeley: University of California Press.

Greenhalgh, Susan. 1990. "Toward a Political Economy of Fertility: Anthropological Contributions." *Population and Development Review* 16: 85–106.

———, ed. 1995. *Situating Fertility: Anthropology and Demographic Inquiry*. Cambridge: Cambridge University Press.

———. 1996. "The Social Construction of Population Science: An Intellectual, Institutional, and Political History of Twentieth-Century Demography." *Comparative Studies in Society and History* 38: 26–66.

———. 2013. "Patriarchal Demographics? China's Sex Ratio Reconsidered." *Population and Development Review* 38: 130–49.

Gürtin, Zeynep B., and Emily Tiemann. 2021. "The Marketing of Elective Egg Freezing: A Content, Cost, and Quality Analysis of UK Fertility Clinic Websites." *Reproductive BioMedicine and Society Online* 12: 56–68.

Hastrup, Anders. 2012. *The War in Darfur: Reclaiming Sudanese History*. London: Routledge.

Hoover, Elizabeth. 2018. "Environmental Reproductive Justice: Intersections in an American Indian Community Impacted by Environmental Contamination." *Environmental Sociology* 4(1): 8–21.

Inhorn, Marcia C. 1994. *Quest for Conception: Gender, Infertility, and Egyptian Medical Traditions*. Philadelphia: University of Pennsylvania Press.

———. 1996. *Infertility and Patriarchy: The Cultural Politics of Gender and Family Life in Egypt*. Philadelphia: University of Pennsylvania Press.

———. 2003. *Local Babies, Global Science: Gender, Religion, and in Vitro Fertilization in Egypt.* New York: Routledge.

———. 2018. *America's Arab Refugees: Vulnerability and Health on the Margins.* Stanford, CA: Stanford University Press.

———. 2020. "Where Has the Quest for Conception Taken Us? Lessons from Anthropology and Sociology." *Reproductive BioMedicine and Society Online* 11: 110–21.

———. 2023. *Motherhood on Ice: The Mating Gap and Why Women Freeze Their Eggs.* New York: New York University Press.

Inhorn, Marcia C., and Pasquale Patrizio. 2015. "Infertility around the Globe: New Thinking on Gender, Reproductive Technologies, and Global Movements in the 21st Century." *Human Reproduction Update* 21(4): 411–26.

Inhorn, Marcia C., and Frank van Balen, eds. 2002. *Infertility around the Globe: New Thinking on Childlessness, Gender, and Reproductive Technologies.* Berkeley: University of California Press.

Inhorn, Marcia C., and Lucia Volk, eds. 2021. *Un-Settling Middle Eastern Refugees: Regimes of Exclusion and Inclusion in the Middle East, Europe, and North America.* New York: Berghahn.

Kahn, Susan Martha. 2000. *Reproducing Jews: A Cultural Account of Assisted Conception in Israel.* Durham, NC: Duke University Press.

Kanaaneh, Rhoda. 2002. *Birthing the Nation: Strategies of Palestinian Women in Israel.* Berkeley: University of California Press.

Kimmerer, Robin Wall. 2013. *Braiding Sweetgrass: Indigenous Wisdom, Scientific Knowledge, and the Teachings of Plants.* Minneapolis, MN: Milkweed Editions.

Kohnert, Dirk. 2023. "On the Impact of the 2023 Sudanese War on Africa and Beyond." June 10. Available at SSRN: https://dx.doi.org/10.2139/ssrn.4473724.

Luna, Zakiya. 2020. *Reproductive Rights as Human Rights: Women of Color and the Fight for Reproductive Justice.* New York: New York University Press.

Maffi, Irene. 2020. *Abortion in Post-Revolutionary Tunisia: Politics, Medicine, and Morality.* New York: Berghahn.

Mezzadri, Alessandra, Susan Newman, and Sara Stevano. 2022. "Feminist Global Political Economies of Work and Social Reproduction." *Review of International Political Economy* 29: 1783–1803.

Morgan, Jennifer L. 2004. *Laboring Women: Reproduction and Gender in New World Slavery.* Philadelphia: University of Pennsylvania Press.

———. 2021. *Reckoning with Slavery: Gender, Kinship, and Capitalism in the Early Black Atlantic.* Durham, NC: Duke University Press.

Munson, Ziad. 2018. *Abortion Politics.* London: Polity.

Murphy, Michelle. 2017. *The Economization of Life.* Durham, NC: Duke University Press.

Pavone, Vincenzo. 2017. "Bio-Identification, Value Creation, and the Reproductive Bioeconomy: Insights from the Reprogenetics Sector in Spain." In *Bioeconomies: Life, Technology, and Capital in the 21st Century*, ed. Vincenzo Pavone and Joanna Goven, 129–60. London: Palgrave Macmillan.

Rao, Smriti. 2021. "Beyond the Coronavirus: Understanding Crises of Social Reproduction." *Global Labour Journal* 12(1): 39–53.

Roberts, Sean R. 2022. *The War on the Uyghurs: China's Internal Campaign against a Muslim Minority*. Princeton, NJ: Princeton University Press.

Sandelowski, Margarete. 1993. *With Child in Mind: Studies of the Personal Encounter with Infertility*. Philadelphia: University of Pennsylvania Press.

Shalhoub-Kevorkian, Nadera. 2022. *Incarcerated Childhood and the Politics of Unchilding*. New York: Cambridge University Press.

Singer, Elyse Ona. 2022. *Lawful Sins: Abortion Rights and Reproductive Governance in Mexico*. Stanford, CA: Stanford University Press.

Strathern, Marilyn. 1992a. *After Nature: English Kinship in the Late Twentieth Century*. Cambridge: Cambridge University Press.

———. 1992b. *Reproducing the Future: Anthropology, Kinship, and the New Reproductive Technologies*. London: Routledge.

Suh, Siri. 2021. *Dying to Count: Post-Abortion Care and Global Reproductive Health Politics in Senegal*. New Brunswick, NJ: Rutgers University Press.

Sultana, Farhana. 2021. "Climate Change, COVID-19, and the Co-production of Injustices: A Feminist Reading of Overlapping Crises." *Social & Cultural Geography* 22: 447–60.

Szreter, Simon. 1993. "The Idea of Demographic Transition and the Study of Fertility Change: A Critical Intellectual History." *Population and Development Review* 19: 659–701.

Thompson, Charis M. 2002. "Fertile Ground: Feminists Theorize Infertility." In *Infertility around the Globe: New Thinking on Childlessness, Gender, and Reproductive Technologies*, ed. Marcia C. Inhorn and Frank van Balen, 52–78. Berkeley: University of California Press.

———. 2005. *Making Parents: The Ontological Choreography of Reproductive Technologies*. Cambridge: MIT Press.

Uehling, Greta Lynn. 2023. *Everyday War: The Conflict over Donbas, Ukraine*. Ithaca, NY: Cornell University Press.

United Nations. 2021. Department of Economic and Social Affairs, Population Division, Expert Group Meeting on the Impact of the COVID-19 Pandemic on Fertility. No. ESA/P/WP/264.

Van de Wiel, Lucy. 2020. *Freezing Fertility: Oocyte Cryopreservation and the Gender Politics of Aging*. New York: New York University Press.

Vanella, Patrizio, Arthur L. Greil, and Philipp Deschermeier. 2023. "Fertility Response to the COVID-19 Pandemic in Developed Countries: On Pre-pandemic Fertility Forecasts." *Comparative Population Studies* 48(January): 19–45.

Vertommen, Sigrid, Vincenzo Pavone, and Michal Nahman. 2022. "Global Fertility Chains: An Integrative Political Economy Approach to Understanding the Reproductive Bioeconomy." *Science, Technology, & Human Values* 47(1): 112–45.

Vertommen, Rodante van der Waal, Sigrid, Michal Nahman, Rishita Nandagiri, Elif Gül, Weeam Hammoudeh, Heba Farajallah and Fatimah Mohamied. 2023.

"Resistance Is Fertile: No Reproductive Justice without Freedom for Palestine." Reprosist, December 19. https://reprosist.org.

Wahlberg, Ayo, and Tine M. Gammeltoft, eds. 2017. *Selective Reproduction in the 21st Century*. London: Palgrave Macmillan.

Wanner, Catherine, ed. 2023. *Dispossession*. London: Routledge.

Ware, Anthony, and Costas Laoutides. 2018. *Myanmar's "Rohingya" Conflict*. Oxford: Oxford University Press.

Weinbaum, Alys Eve. 2019. *The Afterlife of Slavery: Biocapitalism and Black Feminism's Philosophy of History*. Durham, NC: Duke University Press.

Zavella, Patricia. 2020. *The Movement for Reproductive Justice: Empowering Women of Color through Social Activism*. New York: New York University Press.

PART I

In-Fertile Families

The relationship between in-fertility and assisted reproductive technologies (ARTs) has transformed the intimate world of family making, which in the post-IVF era is increasingly understood and imagined in relation to technological assistance. The chapters in this section all focus on in-fertile family formation, including emerging forms of consciousness about how to achieve a pregnancy; whether or not to have children; whether to employ ARTs; and how to acquire the resources, knowledge, and support to use ARTs to create particular family forms. The "IVF turn" in the new reproductive order has led to three particularly salient phenomena. First, the specific choices made in relation to the process of making, or "crafting," family forms offer insights into more general patterns of social and cultural change—a key argument of this volume. Second, IVF technologies are increasingly being normalized and encouraged as a way to make babies in some low-fertility societies that are concerned about their flagging birth rates and the future of their traditional heterosexual families. Third, LGBTQI+ individuals and couples, whose paths to family formation have been transformed by the burgeoning ART sector, are becoming increasingly normative in the new reproductive order—on the one hand, able to consider previously unavailable reproductive possibilities, but on the other, still facing challenging paths to family formation.

This section on ART-assisted family making begins in the Arab world, where fertility rates have plummeted and multiple reproductive technologies have been enlisted to craft the "new Arab family." Yet, a "technological convergence" between contraception and various forms of ART, which may also involve the use of abortion and gender selection, illustrates how the new reproductive order involves not only "new" technologies and practices but also their use in combination with older technologies and values (chapter 1). In Japan, fertility rates have declined so dramatically that women are now being encouraged to engage in an intensive form of "repro-activity" called "*ninkatsu*," or "pursuit of pregnancy," in which IVF and other ARTs are seen as a potential solution to the nation's crisis of "ultra-low" fertility (chapter 2). In the low-fertility societies of southern Europe, Greece stands out for its booming ART sector. Within a cultural context of "repronational familism" that prioritizes family and procreation, "reproductive heterosexism" is nonetheless apparent in the country's ART legislation, which disallows LGBTQI+ family making in the "best interests of the child" (chapter 3). In the United Kingdom, the passage of new legislation has enabled new "reproductive imaginations" for LGBTQI+ people—although the process of imagining parenthood does not always guarantee its outcome for reasons that are complex (chapter 4). One of the major barriers to gay parenthood is economic, as seen in the "spreadsheet fertility" of gay men, who must calculate the immense costs of gestational surrogacy (chapter 5). Having said this, the complex planning involved in pursuing uncertain fertility futures is now a means of imagined family formation that LGBTQI+ people share in common with heterosexual couples in the topsy-turvy landscape of the new reproductive order. In each of these chapters, we see how the rise of ARTs is altering perceptions of family formation, thus revealing some of the core changes in reproductive cause and effect that typify the new reproductive order.

1

Technological Convergence

Creating the New Arab Family through Contraception, Assisted Reproduction, Selective Abortion, and Son Selection

MARCIA C. INHORN

The Arab world is known for its dramatic political revolutions. But one of the "quiet" revolutions occurring across the Arab world involves profound changes in fertility, infertility, and the emergence of reproductive technologies. Over the past three decades, fertility rates have plummeted across the region. By 2012, nearly half of the world's top fifteen fertility declines had occurred in Arab nations (United Nations 2012), reflecting both the increased use of contraceptives and married couples' willingness to have fewer children. Yet, this dramatic fertility decline is not the only reproductive revolution taking place in Arab countries. From Morocco to Saudi Arabia, the Arab world has seen the growth of one of the world's largest in vitro fertilization (IVF) sectors, designed to overcome Arab couples' infertility problems. Infertility treatment via assisted reproductive technologies (ARTs) has been encouraged by Islamic religious authorities (Inhorn and Tremayne 2012), with some governments subsidizing these expensive ARTs for their citizens (Inhorn 2015).

ARTs are not only about treating infertility; they have the power to shape the size of a family and the gender of its offspring. In this regard, two ARTs have also quietly gained traction in Arab countries. One is called "multifetal pregnancy reduction" (MFPR), or simply "fetal reduction," a procedure of selective abortion that may be used in high-order multiple pregnancies (HOMPs) with three or more fetuses, or in any multifetal pregnancy in which one or more of the fetuses has congenital anomalies. The other is preimplantation genetic diagnosis (PGD), a reprogenetic technology designed to diagnose severe genetic disorders in eight-cell IVF embryos, thereby preventing the birth of IVF offspring with life-threatening heritable diseases (Franklin and Roberts 2006). However, in the Arab countries, PGD has increasingly morphed into preimplantation genetic screening of IVF embryos for the purposes of sex selection.

Both MFPR and PGD represent forms of "selective reproduction," defined by medical anthropologists Ayo Wahlberg and Tine Gammeltoft in the following way: "Although they often overlap with assisted reproductive technologies (ARTs), what we term selective reproductive technologies (SRTs) are of a more specific nature: Rather than aiming to overcome infertility, they are used to prevent or allow the birth of certain kinds of children" (Gammeltoft and Wahlberg 2014: 201). Not surprisingly, these selective technologies are controversial. For example, IVF-related practices of fetal reduction and son selection have led to a "bioethical aftermath," in which the potential for skewed sex ratios becomes real when family size and gender composition are no longer left to chance (Inhorn and Tremayne 2016).

This chapter focuses specifically on this *technological convergence*—or the ways in which various reproductive technologies can come together in family building on both an individual and a societal level. In Arab countries, the as-yet-unstudied technological convergence of contraception, assisted reproduction, selective abortion, and son selection is shaping the "new Arab family" (Hopkins 2003)—a small family demonstrating so-called replacement-level fertility of only two children for two parents. Contraceptive technologies are helping Arab couples limit their fertility and control their birth spacing. Assisted reproductive technologies are helping infertile Arab couples overcome their childlessness and conceive IVF offspring. Meanwhile, selective abortion technologies are helping to reduce the risk of high-order IVF pregnancies, thereby producing two children (i.e., twins) in the process. And reprogenetic technologies are helping to reduce genetic disease in IVF embryos, but also assuring the birth of at least one son.

To demonstrate this technological convergence, I draw in this chapter upon more than three decades of anthropological fieldwork in the Arab world, including in Egypt (Inhorn 1994, 1996, 2003), Lebanon (Inhorn 2012), and the United Arab Emirates (UAE) (Inhorn 2015). All of these countries have achieved substantial fertility declines, with Lebanon and the UAE now at or below replacement fertility levels. All three countries have produced highly developed IVF sectors to respond to couples' infertility problems. And for those couples who can afford IVF, selective reproduction is sometimes also taking place to produce the new small Arab family.

The Arab Fertility Decline

The Arab world is often portrayed in popular media, academic circles, and policy reports as a region of high fertility—attributable to men's supposed patriarchal control over women's bodies (Ali 2002) and religiously fueled pronatalism (Inhorn 1996). However, this portrayal of male oppression and hyperfertility is both outdated and inaccurate. Instead, it is important to trace the massive Arab fertility decline—a story that entails a "quiet revolution . . . hiding in plain sight" (Eberstadt and Shah 2012: 43–44).

When total fertility rates (TFRs) were first recorded in Arab countries in the 1975–1980 period, women in seventeen Arab nations had TFRs far exceeding the world average at that time of 3.85 children per woman. Indeed, seven Arab countries—Algeria, Kuwait, Libya, Oman, Saudi Arabia, Syria, and Yemen—had TFRs greater than 7.0, with the highest recorded TFR of 8.58 in Yemen (United Nations 2018). However, by the year 2010, seven of the world's top fifteen fertility declines had occurred in Arab nations (United Nations 2012). As shown in table 1.1, fertility levels had declined by more than 60 percent in each of these countries, with Libya showing the largest fertility reduction of nearly 70 percent.

TABLE 1.1. Arab Countries in the Top Fifteen for Fertility Decline over Thirty-Five Years (1975–2010). Credit: United Nations (2012)

Country	Total Fertility Rate (1975–1980)	Total Fertility Rate (2005–2010)	Difference	Percentage Decline
Libya	7.94	2.67	−4.39	69.9
United Arab Emirates	5.66	1.97	−3.69	65.2
Oman	8.1	2.89	−5.21	64.3
Tunisia	5.69	2.05	−3.64	63.9
Qatar	6.11	2.21	−3.9	63.8
Lebanon	4.23	1.58	−2.66	62.8
Algeria	7.18	2.72	−4.45	62

Today, most Arab nations have TFRs hovering around the world average of 2.3. Only three Arab countries (Egypt, Iraq, and Yemen) have TFRs at 3.0 or above, and only one (Sudan) is above 4.0. Nine Arab countries (Algeria, Jordan, Libya, Oman, Qatar, Saudi Arabia, Syria, the United Arab Emirates, and Yemen) have TFRs that have declined by nearly four births per woman. For example, an Algerian woman in 1980 would have expected to have more than seven children on average. But an Algerian woman today has only two to three—four to five fewer than her mother—as shown in table 1.2.

TABLE 1.2. Decline in Arab Fertility Levels over Forty-Five Years (1975–2020). Credit: United Nations (2012, 2018); World Bank (2023a, 2023b)

Country	Population in Millions (1988)	Population in Millions (2021)	Total Fertility Rate (1975–1980)	Total Fertility Rate (2000–2005)	Total Fertility Rate (2005–2010)	Total Fertility Rate (2010–2015)	Total Fertility Rate (2015–2020)	Total Fertility Rate (2020)
World	5,100	7,890	3.85	2.59	2.53	2.45	2.47	2.3
Algeria	23.9	44.1	7.18	2.38	2.72	2.82	2.65	2.9
Bahrain	0.5	1.46	5.23	2.67	2.23	2.1	2	1.8
Egypt	50.3	109.26	5.5	3.15	2.98	2.79	3.15	3
Iraq	17.6	43.53	6.8	4.75	4.38	4.06	4.27	3.6
Jordan	4	11.15	7.38	3.85	3.64	3.27	3.26	2.9
Kuwait	2.1	4.25	5.89	2.58	2.71	2.6	1.97	2.1
Lebanon	2.8	5.59	4.23	2.01	1.58	1.51	1.7	2.1
Libya	4	6.73	7.94	2.92	2.67	2.38	2.21	2.5
Morocco	23.5	37.08	5.9	2.52	2.38	2.78	2.42	2.4
Oman	1.4	4.52	8.1	3.21	2.89	2.91	2.54	2.7
Qatar	0.4	2.69	6.11	2.95	2.21	2.05	1.88	1.8
Saudi Arabia	15.2	35.95	7.28	3.54	3.03	2.68	2.48	2.5
Sudan	18.9	45.66	6.92	5.25	4.83	4.46	4.43	4.5
Syria	11.7	21.32	7.32	3.67	3.19	3	2.84	2.8
Tunisia	7.9	12.26	5.69	2.04	2.05	2.02	2.15	2.1
United Arab Emirates	1.7	9.36	5.66	2.40	1.97	1.82	1.73	1.5
Yemen	11	32.98	8.58	5.91	4.91	4.15	3.84	3.9

What is most impressive about this Arab fertility decline is that it has occurred even in resource-poor Arab nations. As noted by demographers, most Arab countries have fewer resources (i.e., income, education, urbanization, modern contraception) than the "more developed regions with which their fertility levels currently correspond today" (Eberstadt and Shah 2012: 35). Put another way, the Arab world has achieved its dramatic fertility decline with fewer preexisting resources or advantages. The decline has occurred largely through human agency—namely, the actions of Arab couples wanting fewer children to love and support.

The Rise of Contraception and the "New Arab Family"

How did this massive fertility decline happen? The introduction of family-planning programs and contraception in the Arab world is an important part of this story, along with attitudinal change, or the desire for fewer children on the part of both men and women. New attitudes toward family size and acceptance of contraceptive technologies have led to "the new Arab family" (Hopkins 2003)—namely, a small nuclear family that is the tangible result of the Arab fertility decline.

Contraception came relatively slowly to the Arab world. Egypt, the first country to accept international family planning aid in the 1960s (Stycos and Sayed 1988), had only achieved a contraceptive prevalence rate of 30 percent by the early 1980s. In a survey of eleven Arab countries conducted in 1982, the mean contraceptive prevalence rate was only 19 percent (Lapham and Mauldin 1985). Even in Lebanon, with its low total fertility rate, slightly more than half (53 percent) of Lebanese couples reported using contraceptives. Several Arab countries lacked any form of contraceptive prevalence data, or reported rates that were very low, ranging from 1 to 10 percent (e.g., Algeria, Syria).

By 1985, however, female contraceptive prevalence rates began to increase significantly in several Arab countries, even in the absence of explicit family-planning information or country-wide policies (Lapham and Mauldin 1985). In Jordan, for example—a country with no specific fertility policy (to either raise or lower population growth) and without any direct government family-planning program—the contraceptive prevalence rate nonetheless rose from an average of 40 percent in 1990 to 60 percent in 2009. By then, 82 percent of ever-married Jordanian women aged fifteen to forty-nine had used contraception at some point in their reproductive lives, with the average Jordanian woman able to describe nine different contraceptive methods (Cetorelli and Leone 2012).

It is fair to say that by the beginning of the new millennium, knowledge of contraceptive methods among Arab women had become widespread (Cetorelli and Leone 2012). Surveys showed that between 90 and 98 percent of married Arab women reported knowing about at least one modern method of contraception. In 2010, a survey of the twenty-two Member States of the World Health Organization Eastern Mediterranean Region showed that at least one of seven core components of successful family-planning programs (e.g., integrated services and delivery, promotion of family planning, evaluation and monitoring) were available in 94 percent of the eighteen Member States that responded to the survey (Chikvaidze, Madi, and Mahaini 2012).

In addition, studies conducted in a variety of Arab countries demonstrated men's strong support of female contraception, as well as men's advocacy of male-controlled birth control—not with condoms, which were shown to be negatively perceived in a variety of Arab countries (Kulczycki 2004), but rather through the time-tested method of 'azl (withdrawal, or coitus interruptus) (Myntti et al. 2002). 'Azl has played an important role in the history of Islamic societies (Musallam 1983). Not only does 'azl receive support within the Islamic scriptures as a viable means of male-enacted contraception, but Arab men tend to prefer withdrawal as a "safe" method of family planning that is more "natural" than most female-controlled methods (Myntti et al. 2002).

Between the reproductive efforts of both Arab men ('azl) and Arab women (contraceptives), Arab couples brought into being the new Arab family of two to three children on average. This new Arab family has been in place in some countries since the late 1980s, when contraceptive prevalence rates began to grow. For example, in my own research conducted in 1988–1989 in Alexandria, Egypt, I discovered strong desires on the part of poor urban women to reside in nuclear family households with their husbands and children. Nuclear households allowed poor women some measure of marital privacy and also a space to raise their children free from family (especially in-law) interference. But given small apartment spaces and fragile household economies, women in my study were clear that they and their husbands only wanted two children, no more. They used the Arabic term *"usra"* to describe this small nuclear family, differentiating it from the larger extended family, or *'aa'ila*. Already in the late 1980s, the *usra* had become the well-entrenched norm among the urban Egyptian working poor of my study (Inhorn 1994, 1996).

Similarly, in my 2003 study in Beirut, Lebanon, I found that Lebanese men of all social classes and religious sects were eager to become fathers. Fatherhood, in their view, was one of life's most important joys and masculine ambitions. Yet, with very few exceptions, Lebanese men were adamant that having more than three children was unfeasible and unwise in the current political and economic climate. "Two boys and one girl" was often stated as men's ideal family composition. Yet, some men were insistent that girls were superior to boys in terms of their affection and lifelong commitment to their parents. Thus, they intended to stop at two (or three), even if all of their children were daughters. In other words, the "new Arab man," as I came to call him (Inhorn 2012), also supported this "new Arab family" of two or three children. In general, Arab men, like their wives, also maintained strong preferences for *both* sons and daughters, a desire for "gender balance" that is playing out in the world of Arab assisted reproduction.

The Arab IVF Revolution

Although contraceptive technologies came late to the Arab world, in vitro fertilization (IVF) did not. Less than a decade after the birth of the world's first "test-tube baby," Louise Brown, in England, the Arab world's first test-tube baby, Heba Mohammed, was born in Egypt in 1987 (Inhorn 2003). IVF, the ART used to conceive both children, rapidly globalized in the 1990s, spreading to many parts of the Arab world. For example, Egypt was the first country to open an IVF clinic in 1986, followed by Saudi Arabia and Jordan. By the mid-1990s, Egypt was experiencing an IVF "boom period," with more than seventy IVF clinics eventually opening in Egypt's major cities (Inhorn 2003; International Federation of Fertility Societies 2022). Other Middle Eastern countries soon followed suit. By the mid-2000s, the Middle East boasted one of the largest and most successful IVF sectors in the world (Inhorn and Patrizio 2015). As shown in table 1.3, among the forty-eight countries performing the most

TABLE 1.3. Arab Countries Performing the Most
ART Cycles per Capita. Credit: Adamson (2009)

Country	Rank in Top 48
Lebanon	6
Jordan	8
Tunisia	25
Bahrain	28
Saudi Arabia	31
Egypt	32
Libya	34
United Arab Emirates	35

ART cycles per million inhabitants in 2009, eight Arab nations could be counted. Today, more than a dozen Arab nations host IVF clinics, with the largest numbers found in Egypt (110), Qatar (sixty-six), Saudi Arabia (fifty), Libya (forty), and Jordan (thirty-five). Yet, even the smallest Arab nations today host vibrant IVF sectors—for example, Lebanon (twenty), Kuwait (fifteen), Tunisia (twelve), and the UAE (ten) (International Federation of Fertility Societies 2022). This burgeoning Arab IVF sector is somewhat surprising given the high cost of this technology. On average, a single cycle of IVF costs one thousand to thirty-five hundred dollars in countries such as Lebanon and Egypt, but can range from six to twelve thousand dollars in wealthier Arab Gulf nations such as the UAE.

This Arab IVF revolution could not have happened without Islamic support (Inhorn 2003; Serour 2008). On March 23, 1980, the grand shaykh of Egypt's renowned religious university, Al Azhar, issued the first widely authoritative *fatwa* on assisted reproduction—only two years after Louise Brown's birth in England, but a full six years before the opening of Egypt's first IVF clinic. Nearly fifty years on, this original Al-Azhar *fatwa* has proved to be quite authoritative and enduring across the Sunni Muslim world (i.e., about 90 percent of the world's Muslims). It has been reissued many times in Egypt, and subsequently reaffirmed by *fatwa*-granting authorities and institutes in other parts of the Sunni Muslim world, from Morocco to Malaysia.

In general terms, Islamic religious authorities have been permissive in authorizing the use of ARTs among Muslim IVF physicians and their patients. Their *fatwas* on ARTs have allowed not only IVF but also intracytoplasmic sperm injection (ICSI), a variant of IVF used for male infertility; cryopreservation (freezing of sperm, eggs, and embryos); preimplantation genetic diagnosis (PGD) for couples at high risk of genetic disorders in their offspring; and IVF via uterine transplantation, with Saudi Arabia being the first country in the world to attempt this form of organ transplantation (Fageeh et al. 2002). However, Sunni religious authorities have not condoned every ART, and especially not the use of third-party reproductive assistance. In IVF clinics in Sunni-majority countries, sperm donation, egg donation, embryo donation, and surrogacy are religiously prohibited, translating into a ban on the clinical practice of third-party reproductive assistance that has held sway across the Sunni world since 1980 (Inhorn and Tremayne 2012).

The Rise of Selective Technologies in the Arab World

Despite this prohibition on third-party reproduction, Islamic religious leaders have generally condoned selective reproductive technologies, especially if they can help to reduce the various risks of IVF pregnancies and births. MFPR, or fetal reduction, is a case in point. In the Arab world, many women undergoing IVF experience high-order multiple pregnancies (HOMPs), because multiple embryos (i.e., three, four, and sometimes more) are transferred to women's wombs in an attempt to achieve an IVF pregnancy in a single cycle, usually because of the high costs (emotional, physical, and financial) of IVF repetition. Yet, current international guidelines advise the transfer of only one or two embryos for women under the age of thirty-five, because pregnancies with multiple fetuses are always high risk. Infants born as part of a multiple pregnancy are often premature and face increased risks of cerebral palsy, cognitive delays, and perinatal death (International Federation of Fertility Societies 2019).

Given these risks, women in the Arab world who experience multifetal pregnancies are often medically advised to undergo MFPR, a form of selective abortion. In MFPR, potassium chloride solution is injected under ultrasound guidance into one or more of the fetal hearts, causing the heart to stop beating and leading to fetal demise. From a medical standpoint, MFPR is a way to diminish risk by "reducing" an HOMP to a more manageable pregnancy with one or two fetuses. From a religious standpoint, MFPR has been allowed by most Islamic religious authorities because it is deemed a form of "therapeutic" abortion, necessary to save the life of a mother and at least one or two of her fetuses. In general, abortion is highly restricted across the Arab world, with only one country, Tunisia, allowing full legal access to abortion. In all other Arab countries, abortion is criminalized to varying degrees, with thirteen countries having abortion laws described as "very restrictive" (Hessini 2007). In these countries, abortion is allowed only in cases in which a pregnant woman's life is in jeopardy. Having said this, abortions are widely practiced across the Arab world, with one in every ten pregnancies ending this way (Hessini 2007). Perhaps this is the case because Islam considers life to begin at the moment of "ensoulment," not conception—with ensoulment defined as occurring between 40 and 120 days of gestation, depending upon the legal school.

Given that life is not defined as beginning at the moment of IVF conception, it is perhaps not surprising that MFPR is practiced widely in Arab IVF clinics. Undergoing MFPR is never easy, especially for those couples who have waited years for a successful IVF pregnancy. In my research in Egypt, Lebanon, and the UAE, I met many women who were making this agonizing decision to "reduce" their multifetal pregnancies, especially women carrying triplets, quadruplets, and more. Women often considered MFPR to be excruciating—physically, emotionally, and morally. Yet, I never met a woman who refused MFPR when it was advised by her physician. Many women, in fact, were relieved to "reduce" a high-order pregnancy, especially of four or five fetuses, down to two. Women often rationalized that fetal reduction would increase the chances of their remaining twins being born alive, healthy, and free from physical and cognitive disabilities. Furthermore, the birth of twins was seen as achieving ideal family size goals within a single IVF pregnancy. In other words, through this particular "HOMP-MFPR nexus" (Inhorn 2017), a selective abortion technology was being used to modify the results of an IVF pregnancy in order to create the new, small, *healthy* Arab family.

Whereas MFPR effectively culls IVF fetuses from women's wombs, PGD is a technology designed to cull IVF embryos before they ever reach women's wombs. To be exact, PGD is performed on eight-cell embryos so that only disease-free ones are transferred into a woman's uterus as part of an IVF cycle. PGD is also used to sex embryos, with the intent of preventing X-linked genetic disorders, such as hemophilia and Duchenne muscular dystrophy (Bhatia 2018).

In the Muslim world, Islamic authorities have generally accepted the use of PGD for the prevention of genetic disease, including those diseases carried in the female chromosomes. However, PGD for the sole purpose of sex selection has become a major area of Islamic controversy. Sex selection against girls—including female infanticide—has a long history of moral opprobrium in Islam, with the Prophet Muhammad specifically condemning this pre-Islamic practice (Zavis 2018). Thus, the notion that Muslim parents might eliminate daughters has always been viewed as anathema in the religion.

The issue of technologically assisted sex selection was debated in 1983—seven years before PGD's existence—in a conference on "Reproduction in Light of Islam" organized by the Islamic Organization for Medical Sciences (Shabana 2017). At the end of the conference, a statement condemning sex selection was issued, and was reaffirmed by the Islamic Fiqh Council of the Muslim World League once PGD became clinically available. According to these authorities, PGD-assisted sex selection should only be used in cases of medical necessity, when genetic diseases are affecting embryos of either sex (Shabana 2017).

However, *fatwas* allowing "gender selection" and "family balancing" have been issued, including from Egypt's famous religious university, Al Azhar. Although sex selection on the "community" level has been viewed as dangerous, sex selection on the "individual" level has been deemed appropriate in cases where a couple has born children of only one sex. As a result of these permissive *fatwas*, IVF clinics in at least ten Arab countries have been offering PGD for sex selection since the early 2000s (Kilani and Hassan 2002; Serour 2008). In most cases, sex selection is being chosen to produce sons, not daughters.

But why son selection? As shown in a recent multicountry survey, the belief that sons are socially mandatory within family life is widespread across the Arab world and is upheld by traditional patriarchal values (El Feki, Heilman, and Barker 2017). Even if Arab parents say they love their daughters and prefer them as lifelong companions (Inhorn 1996, 2012), they still "need" their sons to complete their families and ensure the reproduction of the patrilineage. Sons are expected to contribute to family labor and maintain family assets and are widely regarded as a family's social safety net, guaranteeing the financial support of their aging parents (Inhorn 2012; Kanaaneh 2002; Obermeyer 1996, 1999; Zavis 2018). Given these social realities, ensuring the birth of at least one son is vital to most Arab families. Arab couples wanting to "plan" their small families, while still ensuring the birth of a son, thus face a major predicament, especially when one or more daughters have already been born. PGD-assisted son selection may represent an individual Muslim couple's solution to this predicament, as well as a Muslim society's technological tool to enact male-centric norms.

Of the many Arab countries now performing PGD for son selection in IVF clinics, the UAE can be counted. In 2007, PGD was introduced in the UAE for sex-linked genetic diagnosis, which was deemed a medical priority in a nation with one of the highest frequencies of genetic disease in the world (Al-Gazali 2005; Al-Gazali et al. 1997). By 2010, PGD was formally recognized as one of the legal ART practices in UAE's federal ART law, which was enacted that year (Inhorn 2015). Yet, by then, it had already become clear that new demand for PGD had little to do with genetic diagnosis. In a study I conducted in 2007 in the UAE's largest IVF clinic, I began to meet Emirati couples who were clearly not infertile, but who wanted a son after the birth of one or more daughters. Their PGD-assisted son selection—usually performed in secrecy without others' knowledge—seemed to be occurring as an intentional form of family planning among Emirati professional couples, especially those who wanted only two children, having already birthed a daughter.

A decade on, son selection in the UAE is no longer a secret. In a follow-up interview I conducted with one of the UAE's most well-regarded IVF physicians, he reported an alarming new trend of son selection—not only among his Emirati patients but also among South Asian couples, who constitute the single largest expatriate population in the UAE (Vora 2013). As this physician explained to me,

> There is a lot of demand among "locals" and Indians, and the Indians more than among the Emiratis. They seem even more interested in getting a boy! [Another IVF physician] offers it to *all* of his patients, and 60 to 70 percent of them do PGD. Here, if the couple brings it up, then we

have a discussion. The only times I recommend PGD are for recurrent miscarriages, where there could actually be some genetic translocations, and then this is the correct thing to do. Also for repeated, unexplained IVF failures, we offer it then. But some couples ask for sex selection. We're not doing PGS [preimplantation genetic screening] often, maybe only five to six cycles a month. But [my colleague] is doing forty to fifty cycles of PGS a month, and then you could really start running into problems of gender imbalance. Ninety percent will want to select for boys, and only 10 percent for girls. Among Arabs and Indians, all will want a boy, I'm afraid.

In fact, many Emirati IVF clinics now openly advertise gender selection as part of their services, even if they cast the technology as a form of "family balancing" and "enhancement" (Krolökke and Kotsi 2018). In the UAE's booming IVF sector, clinicians often speak about the "need" for sons as the major determinant of sex selection. Moreover, this need for sons is justified, according to them, because Middle Eastern couples today want a "smaller, yet nevertheless balanced, family" (Krolökke and Kotsi 2018: 13).

Arab Technological Convergence and Its Bioethical Aftermath

The emergence of fetal-reductive MFPR and sex-selective PGD in the Arab IVF sector has not arisen out of nowhere. These selective technologies have occurred amidst the massive Arab fertility decline, facilitated by the use of contraception. Today, most Arab nations are close to achieving replacement fertility, as shown in table 1.2. However, this massive Arab fertility decline has brought with it a demand for newer smaller families, sometimes created through the use of selective technologies.

Already, the coming of PGD to the Arab world has reinscribed age-old son preferences, which, prior to the advent of this technology, had been shown to be in decline. For example, Demographic and Health Surveys conducted back in the mid-1990s showed that son preference was not pronounced in the Arab world. Equal treatment of boys and girls was found in almost every aspect of child health (Obermeyer and Cardenas 1997), and the impact of son preference on fertility levels was deemed negligible (Obermeyer 1996). However, much has changed over the ensuing decades, as IVF and PGD have made their way across the region, fueling renewed son preference along the way.

In the Arab world, the potential bioethical aftermath of PGD includes four major consequences. First, the increased prevalence of PGD-assisted son selection in the Arab world could exacerbate daughter discrimination, even leading to the endangerment of already-born girl children. As anthropologist Elisabeth Croll (2000) once argued in her book *Endangered Daughters: Discrimination and Development in Asia*, an overarching focus on son preference hides the insidious countereffect of daughter discrimination, including the fact that millions of girls around the world do not survive into adulthood. Because PGD promotes son selection, it invariably contributes to daughter discrimination, and especially toward "extra" daughters born in a family who are considered superfluous by their parents. These societal increases in sexism and tangible forms of gender discrimination and endangerment are perhaps the most insidious effects of PGD (Klitzman 2016).

Second, if PGD comes to be routinized in prenatal practice, particularly in Arab countries with well-developed IVF infrastructures, we may begin to see the distortion of natural sex ratios at birth—a phenomenon that has already happened quite profoundly and well beyond government control in large swaths of Asia (Hesketh, Lu, and Zhu 2011). Where sex-selective technologies and abortion are readily available, such as in China, India, South Korea, and Vietnam (Croll 2000), distorted sex ratios have invariably followed. If PGD is increasingly used in Arab countries for the purposes of son selection, then the result will be a fundamental gender imbalance, altering the demography of Arab countries, and potentially other Muslim countries across the world.

Third, PGD may be promoted as a more "humane" method of sex selection, reducing the incidence of sex-selective abortions. Although ultrasound-guided, sex-selective abortions have not been widely documented within the Middle East's own illicit abortion landscape (Hessini 2007), sex-selective abortion is widely practiced across most parts of Asia (e.g., Bhatia 2018; Croll 2000; Gammeltoft and Wahlberg 2014; Hesketh, Lu, and Zhu 2011). Eventually, in the Arab world, PGD may come to be promoted as a more "acceptable" form of sex selection, one that does not depend upon the destruction of the female fetus through abortion (Van Balen and Inhorn 2003).

Finally, as a reprogenetic technology, PGD may lead humans down the "slippery slope" of "designer" babies and eugenic removal of the "unfit" (Klitzman 2016). Choosing embryos of only one sex, culling embryos of the other sex, and eliminating all embryos with perceived genetic defects are selective reproductive practices that ensure the births of some children rather than others (Gammeltoft and Wahlberg 2014). Arab societies will need to grapple with these conundrums, especially now that gender selection has been permitted by some Muslim religious authorities to "balance" the family on the individual level.

Conclusion

As this chapter shows, revolutionary changes in the use of reproductive technologies are creating the new Arab family. The uptake of *contraceptive technologies* by Arab couples wanting smaller families has led to dramatic fertility declines. The use of *assisted reproductive technologies* by infertile Arab couples wanting to become parents has led to the growth of a booming IVF sector. And the turn to *selective reproductive technologies* by Arab couples desiring the birth of healthy IVF offspring has led to increasing practices of abortion and sex selection. This technological convergence in the Arab world has had profound demographic, societal, and bioethical implications. Yet, it is a reproductive revolution "hiding in plain sight" (Eberstadt and Shah 2012), with little acknowledgment in scholarly, policy, or media circles.

In considering changing in-fertilities in the twenty-first-century new reproductive order, it seems important to reflect upon the ways in which diverse reproductive technologies converge over time, affecting the fertility trends of whole regions. As this chapter on the Arab world has shown, family size and sex of offspring are being shaped—for better and for worse—through a technological convergence of contraception, assisted reproduction, selective abortion, and son selection. The result is a new, small, "gender-balanced" Arab family—created through human agency, child desire, and the convergence of multiple reproductive technologies.

REFERENCES

Adamson, G. David. 2009. "Global Cultural and Socioeconomic Factors That Influence Access to Assisted Reproductive Technologies." *Women's Health* 5: 351–58.

Al-Gazali, L. I. 2005. "Attitudes toward Genetic Counseling in the United Arab Emirates." *Community Genetics* 8: 48–51.

Al-Gazali, L. I., A. Bener, Y. M. Abdulrazzaq, R. Micallef, A. I. Al-Khayat, and T. Gaber. 1997. "Consanguineous Marriages in the United Arab Emirates." *Journal of Biosocial Science* 29: 491–97.

Ali, Kamran Asdar. 2002. *Planning the Egyptian Family: New Bodies, New Selves.* Austin: University of Texas Press.

Bhatia, Rajani. 2018. *Gender before Birth: Sex Selection in a Transnational Context.* Seattle: University of Washington Press.

Cetorelli, Valeria, and Tiziana Leone. 2012. "Is Fertility Stalling in Jordan?" *Demographic Research* 26: 293–318.

Chikvaidze, P., H. H. Madi, and R. K. Mahaini. 2012. "Mapping Family Planning Policy and Programme Best Practices in the WHO Eastern Mediterranean Region: A Step towards Coordinated Scale-up." *Eastern Mediterranean Health Journal* 18: 1–9.

Croll, Elisabeth. 2000. *Endangered Daughters: Discrimination and Development in Asia.* New York: Routledge.

Eberstadt, Nicholas, and Apoorva Shah. 2012. "Fertility Decline in the Muslim World: A Demographic Sea Change Goes Largely Unnoticed." *Policy Review* 173: 29–44.

El Feki, Shereen, Brian Heilman, and Gary Barker, eds. 2017. *Understanding Masculinities: Results from the International Men and Gender Equality Survey (IMAGES)— Middle East and North Africa.* Cairo: UN Women and Promundo.

Fageeh, W., H. Raffa, H. Jabbad, and A. Marzouki. 2002. "Transplantation of the Human Uterus." *International Journal of Gynecology & Obstetrics* 76: 245–51.

Franklin, Sarah, and Celia Roberts. 2006. *Born and Made: An Ethnography of Preimplantation Genetic Diagnosis.* Princeton, NJ: Princeton University Press.

Gammeltoft, Tine, and Ayo Wahlberg. 2014. "Selective Reproductive Technologies." *Annual Review of Anthropology* 43: 201–16.

Hesketh, Therese, Li Lu, and Zhu Wei Zing. 2011. "The Consequences of Son Preference and Sex-Selective Abortion in China and Other Asian Countries." *Canadian Medical Association Journal* 183: 1374–77.

Hessini, Leila. 2007. "Abortion and Islam: Policies and Practice in the Middle East and North Africa." *Reproductive Health Matters* 15: 75–84.

Hopkins, Nicholas S., ed. 2003. *The New Arab Family.* Cairo: American University Press.

Inhorn, Marcia C. 1994. *Quest for Conception: Gender, Infertility, and Egyptian Medical Traditions.* Philadelphia: University of Pennsylvania Press.

———. 1996. *Infertility and Patriarchy: The Cultural Politics of Gender and Family Life in Egypt.* Philadelphia: University of Pennsylvania Press.

———. 2003. *Local Babies, Global Science: Gender, Religion, and in Vitro Fertilization in Egypt.* New York: Routledge.

———. 2012. *The New Arab Man: Emergent Masculinities, Technologies, and Islam in the Middle East*. Princeton, NJ: Princeton University Press.

———. 2015. *Cosmopolitan Conceptions: IVF Sojourns in Global Dubai*. Durham, NC: Duke University Press.

———. 2017. "Wanted Babies, Excess Fetuses: The Middle East's in Vitro Fertilization, High-Order Multiple Pregnancy, Fetal Reduction Nexus." In *Abortion Pills, Test Tube Babies, and Sex Toys: Emerging Sexual and Reproductive Technologies in the Middle East and North Africa*, eds. L. L. Wynn and Angel Foster, 99–111. Nashville, TN: Vanderbilt University Press.

Inhorn, Marcia C., and Pasquale Patrizio. 2015. "Infertility around the Globe: New Thinking on Gender, Reproductive Technologies, and Global Movements in the 21st Century." *Human Reproduction Update* 21: 411–26.

Inhorn, Marcia C., and Soraya Tremayne, eds. 2012. *Islam and Assisted Reproductive Technologies: Sunni and Shia Perspectives*. New York: Berghahn.

———. 2016. "Islam, Assisted Reproduction, and the Bioethical Aftermath." *Journal of Religion and Health* 55: 422–30.

International Federation of Fertility Societies' Surveillance (IFFS). 2022. "Global Trends in Reproductive Policy and Practice, 9th Edition." *Global Reproductive Health* 7(3): e58.

Kanaaneh, Rhoda Ann. 2002. *Birthing the Nation: Strategies of Palestinian Women in Israel*. Berkeley: University of California Press.

Kilani, Z., and L. Haj Hassan. 2002. "Sex Selection and Preimplantation Genetic Diagnosis at the Farah Hospital." *Reproductive BioMedicine Online* 4: 68–70.

Klitzman, Robert. 2016. "Struggles in Defining and Addressing Requests for 'Family Balancing': Ethical Issues Faced by Providers and Patients." *Journal of Law, Medicine & Ethics* 44: 616–29.

Krolökke, Charlotte, and Filareti Kotsi. 2018. "Pink *and* Blue: Assemblages of Family Balancing and the Making of Dubai as a Fertility Destination." *Science, Technology, & Human Values*: 1–21.

Kulczycki, Andrej. 2004. "The Sociocultural Context of Condom Use within Marriage in Rural Lebanon." *Studies in Family Planning* 35: 246–60.

Lapham, Robert J., and W. Parker Mauldin. 1985. "Contraceptive Prevalence: The Influence of Organized Family Planning Programs." *Studies in Family Planning* 16: 117–37.

Musallam, Basim F. 1983. *Sex and Society in Islam: Birth Control before the Nineteenth Century*. Cambridge: Cambridge University Press.

Myntti, Cynthia, Abir Ballan, Omar Dewachi, Faysal El-Kak, and Mary E. Deeb. 2002. "Challenging the Stereotypes: Men, Withdrawal, and Reproductive Health in Lebanon." *Contraception* 65: 165–70.

Obermeyer, Carla Makhlouf. 1996. "Fertility Norms and Son Preference in Morocco and Tunisia: Does Women's Status Matter?" *Journal of Biosocial Science* 28: 57–72.

———. 1999. "Fairness and Fertility: The Meaning of Son Preference in Morocco." In *Dynamics of Values in Fertility Change*, ed. Richard Leete, 275–92. Oxford: Oxford University Press.

Obermeyer, Carla Makhlouf, and Rosario Cardenas. 1997. "Son Preference and Differential Treatment in Morocco and Tunisia." *Studies in Family Planning* 28: 235–44.

Serour, Gamal I. 2008. "Islamic Perspectives in Human Reproduction." *Reproductive BioMedicine Online* 17: 34–38.

Shabana, Ayman. 2017. "Empowerment of Women between Law and Science: Role of Biomedical Technology in Enhancing Equitable Gender Relations in the Muslim World." *Hawwa: Journal of Women in the Middle East and the Islamic World* 15: 193–218.

Stycos, J. Mayone, and Hussein Abdel Aziz Sayed. 1988. *Community Development and Family Planning: An Egyptian Experiment*. Boulder, CO: Westview Press.

United Nations. 2012. *World Population Prospects: The 2012 Revision*. Volume 1, *Comprehensive Tables*. New York: United Nations.

———. 2018. *World Population Prospects: The 2017 Revision*. New York: United Nations.

Van Balen, Frank, and Marcia C. Inhorn. 2003. "Son Preference, Sex Selection, and the 'New' New Reproductive Technologies." *International Journal of Health Services* 33: 235–52.

Vora, Neha. 2013. *Impossible Citizens: Dubai's Indian Diaspora*. Durham, NC: Duke University Press.

Wahlberg, Ayo, and Tine Gammeltoft, eds. 2018. *Selective Reproduction in the 21ˢᵗ Century*. London: Palgrave Macmillan.

World Bank. 2023a. "Fertility Rate, Total (Births per Woman)." Accessed May 15, 2024. https://data.worldbank.org.

———. 2023b. "Population, Total." Accessed May 15, 2024. https://data.worldbank.org.

Zavis, Monika. 2018. "The Issue of the Sex of a Conceived Child in Islam: From the Pre-Islamic Conceptions to the Current Methods of Genetic Selection of the Sexes." *Spirituality Studies* 4(2): 8–15.

2

Pursuit of Pregnancy

Assisted Reproduction and Women's Repro-Activity in Japan

NANA OKURA GAGNÉ

Like other East Asian societies experiencing rapid changes in education, employment, and family structure, Japan is in the midst of a demographic transformation, marked as an aging, "ultra-low-fertility" nation. The number of women in the workforce has risen dramatically, and marriage has become increasingly delayed, affecting the timing and tempo of childbearing. This trend comes with a growing awareness of medical infertility and a growing demand for treatments, with a nearly fivefold increase in assisted reproductive technology (ART) usage between 2000 and 2020, and one in 4.4 Japanese couples using some form of infertility treatment (Ministry of Health, Labour, and Welfare 2022a: 2). As a result, marriage and reproduction are increasingly more precarious, while desires for family take on new urgency and intensity. And even as public attention is being drawn to the "crisis" of the declining birth rate, there is an intense and growing private struggle in starting a family that is deeply tied to individual and social ailments of contemporary Japan.

Despite these economic, demographic, and social changes, modern norms of gender and family persist. Moreover, new reproductive technologies have been normalized and encouraged as a way to have a "natural" family. The increasing knowledge of infertility provides women with new options for reproductive practices, while also putting the onus on women to demonstrate their *repro-activity*, or efforts to complete all of the requisite steps for achieving a "natural" family via ARTs. These steps include planning to find a marriage partner before one's reproductive window closes; enhancing one's fertility through mental and physical health; and making the decision to pursue fertility treatments if needed.

Altogether, these social changes involving new perceptions of fertility and infertility have produced an increasingly diversified field of new discourses and practices around planning for family and treating infertility, accompanied by new feelings of responsibility vis-à-vis a personalized logic of "reproductive cause and effect" that puts the burden of reproductivity on the choices of women. Yet, for many women, (re)defining their pursuits through new discourses of fertility and infertility also fuels a new sense of agency and active control over one's body, one's health, and couples' relationships in ways that were not available to women of earlier generations. Taken together, Japan's fertility challenges reveal an ongoing structural phenomenon that resonates with the emergence of the new reproductive order in societies across the world. In short, ARTs are not only a response to fertility concerns; the fact that ARTs are now widely available also impacts the way women imagine, desire, pursue, and embody repro-activity.

This chapter examines the emergent discourse and practice of infertility treatments, popularly called the "active pursuit of pregnancy" (*ninkatsu*) in Japan. Based on ethnographic research and interviews with sixty women and twelve men undergoing infertility treatment in the Tokyo and Kansai metropolitan regions in 2017 and 2023, I analyze how *ninkatsu* as a discourse and practice has emerged alongside medical and social discourses about infertility (*funin*). Specifically, this chapter explores how the discourse and practice of *ninkatsu* has emerged and how women situate themselves within the new reproductive order, represented by *ninkatsu*, and the possibilities of ART in a society that retains strong gender and family norms and ideals. Furthermore, I examine how the discourse and practice of *ninkatsu* both enables and delimits possibilities for women in Japan.

By situating these women's desires and subjectivities within the context of medical and social discourses of infertility, I argue that while ART is both enabling and delimiting—and even dehumanizing—as a technology of reproduction, *ninkatsu*'s holistic and amorphous discourse and practice challenge and redefine previous notions of the female body, family planning, and pregnancy, while encouraging women to take control of their bodies, lifestyles, and plans for the future—even in the face of unexpected negative outcomes. Specifically, while the women I interviewed described prolonged ART processes and new kinds of private struggles, their pursuit of pregnancy in the form of *ninkatsu* gives them a unique form of agency—what I characterize as repro-activity—the ability to acknowledge their bodies and desires, as well as to confront and control their own health, reproductive potential, personal trajectories, and family life plans in ways that did not exist before.

Analyzing how these women frame their experiences of ART within this broader concept of *ninkatsu* highlights both the challenges, limits, and struggles and a sense of agency and control in a situation where they would have had little such control in the past. As a result, rather than simply reflecting either traditional or neoliberal gender expectations, women's aspirations for and practices of *ninkatsu* reveal a particular repro-activity that reflects a new logic of gendered agency underlying individual reproductive desires amid contemporary economic and sociocultural challenges. Moreover, this repro-activity expands gendered agency in relation to fertility far beyond the establishment of pregnancy per se, and into many other aspects of women's identities, relationships, and life trajectories.

Family Formations and Fertility Treatments in Japan

Historically speaking, under the *ie* (family lineage) system, the continuation of the family lineage/business was of primary importance, and thus "the quality of offspring" rather than infertility was of primary concern (Lock 2005: 485). Up until the Meiji period (1868–1912), family formations—such as getting married and divorced and having and raising children—were flexible and not strictly bound by biological ties. For example, families engaged in trial marriage, frequent divorce, and various forms of adoption outside of the family (Ono and Sanders 2009). Furthermore, fertility was bound in different ways with the maintenance of the *ie* and nationalist ideologies of pronatalism (Lock 2005). Moreover, Japanese society has long held the fatalistic idea that a "child is a gift" (*sazukarimono*), not something actualized through planning and proactive effort. Thus, while infertile women faced challenges, the concepts of infertility as "fate" or as one's "bodily constitution" (*taishitsu*) relieved women from the heavy burden of feeling responsible for infertility and making long investments in their pursuits of pregnancy.

However, with the dismantling of traditional lineage frameworks and nationalist pronatalist policies in the postwar period, there emerged new ideals for childbearing and new meanings for family, including a rise in love marriages and nuclear families in a context of increasing democratization and economic prosperity. More recently, since the 1990s, the generally stagnant economy, alongside increasing female education rates, increased labor participation rates among women, higher costs of education and insufficient childcare, and rising burdens of caregiving for aging parents have all played into the phenomena of delayed marriage or lifelong singlehood, and lower birth rates (Atoh 2001). The birth rate dropped from 4.54 in 1947 to less than 2.0 in 1975 to 1.3 in 2021, placing Japan in the vanguard of rapidly aging and low-fertility societies (Ogawa 2011; Tanaka-Naji 2009; see figure 2.1).

Another notable change has been the increasing number of never-married women and men, which has risen sharply among all age groups since the 1980s. While this trend is mirrored in many other postindustrial countries, the Japanese case differs from Euro-American counterparts in that adults continue to express a desire to marry even as marriage rates decline (Atoh 2001). Thus, the increased prevalence of singlehood does not simply imply a declining interest in marriage or children. Moreover, despite the changing realities of marriage and childbirth, the postwar coupling of marriage and childbirth as an ideal persists (Roberts 2016). This ideal is evident in low levels of out-of-wedlock childbirth and in the strong preference for marriage once a child is conceived; otherwise, abortion is preferred (Hertog 2009). At the same time, a variety of factors, including increasing numbers of women pursuing careers and rising challenges of finding an appropriate marital partner, have contributed to a growing trend of delaying childbirth, with roughly 20 percent of couples planning to have their first child after the age of thirty-five (Kubo 2009; Castro-Vázquez 2015).

These factors contribute to a growing attention to "social infertility"[1]—referring to the individual lifestyle factors and social and economic conditions that lead to declining fertility rates and, in many cases, to medical infertility requiring ART treatments. Between 2007 and 2020, Japan saw a nearly fivefold increase in ART usage, and a 2022 survey estimated that one in 4.4 couples resorts to some form of infertility treatment in Japan (Ministry of Health, Labour, and Welfare 2022a: 2; see figure 2.2). It was

**Total Fertility Rate of Japan
(1947-2021)**

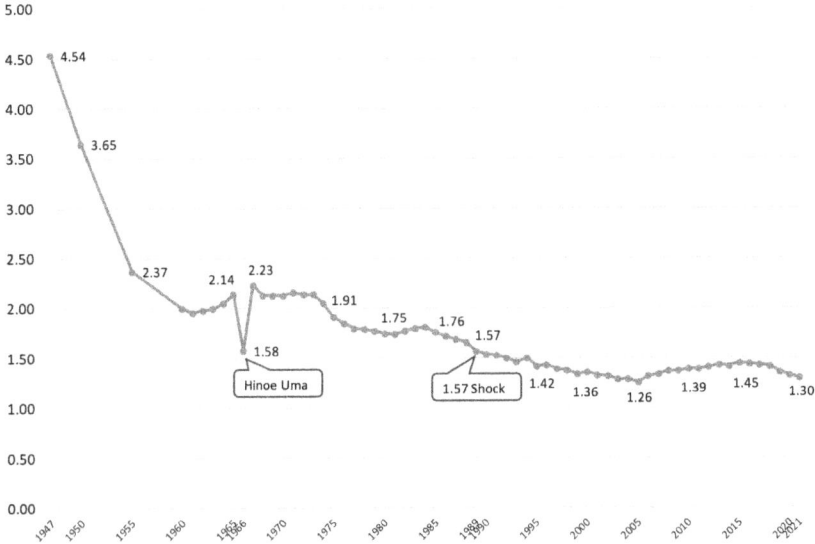

Figure 2.1. Total Fertility Rate of Japan (1947–2021). Credit: Ministry of Health, Labour, and Welfare (2022b)

**Numbers of Neonate Births by IVF, ICSI, and FET in Japan
(1985-2020)**

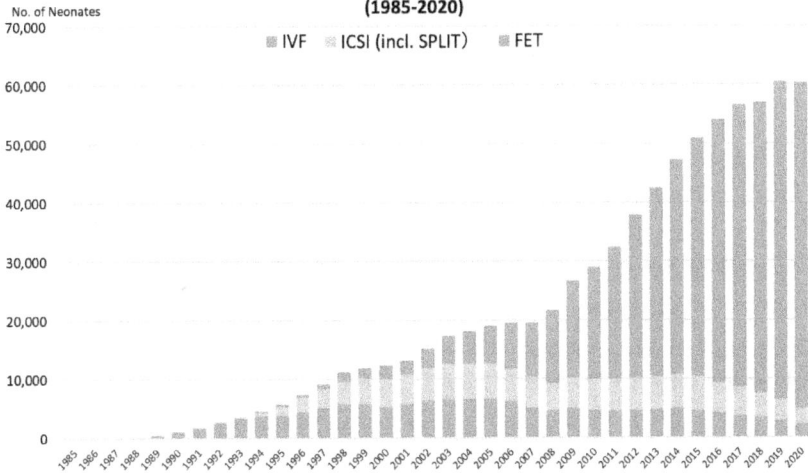

Figure 2.2. Numbers of Neonate Births by In Vitro Fertilization (IVF), Intracytoplasmic Sperm Injection (ICSI), and Frozen–Thawed Embryo Transfer (FET) in Japan. Credit: Adapted from Japan Society of Obstetrics and Gynecology (2022)

in this context of a rapidly growing medical field of infertility treatments and intensifying public awareness of Japan's demographic crisis that the term *"ninkatsu"* gained traction in the early 2010s, eventually becoming a popular shorthand to describe proactive engagement toward fertility goals. By rendering private desires and efforts into a publicly recognizable endeavor, this term also indexes a new reproductive order, in which the meaning of infertility is no longer merely individual: it reveals a shared, social, national, and structural condition in Japan.

The Development of ART and the Birth of *Ninkatsu*

Medical professionals and social commentators have long expressed an urgent need for research into the causes of infertility and emphasized the essential role of ART in meeting Japan's demographic "deficit." Indeed, Japan has become one of the world's leading ART providers per capita, with more than 620 registered fertility clinics across the country as of 2020 (Nomura Research Institute 2021). It is estimated that between 15 and 20 percent of women in Japan will experience infertility (Kubo 2009), and a Benesse survey shows that as of 2009, 41.5 percent of women over the age of thirty-five who gave birth received some form of infertility treatment (Shirakawa and Tsunemi 2012: 320). This high rate reflects the increased desire for children and an awareness of infertility among women in their thirties and forties in Japan, and the increased access to ART treatments from around this time. Less than a decade later, a 2020 survey found that one in 13.9 children from women of all ages (7.19 percent) born in Japan were conceived via in vitro fertilization (IVF) (Japan Society of Obstetrics and Gynecology 2020).

It is within this context of working women's unmet desires for biological children, amid the burgeoning ART market, that the term *"ninkatsu"* emerged. The term has been traced to an early publicity campaign by the pharmaceutical company Merck in 2009, which collaborated with the women's magazine *FRaU* for a 2011 special issue on women's pursuit of pregnancy (Fassbender 2022). However, it gained sudden popularity beginning in 2011 through publications by Shirakawa Tōko, a female journalist who advocates women's work and life balance, and it became the most popular word of 2011 in the Nikkei Women's Online Survey (see figure 2.3).

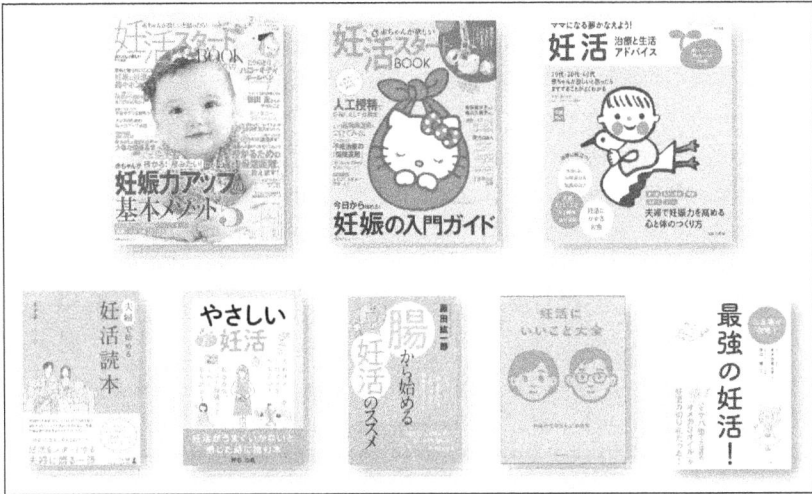

Figure 2.3. Various *Ninkatsu*-Related Books

"*Ninkatsu*" is one of many terms that have emerged in Japan in recent years that emphasize "active pursuit" of key life goals, marked by the suffix "-*katsu*." "*Ninkatsu*" means the "pursuit of pregnancy," which follows in the tradition of other terms such as "*shūkatsu*," "job hunting" (circa 2000), and "*konkatsu*," "marriage hunting" (circa 2007). The use of the suffix "-*katsu*" reveals how those life events are no longer considered to happen "naturally," but must instead be achieved through determination and deliberate effort. Echoing Marcin Smietana's concept of "spreadsheet fertility" in chapter 5 of this volume, "*ninkatsu*" expresses the increasingly recognizable perception that one must consciously plan and invest effort to achieve one's reproductive goals in life. As a result, whether it be getting a job, getting married, or getting pregnant, individuals' active pursuit of these goals is understood to require more conscious and strategic planning (e.g., Dalton and Dales 2016).

One of the novel aspects of the *ninkatsu* discourse is its increasing public legitimacy. This marks a significant shift in the way fertility is perceived, by both deindividualizing it and to a certain extent debiologizing it. As many feminist reproductive scholars have pointed out, issues of pregnancy and infertility, including the use of ARTs, are conventionally considered private, intimate familial matters that are not discussed openly in the media nor in social or even familial contexts. However, with the rising number of women who are struggling to combine work and family, as well as the increasing media attention to *ninkatsu* since 2010, more and more public figures and individuals are breaking this taboo and openly announcing their engagement in *ninkatsu*.

One of the pioneers to publicize *ninkatsu* is Riko Higashio, a professional golfer and media personality. In 2012 she published the book *Not Infertility, but TGP (Trying to Get Pregnant)*, in which she questions the use of the Japanese term "*funin*," meaning "infertility," as negative and disempowering to women (see figure 2.4). Motivated by a desire to change public perceptions of infertility and to empower women to be more positive and agentive about their active pursuit of pregnancy, Higashio kept a blog detailing her treatments and offering healthcare advice, while using media appearances to encourage a public conversation about infertility and how to support women struggling to overcome it.

Echoing Higashio's activism, my informants preferred the term "*ninkatsu*" rather than "*funin* treatments" to describe their pursuits, with many problematizing the negative connotation of the latter. Although the term "*ninkatsu*" is used ambiguously by women themselves, it has become a powerfully multivalent concept. Some see it as an initial step toward family planning or active involvement in medical infertility treatments, while others see it as readjusting/balancing their working lives and pursuing more holistic treatments such as dietary changes and exercise or traditional Chinese medicines. One informant in her late thirties explained, "I experienced 'facing my body' for the first time in my life," which gives the vantage point of "thinking about 'our future.'" Many also emphasize the importance of "stress reduction" and "not taking things too seriously," citing that "pregnancy is harder than you think. . . . So, it is important to create a good environment for your fertility while taking trips and changing your mood by reducing stress and improving overall health." Moreover, though it is not technically a legal term, some women use "*ninkatsu*" as a socially acceptable reason to leave work temporarily, reduce working hours, or reduce the frequency of social outings with friends and colleagues. Some companies have even instituted special leave days for *ninkatsu*-related activities under the more recent label "*ninkyū*" ("pregnancy-pursuit leave") or created

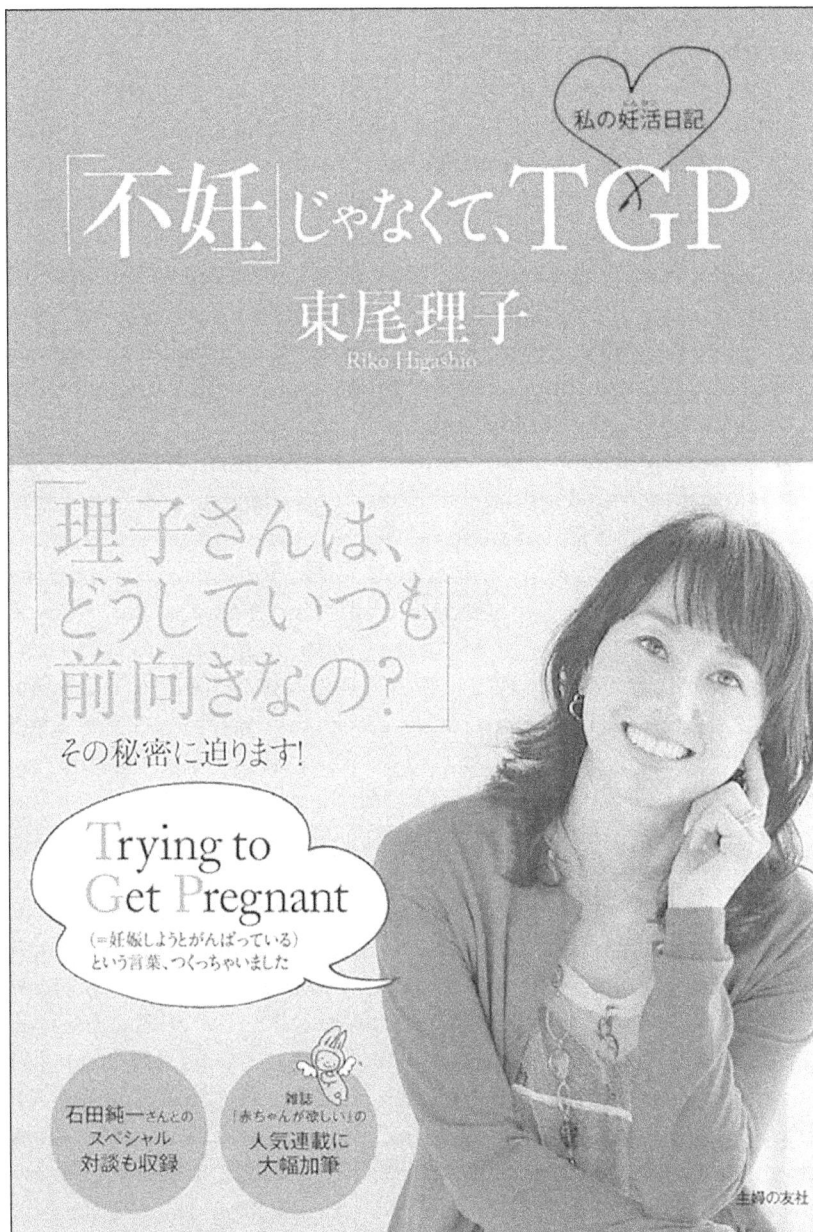

Figure 2.4. Riko Higashio's Best-Selling Book, *Not Infertility, but TGP (Trying to Get Pregnant)* (2012)

a new broad category of leave days for women under the term "*f-kyū*" ("female leave") (Inoue 2014).

Some might conflate *ninkatsu* with *funin* and view *ninkatsu* as just another pronatalist ideology imposed from the top (men) to compel women to have more children. Indeed, the increased media attention to infertility has produced new anxieties in society. For example, a public debate was triggered by a program, aired by the public broadcaster NHK in 2014,[2] which seemingly reduced women's reproductive challenges to female biology, typified by worried references to the "aging of eggs" (Tanaka 2018). In these ways, it is possible to imagine *ninkatsu* as a reactive response and another permutation of a patriarchal effort to govern women's reproductive choices.

Yet, from a different perspective, the *ninkatsu* discourse stands apart from government-led reproductive health campaigns in its bottom-up and progressive rather than reactionary messages to women. This feature of *ninkatsu* becomes even clearer when we look more closely at the motivations of women who are/were pursuing *ninkatsu*. For those in *ninkatsu*, it is thus not simply a matter of finding and pursuing technological treatment but rather it is deliberately more encompassing, cultivating the idea of "consciously and proactively preparing to get pregnant" in its broadest sense (see Shirakawa and Tsunemi 2012; see also Smietana's description of crafting fertility pursuits as "artisanal" in chapter 5). As one informant explained, "While medical treatment can take a long time between cycles, there is still a lot we can do for our body during those empty periods. I was happy to work on it, thinking, 'I'm going to review my lifestyle and clean up my body and mind so that it will be easier to have a baby!'" In this sense, *ninkatsu* reflects more of the consciousness of women on the ground rather than men at the top.

In her pioneering anthropological study on pregnancies in Japan and Israel, Tsipy Ivry (2009: 11) characterizes the core ethos of the Israeli repro-medical regime as "geneticism," pointing to its heavy emphasis on the prenatal diagnosis of inborn genetic and chromosomal abnormalities and the liberal use of selective reproduction. In contrast, Ivry refers to the corresponding Japanese regime of "environmentalism," in which the maternal environment takes central place. Due to the mainstreaming of *ninkatsu* as a discourse and practice, this emphasis on what could be called "cultivating environments" extends to pre-pregnancy preparation and to women who start reflecting on and reconsidering their health and work lives. Moreover, *ninkatsu* writers call on young women to be more proactive in their pursuits of career and family, suggesting that they study employment rules and women's rights, such as maternity leave and child-raising leave policies. It is also important to note that most *ninkatsu* writers and nonprofit-organization infertility specialists/counselors are themselves women who suffered from involuntary childlessness. Indeed, this empathetic motivation to help others is another aspect of women experiencing infertility in Japan, as many who struggled but could not conceive end up trying to support others in similar situations.

The Context of ARTs in Japan

The rising use of ARTs and the popularity of *ninkatsu* do not mean that infertility technologies have become embraced uncritically in Japan. In my fieldwork, many informants waited two or three years before they even considered consulting doctors. Even as the new possibilities enabled by ARTs became increasingly heralded as potential solutions for couples facing unwanted childlessness, such discourses are also colored by fears of ARTs becoming a handmaiden for eugenics by encouraging genetic screening and creating "designer babies" and even undermining the value of life (Kato and Sleeboom-Faulkner 2011: 510; Kubo 2009: 25; Lock 1998, 2005). Thus, reproductive technology in Japan is not embraced simply as empowering or modern, and there is continued skepticism toward the "pill" (Jitsukawa and Djerassi 1994), as well as a reluctance to undergo C-sections. In other words, despite Japan's reputation as a technology-loving society, reproductive technology is increasingly normalized, but it is not fetishized (see also Lock and Kaufert 2001).[3]

The Japan Society of Obstetrics and Gynecology (JSOG) has protested the use of ARTs, since their inception, for creating "non-normative" family structures (Tsuge 2005). Such "non-normative" families include single-parent families where a child is raised without a legal father or without a legal mother, as well as cases where children are the product of a third party, such as surrogacy or gamete donation (Lock 2005). While critics see this as stemming from a conservative, heteronormative ideology of family, physicians explain that these guidelines are under-girded by a desire to prevent commercializing ART practices (i.e., paid surrogacy and gamete donation), to avoid the coercion of donors, and to prevent "potential confusion and complications in the relationship between parent and child" (Shimazono and Hibino 2013: 341).

The stance of the powerful medical organization JSOG is also re-flected in the restrained and incremental practice of ARTs. First, the very possibility of the use of ARTs is limited to legally married indi-viduals, and donor insemination, egg donation, and surrogacy are generally prohibited. Second, even within this limited context of use, infertility specialists usually begin with basal thermometers and certain medications (such as clomiphene to induce ovulation) to encourage couples to use "rhythm methods" before moving on to intrauterine in-semination (IUI) or IVF.

Despite the normative power of medical organizations like JSOG, it would be misleading to explain the use and meaning of ARTs sim-ply in terms of institutional pressures, technological availability, or cultural "traditionalism." For example, many refrain from pursuing a wider range of ARTs, such as gamete donation or surrogacy, not nec-essarily due to conservative ideas about family per se but rather due to legal constraints and the increasing desire to carry one's own child with one's chosen partner.

Altogether, the Japanese case reveals that institutional access and so-cial attitudes regarding ARTs, and pregnancy more generally, emerge from the ambivalent juxtaposition of seemingly opposing desires on the part of women—to both pursue careers and find their own mari-tal partners and have their own children—amid changing socioeco-nomic milieus. Modern changes in workways and family formations have enabled individual women to aspire to achieve it all, but they have nonetheless created new tensions that ARTs have simultaneously exac-erbated and mitigated.

Ninkatsu in Practice

While women commonly left the workforce before or upon marriage until the 1980s, all of the women I interviewed worked continuously after marriage. For many, this is one reason why it was difficult to suddenly start thinking about a child during their busy working lives: they worked hard during their twenties and delayed marriage and child-birth altogether, unintentionally neglecting their reproductive health (including OB/GYN exams), and some later discovered previously unknown fertility problems. Recognizing such challenges, *ninkatsu* is meant to be a wake-up call to get women thinking more proactively about their health and life goals.

In this way, using the term "*ninkatsu*" rather than "ARTs" or "infertil-ity treatments" is more holistic as it can be a long-term activity for many women who aspire to get pregnant. Most of my informants explained that through *ninkatsu* they started to pay attention to their neglected bodies and feelings of stress and aspired to become healthy. Many women see being infertile as meaning that "their body has something wrong with it" and is "somehow unhealthy." In other words, they link the idea of being healthy with being "naturally fertile," and thus improving their overall health is seen as a key dimension of *ninkatsu*.

For example, one informant, Ishizuka-san, started seeing a gynecolo-gist at the age of thirty after two years of trying unsuccessfully to get pregnant. After going through a miscarriage, she explained how she tried everything she could, including diet changes, monitoring her basal temperature, acupuncture, and traditional Chinese medicines, as well as reducing working hours and pursuing psychological counseling for stress reduction. As she and her husband had been working full-time, she realized how much they had neglected their health and bodies.

For other informants, especially those who work night shifts, *ninkatsu* is impossible to start. Due to the nature of their work and their reversed night and day lifestyles, they felt that they could not possibly get preg-nant. One informant, Tayama-san, worked as a caregiver at a hospital. Working nights, she had an unhealthy lifestyle and disrupted hormone levels. When she consulted with a clinician, he told her that if she left the situation as it was, her disrupted hormone levels would become her normal state. Tayama-san told her boss about her future family concern and switched to being a home caregiver so she no longer needed to work night shifts. After changing her job, she was finally able to think about her own health and pursue family planning more actively.

In these ways, the term "*ninkatsu*" is a multivalent touchstone for a variety of attitudes toward pursuing pregnancy, but in all cases, it symbolizes women's proactive determination to take control of their (re-productive) bodies. Though some were not able to begin *ninkatsu* due to workplace conditions, knowledge of their infertility challenges and the increasing public awareness of infertility brought about by the discourse of *ninkatsu* encouraged them to find ways to rebalance their lives and take control over their health. For these women, the fact that they can begin investing in *ninkatsu* is the first step toward repro-activity, and it can also encourage them to rethink everyday stress and the biologically and psychologically damaging work/life balance that so many women take for granted. Thus, *ninkatsu* also resituates notions of infertility within the broader idea of a healthy lifestyle.

Women who pursue *ninkatsu* continue to face challenges. When speaking about her single female friends in their late thirties and early forties, Shibata-san, an infertility counselor, described "a new form of in-equality" emerging in society between two groups of women: women in their twenties who have children early without planning, and women in their late thirties and forties who planned to pursue careers, get married, and have children, but then confront infertility. Pointing to the idea that childbearing is something that simply happened "naturally" in the past but is not happening naturally anymore, despite how many women want children, she suggests that this inequality "did not really exist before, as women never really faced infertility and did not have much reproductive knowledge." Of course, women did experience infertility, and divorce due to infertility was not uncommon in prewar generations. However, infer-tility was understood not as a medical problem that could be managed but rather as a matter of an individual's "constitution," over which one had no control. Moreover, in earlier generations, a majority of women tended to marry and start families at a younger age, which gave them a naturally longer reproductive window to achieve pregnancy, even if they had (unrecognized) infertility difficulties.

Mita-san is another informant who faced *ninkatsu* challenges. Despite undergoing fertility treatments for five years, she has been unable to con-ceive. Mita-san had a corpus luteum deficiency, and her husband strug-gled with obstructive azoospermia. As a result, Mita-san went through four rounds of egg retrieval and four cycles of frozen embryo transfers, while her husband underwent micro-dissection testicular sperm extrac-tion. To cover the costs of these expensive treatments, she cut down on other things like dietary supplements and oriental medicines. IVF became her entire world, to the extent that she ended up ignoring various other aspects of *ninkatsu*. Mita-san advised those struggling with *ninkatsu* not to give up due to financial reasons, as money, unlike one's biological clock, can always be earned back.

Situating these women's desires and subjectivities within the context of medical and social discourses of infertility, my informants expressed that "people who had children naturally and people from older generations tend to think that 'if you try hard naturally and cannot conceive, you should just give up.'" Faced with such sentiments, many women refused to see themselves denied the pursuit of their desire for children. Their responses echo Lock's findings among women in the 1990s of "a widely shared sentiment that, if nature can be perfected through technology, then there is nothing inherently wrong with its use" (Lock 1998: 486). Here, the intentions and goals of reproductive technology supersede the moral questions regarding its use.

At the same time, *ninkatsu*'s increasing legitimacy, coupled with the lack of other options, such as adoption,[4] donor insemination, egg donation, and surrogacy, leaves some Japanese women pursuing the same treatments over and over, which can lead to protracted physical, financial, and mental hardship. In this sense, the new reproductive order of the *ninkatsu* movement also reflects how infertility treatments are caught up in similar stratified, commercialized, and precarious conditions, as seen in other societies addressed in this volume, thereby creating distinctions between women who can devote time and money to *ninkatsu* and those who cannot. Nonetheless, given their new desires, challenges, and strategies, my informants' aspirations resonate with Jenkins and Inhorn's (2003) characterization of women pursuing ART as "reproductive agents" who resist being defined and constrained by their biological infertility, but instead actively pursue infertility treatments in spite of the challenges.

Conclusion

As pioneering works on the anthropology of reproduction by Jordan (1978), Davis-Floyd (1992), and others have shown, "birth—in both biomedical and local birthing systems—constitutes a cultural production"

(Sargent and Gulbas 2011: 291). Echoing the concepts of fertility as a "reprolens" or "optic" (Inhorn 2020; Franklin 2022), ARTs constitute a nexus of biotechnical possibilities of human reproduction and socio-cultural norms and values of family, which are played out on the legal stage of bioethics discourse, the biomedical stage of infertility treatment, and the private backstage of personal psychological, physiological, and emotional struggles by individual women and men and their families.

In this sense, the term *"ninkatsu"* has transformed from a pharmaceutical marketing term to a media buzzword indexing a new public awareness of infertility to a widespread and explicit discourse of repro-activity that combines individual, familial, and social concerns about fertility precarity from a grassroots perspective. In their rescripting of not only the causes of infertility but the very nature of reproductive cause and effect—e.g., through its denaturalization, deindividualization, and demedicalization of the causes and solutions of unwanted childlessness—*ninkatsu* confirms the arrival of a new reproductive order combining individual effort with technological intervention.

As this chapter argues, the discourse of *ninkatsu* offers us yet another example of a fertility figuration, calculation, or optic through which to understand broad forces of social change—and to chart a new reproductive order based on an altered model of reproductive cause and effect. The emergence of this repro-activity reveals that in contrast to the prewar and wartime family, postwar women's lives in Japan are no longer dictated by the needs of the nation or their extended families, but rather by the work they can do to make their own families. At the same time, as more women pursue higher education and careers, childbirth has also become something that does not happen "naturally." In other words, the increase in the number of working women, unmarried women, and divorcees did not really encourage a desire for radically different lifestyles. Rather, the concepts of a child-centered family and responsible parenthood remain central among women whose own lives diverge from this model. Therefore, the transformation of social discourses of motherhood alongside rapid socioeconomic changes over the past century have given birth to new desires and new options for women. And yet, as women's social roles and workways have transformed dramatically in the past several decades, the "cultural production of birth" has fallen out of step with women's biological realities.

The transition from passively expecting a "naturalistic" pregnancy and childbirth to actively struggling for these ideals, combined with the tantalizing hope of new technologies of fertility, can push women to a breaking point. And yet, through this striving and through new discourses like *ninkatsu*, the private desires of such women assume a new, proactive form of reproductivity that has heretofore not existed in Japan. This socially legitimated, holistic pursuit of pregnancy as a repro-activity is changing the medical, technological, and social landscape of reproduction: a new generation of women taking control of the childbearing process from start to finish.

Acknowledgments

This research was supported by the Chinese University of Hong Kong's Direct Grant and the Research Grants Council of Hong Kong's Early Carrier Scheme.

NOTES

1 See Weston Vollenhoven (2002) and Lombardi (2016) for examples of discussions on how different social factors intertwine with infertility issues.

2 "I Want to Have a Baby, but I Can't: The Impact of Egg Aging" in *Close-up Gendai* (February 14, 2012) and *NHK Special* (June 23, 2012)

3 Feminist and disability-rights groups tend to caution against ART or any use of technological intervention that will affect women's "natural" bodies or the process of "natural" conception (Izumi 2015; Ogino 2011). As a result, while ARTs have achieved rapid technological progress and utilization under the banner of "saving women who cannot bear children" (Izumi 2015), many feminist groups see ARTs as a "blatant and direct manipulation and intervention" of a woman's reproductive body (Ogino 2011: 32).

4 Historically, adoption of adults (usually male) to take over a family business or carry on a lineage was common, but adoption of young children was uncommon. In contemporary Japan, giving up children for adoption is rare, and adopting young children is an arduous process with very strict criteria regarding adoptive parents' age, marital status, housing, income, etc. (see Nobe 2012).

REFERENCES

Atoh, Makoto. 2001. "Very Low Fertility in Japan and Value Change Hypotheses." *Review of Population and Social Policy* 10: 1–21.

Castro-Vázquez, Genaro. 2015. "Late-in-life Childbearing (*kōrei shussan*) in Contemporary Japan." *Culture, Health & Sexuality* 17(10): 1221–36.

Dalton, Emma, and Laura Dales. 2016. "Online *Konkatsu* and the Gendered Ideals of Marriage in Contemporary Japan." *Japanese Studies* 36(1): 1–19.

Davis-Floyd, Robbie. 1992. *Birth as an American Rite of Passage.* Berkeley: University of California Press.

Fassbender, Isabel. 2022. "Family Planning and Life Planning in Contemporary Japan: The 'Active Pursuit of Pregnancy' (*Ninkatsu*) Phenomenon and Its Stakeholders." *Contemporary Japan* 34(2): 228–44.

Franklin, Sarah. 2022. *Embodied Progress: A Cultural Account of Assisted Conception,* 2nd ed. London: Routledge.

Hertog, Ekaterina. 2009. *Tough Choices: Bearing an Illegitimate Child in Japan.* Stanford, CA: Stanford University Press.

Higashio, Riko. 2012. *Funin janakute, TGP (Trying to Get Pregnant)* [Not Infertility, but TGP (Trying to Get Pregnant)]. Tokyo: Shufunotomosha.

Inhorn, Marcia C. 2020. "Where Has the Quest for Conception Taken Us? Lessons from Anthropology and Sociology." *Reproductive BioMedicine and Society Online* 10: 46–57.

Inhorn, Marcia, and Daphna Birenbaum-Carmeli. 2008. "Assisted Reproductive Technologies and Culture Change." *Annual Review of Anthropology* 37: 177–96.

Inoue, Osamu. 2014. "*Saibāējento, Josei Shain no 'Ninkatsu' Shien*" [CyberAgent's 'Ninkatsu' Support for Female Employees]. *Nikkei Business Online,* April 25.

Ivry, Tsipy. 2009. *Embodying Culture: Pregnancy in Japan and Israel.* New Brunswick, NJ: Rutgers University Press.

Izumi, Hiroe. 2015. "Seishoku Hojo Iryo to Kazoku" [Assisted Reproductive Technologies and Family]. *Annals of Family Studies* 40: 1–5.

Japan Society of Obstetrics and Gynecology. 2020. "ART ētabukku" [ART Databook]. Tokyo: JSOG.

———. 2022. "Taigaijusei, Haiishoku to-no Rinshō Jisshi Seiseki" [Data on Clinical Implementation of IVF, Embryo Transfer, etc.]. Tokyo: JSOG.

Jenkins, Gwynne, and Marcia C. Inhorn. 2003. "Reproduction Gone Awry: Medical Anthropological Perspectives." *Social Science & Medicine* 56(9): 1831–36.

Jitsukawa, Mariko, and Carl Djerassi. 1994. "Birth Control in Japan: Realities and Prognosis." *Science* 265: 1048–51.

Jordan, Brigitte. 1978. *Birth in Four Cultures: A Crosscultural Investigation of Childbirth in Yucatan, Holland, Sweden, and the United States.* Montreal: Eden Press Women's Publications.

Kato, Masae, and Margaret Sleeboom-Faulkner. 2011. "Dichotomies of Collectivism and Individualism in Bioethics: Selective Abortion Debates and Issues of Self-Determination in Japan and 'the West.'" *Social Science & Medicine* 73(4): 507–14.

Kubo, Harumi. 2009. "Epidemiology of Infertility and Recurrent Pregnancy Loss in Society with Fewer Children." *Japan Medical Association Journal* 52(1): 23–28.

Lock, Margaret. 1998. "Perfecting Society: Reproductive Technologies, Genetic Testing, and the Planned Family in Japan." In *Pragmatic Women and Body Politics,* ed.

Margaret Lock and Patricia A. Kaufert, 206–39. Cambridge: Cambridge University Press.

———. 2005. "Preserving the Moral Order: Responses to Biomedical Technologies." In *A Companion to the Anthropology of Japan*, ed. Jennifer Robertson, 483–500. Malden, UK: Blackwell Publishing.

Lock, Margaret, and Patricia A. Kaufert. 2001. "Menopause, Local Biologies, and Cultures of Aging." *American Journal of Human Biology* 13(4): 494–504.

Lombardi, Lia. 2016. "Reproductive Technology in Italy between Gender Policy and Inequality: Can We Speak of 'Social Infertility'?" *AG About Gender: International Journal of Gender Studies* 5(9): 1–18.

Ministry of Health, Labour, and Welfare. 2022a. "Funin Chiryō to Shigoto no Ryōritsu Sapōto Handobukku" [Handbook on Support for Balancing Work and Fertility Treatment]. Tokyo: MHLW.

———. 2022b. *White Paper on Health, Labour, and Welfare*. Tokyo: MHLW.

Nobe, Yoko. 2012. "Naze Yōshi-engumi wa Funin Tōjisha ni Sentaku Sarenainoka? 'Ketsuen' to 'Kosodate' ni Kansuru Imizuke o Chūshin ni" [Why Is Adoption Not an Option for Infertile Couples? The Implications Regarding "Blood Relations" and "Childbearing"]. *Japanese Journal of Research on Household Economics* 93: 58–66.

Nomura Research Institute. 2021. "Funin Chiryō no jittai ni kansuru chōsa kenkyū: Saishū hōkokusho" [Survey Research on Current Use of Fertility Treatment: Final Report]. https://www.mhlw.go.jp.

Ogawa, Naohiro. 2011. "Population Aging and Immigration in Japan." *Asian and Pacific Migration Journal* 20(2): 133–67.

Ogino, Miho. 2011. "Seishoku ni Okeru Shintai no Shigenka to Feminizumu: Nihon to Amerika o Chushin Ni" [The Resourcization of the Body and Feminism in Reproduction: Examples from Japan and the USA]. *Death and Life Studies* 15: 27–51.

Ono, Hiromi, and James Sanders. 2009. "Divorce in Contemporary Japan and Its Gendered Patterns." *International Journal of Sociology of the Family* 35(2): 169–88.

Roberts, Glenda. 2016. *Japan's Evolving Family: Voices from Young Urban Adults Navigating Change*. Honolulu, HI: East-West Center.

Sargent, Carolyn, and Lauren Gulbas. 2011. "Situating Birth in the Anthropology of Reproduction." In *A Companion to Medical Anthropology*, ed. Merrill Singer and Pamela Erickson, 289–303. London: Blackwell.

Shimazono, Susumu. 2011. "The Ethical Issues of Biotechnology: Religious Culture and the Value of Life." *Current Sociology* 59(2): 160–72.

Shimazono, Yosuke, and Yuri Hibino. 2013. "Japanese Infertility Patients' Attitudes towards Directed and Non-Directed Oocyte Donation: Analysis of a Questionnaire Survey and Implications for Public Policy." *Asian Bioethics Review* 5(4): 331–43.

Shirakawa, Tōko, and Yōhei Tsunemi. 2012. *Joshi to Shūkatsu: 20 Dai Kara no "Shū, Nin, Kon" Kōza* [Women and Job-Hunting: A Job, Pregnancy, and Marriage Course from Their Twenties]. Tokyo: Chuo Koron Shinsha.

Tanaka, Sigeto. 2018. "Unscientific Visual Representations Used for the 'Egg Aging' Campaign in 2010s Japan." Unpublished Paper.

Tanaka-Naji, Hiromi. 2009. "Stated Desire versus Actual Practice: Reviewing the Literature on Low Fertility Rates in Contemporary Japanese Society." *Japanese Studies* 29(3): 415–30.

Tsuge, Azumi. 2005. "How Society Responds to Desires of Childless Couples: Japan's Position on Donor Conception." *Bulletin of Institute of Sociology and Social Work*, Meiji Gakuin University 35: 21–34.

3

Reproductive Heterosexism

Assisted Reproduction and Family Making in the
"Best Interests of the Child" in Greece

VENETIA KANTSA

A few days before the second round of national elections on June 25, 2023, the leader of Greece's main right-wing New Democracy Party and aspiring next prime minister, Kyriakos Mitsotakis, announced his plan to introduce a Ministry of Family to address demographic issues and family policies. Immediately following his party's election victory, the new Ministry of Social Cohesion and Family was formed with its first minister, Sofia Zacharaki, declaring its intention to work on "strengthening the family" and on the "harmonization that must exist between professional and family life," with "supporting children . . . at the 'heart' of this effort" ("Social Cohesion" 2023).

Greece has been largely described as a society where kinship and family relations play a crucial role in the definition of gender identities, with full adult status for both women and men obtained through marriage and childbearing or the acquisition of children (*apoktisi pedion*) (Loizos and Papataxiarchis 1991; Papataxiarchis 2013). Parenthood, and especially motherhood, has persistently served as a metaphor for the nation's continuity and integrity, appropriated by both the state and the church (Halkias 2004; Paxson 2004, 2006; Athanasiou 2006; Kantsa 2006, 2013). Assisted reproductive technologies (ARTs) are viewed as means to fulfill personal goals and address state concerns regarding the country's low fertility and birth rates.

The case of Greece presents a specific set of contrasts that illustrate not only the role of ARTs in shifting traditional ideas about parenthood, procreation, and family but also how these changes affect different sectors of society. Although, as this volume argues, ARTs help us understand the new reproductive order and altered logics of reproductive cause and effect, we can also use the "reprolens" of ARTs (Inhorn 2020) to look within specific regional contexts at the situated fertility transitions taking place—or not—at a more granular level. A generally permissive legal framework allowing high levels of access to ARTs, combined with extensive fertility services, has established Greece as one of Europe's leading "reprohubs" (Inhorn 2015). Yet, access to ARTs is granted legally only to heterosexual couples and single women, while lesbians may use ARTs only in their capacity as single women. Drawing from a cultural context of *repronational familism*—in which family and procreation are highly valued, and fertilities and infertilities are often embedded in prevalent conceptualizations of gender, kinship, and sexuality—this chapter shows how the simultaneous coexistence of *reproductive heterosexism*—or traditional heterosexual family norms, which are valorized in Greek society—both allow and contain lesbian motherhood, revealing complex and ambivalent modes of reproduction.

In view of these modern biotechnological developments, the challenge faced by the social sciences is to study the ways in which "new" answers may be provided to "old" questions in relation to life and death, the individual and kinship, and society and technology (Strathern 1992, 2005; Edwards 2000; Edwards et al. 1999 [1993]; Edwards and Salazar 2009; Franklin and Ragoné 1998; Franklin 2013). Thus, despite the fact that technological developments are acquiring an increasingly global dimension, anthropological studies show that the individual, kinship, genealogy, and conceptualization of the limits of life and death vary significantly across different cultural contexts (Inhorn and Birenbaum-Carmeli 2008). ARTs are a good example of how a technique offering "new" ways to answer "old" questions about parenthood, family, fertility, and continuity has spread quickly around the globe and gained local acceptance in many societies, including in Greece. As this chapter will show, ARTs have changed the ways in which relatedness is now perceived in Greece. Yet, at the same time, ARTs have reinforced more "traditional" conceptualizations of reproduction in Greece, including heterosexist values that are being justified in the "best interests" of the ART-conceived child.

The (In)FERCIT Study

The research material for this chapter derives mainly from a research project called (In)Fertile Citizens: On the Concepts, Practices, Politics, and Technologies of Assisted Reproduction in Greece: An Interdisciplinary and Comparative Approach ([In]FERCIT). I served as principal investigator of (In)FERCIT, which spanned three years between September 2012 and September 2015 and was funded by the European Social Fund and the General Secretariat of Research and Technology, Greece, and conducted by the Lab of Family and Kinship Studies, Department of Social Anthropology and History at the University of the Aegean. The project aimed to offer a detailed, multisited ethnographic account of assisted reproduction concepts, practices, politics, and technologies in Greece, relate them to legal issues and human rights on in-fertility and reproduction, and provide a comparative perspective that would associate the Greek project with similar research conducted in Spain, Italy, Bulgaria, Turkey, Cyprus, and Lebanon.

Using an array of methodologies—quantitative, qualitative, participant observation, and legal archival documentation—this interdisciplinary anthropological and legal project revolved around four clusters of research: (1) shifting concepts of kinship, relationships, parenthood, and personhood in the context of social and technological transformations and nature/culture/technology perceptions; (2) practices of reproduction in relation to gender, sexuality, age, religion, and ethnicity; (3) politics of in-fertility, "reproductive citizenship," and cross-border reproduction across different states; and (4) reproductive technologies and networks on local and global levels. Ultimately, the project aimed to provide an account that would transcend permissive versus restrictive discourse on reproductive citizenship and reconsider the specific cultural contexts in which such discourses emerge, particularly local-global exchanges and social-technological networks (Kantsa 2015; Chatjouli, Daskalaki, and Kantsa 2015; Kantsa, Papadopoulou, and Zanini 2015). In addition, the study drew upon present demographic data from Eurostat, the current legal context in Greece, and ongoing ethnographic research on assisted reproduction.

Assisting Reproduction in Greece

The first Greek child born from in vitro fertilization (IVF) came into the world only four years after the birth of Louise Brown (the first "test tube baby" in the history of humankind), and was born in Greece on January 20, 1982, with the participation of the British obstetrician Patrick Steptoe and a team of Greek doctors. In the years that followed, the new IVF method was disseminated by doctors trained in the country or abroad, mainly in the United States and the United Kingdom (Kantsa 2014). In an interview, Themis Mantzavinos, former associate professor of obstetrics-gynecology at the University of Athens, president of the Panhellenic Association of Doctors of Assisted Reproduction, and one of the first proponents of this method of assisted reproduction in Greece, spoke about IVF with enthusiasm, also crediting his mentor, Howard Jones, managing director of the Jones Institute Foundation in Reproductive Medicine in Norfolk, Virginia, and a pioneer in the method of assisted reproduction in the United States: "Well, as this wise man [Howard Jones] used to say, this method came to stay. It will stay and will improve. It will improve. And we really see it. Every year we see things happening, that is, the various developments that even in our imagination [didn't exist]." This excerpt from my interview with Dr. Mantzavinos, carried out in 2013 in person in Athens, is characterized by an inherent faith in the future and the possibilities of continuous development of the method. According to Mantzavinos, assisted reproduction creates expectations, offers hope, and opens new futures.

Similarly, Vassilis Tarlatzis, emeritus professor of obstetrics-gynecology and human reproduction at Aristotle University of Thessaloniki and former president of the European Society of Human Reproduction and Embryology (ESHRE), as well as the International Federation of Fertility Societies (IFFS), points out that the increase in the number of IVF clinics is directly related to the continuous emergence of new techniques in the field of assisted reproduction. In a 2013 interview in person in Thessaloniki, he said, "Cryopreservation readily opened up new possibilities because multiple attempts were feasible with only one egg retrieval. Then came the use of eggs from a third donor. The population in need for assisted reproduction expanded because they were women who, either from birth or epigenetically, did not have ovarian function. Later, in 1992, microinsemination [intracytoplasmic sperm injection (ICSI)] was introduced. . . . So, the demand increased a lot, so in order to meet the demand, the centers also increased. This is a global phenomenon." According to ESHRE's European IVF Surveillance Consortium (IEC), there were more than fifty IVF clinics and medical centers in 2006 for a population of ten million people (De Mouzon et al. 2010), distributed among the major Greek cities. According to the same organization, the number of these clinics rose to seventy-six in 2012 (Calhaz-Jorge et al. 2016), but then declined over the years to forty-three in 2018 (Wyns et al. 2022). Today there are forty-seven licensed assisted reproduction facilities in Greece, dispersed over eight cities (National Authority of Assisted Reproduction 2023). These figures illustrate the rise of assisted reproduction clinics at the beginning of the twenty-first century, their significant decline during the Greek financial crisis beginning in 2008, and their recent stabilization.

The legislative framework that regulates the operation of these clinics and centers took shape almost twenty years after the introduction of ARTs in Greece, at the dawn of the twenty-first century. These laws were designed to answer the pressing questions posed by the adoption of ARTs in the county. The first legislative framework was introduced by law 3089 (2002), Medical Assistance in Human Reproduction, which tried to compensate for the previous legal vacuum and introduced amendments to the Civil Code on issues of kinship and inheritance. The law defined kinship as a social-sentimental relationship, where choice and the desire for the child take priority over biological relationships. The law empowered married people, nonmarried couples, and single women alike with rights to reproductive technologies. More specifically, the law permitted the use of fertilized eggs for research or therapeutic reasons, permitted surrogate motherhood, and permitted posthumous conception, but imposed donor anonymity for both egg and sperm donors. Donors may be no older than thirty-five and forty, for women and men, respectively, while recipient women may not be older than fifty.

The subsequent law 3305 (2005), Application of Methods of Medically Assisted Reproduction, focused on the applications of medically assisted reproduction and issues of "national health." It defined the biomedical dimensions of the 2002 law, provided the context for research on gametes and fertilized embryos, defined the terms for the establishment and operation of IVF clinics and cryopreservation banks, set the terms for the establishment of an independent National Authority for Medically Assisted Reproduction, and legislated punitive and administrative sanctions against the breach of the 2002 and 2005 laws. Its thirty articles are structured around two main principles: first, the application of medically assisted reproduction methods in a way that secures respect for individual freedom, the right to personhood, and the satisfaction of the desire to acquire descendants, taking into account the possibilities of medicine and biology and the principles of bioethics; and second, a concern that during the application of the aforementioned methods, the interest of the child to be born is to receive primary consideration. Following these two principles, the Greek legal context permitted preimplantation genetic diagnosis, embryo freezing, anonymous sperm donation, anonymous egg donation, embryo donation, surrogacy, research on genetic material (donated gametes and fertilized embryos), and the free transportation of genetic material and fertilized eggs from and to other European countries, thus forming one of the most "permissive" profiles among European countries, one that illustrates the uneasy mix of ethics and politics (Pennings 2004).

Law 4272 (2014) introduced minor changes in the context of a broader law on organ donation, while the most recent Law 4958 (2022), Reforms to Medically Assisted Reproduction and Other Emergency Adjustments, voted on by the Greek Parliament in July 2022, introduced a number of measures to facilitate the acquisition of children through assisted reproduction. The law extends the age limit for women from fifty to fifty-four, permits oocyte cryopreservation for social and not only medical reasons, removes cryopreservation time restrictions, and provides as an option donor anonymity, which is no longer mandatory.

Not surprisingly, the enactment of this series of increasingly permissive laws led to a boom in IVF cycles across Greece. The National Authority of Assisted Reproduction (2018) revealed that the number of ART cycles in 2015 was 30,728, of which 4,127 were carried out by transport of cryogenically preserved embryos and 4,768 by donation of eggs. This represented a growth rate of 28 percent and 41 percent, respectively, since 2014. The National Authority concluded, "According to these results, it can be stated that in Greece there is an oversupply of assisted reproduction methods since we know that globally the application of medically assisted reproductive technologies reaches 1,000 cycles per 1,000,000 inhabitants per year, whereas here we are approaching 3,500 cycles." This "oversupply" of assisted reproduction methods in Greece continues today (Wyns et al. 2022).

The Booming Greek ART Sector

This Greek ART boom must be understood within the growing medicalization of reproduction in the country. Indeed, the medicalization of reproduction has been a target of ethnographic research in Greece since the 1990s, having focused initially on issues related to pregnancy and birth (Georges 2008; Trakas 2013; Chatjouli 2012). The cultural value attributed to parenthood, the highly medicalized context of reproduction, and the highly "permissive" ART legal framework in Greece provided a fertile ground for the establishment of a reproductive "industry," particularly in the private sector. In such a context, ARTs have become another "natural" way to reproduce, further normalizing the problem of involuntary childlessness after its reconceptualization in biomedical terms and further reproducing the dominant biopolitical regime of heteronormative-conjugal family making.

At the same time, Greece has established itself as a fertility destination. According to one report, published in 2020, Greece has managed "to attract more patients and from being in the 5th or 6th place in the list of European destinations for cross-border fertility travel, Greece has climbed in the 3rd place, 'threatening' to overtake the Czech Republic and figure out in the 2nd place after Spain" (Kavakas 2020). In a study based on fourteen open-ended interviews with Greek assisted reproduction professionals and 130 questionnaires from those who visited these centers from other countries, Anastasia Paraskou and Babu P. George (2017) concluded that Greece's eminence in the "reproductive tourism" market is due mainly to its high success rate, permissive legal framework, and comparatively low costs.

Thus, assisted reproduction is presented in Greece not only as hope for one's individual future constituted through personhood and kinship relations but also as hope for the nation's future—a guarantee of its very existence not only demographically (*to demografiko*), as the Greek population shrank by at least five hundred thousand between 2010 and 2020

(European Parliament 2021), but also economically. In this context, experts who cure infertility act as agents of hope. As some of them emphatically stated in interviews, "We give you hope"; "We allow you to hope."

Athena Athanasiou argues persuasively, "In the face of a dwindling population, the *self-interest* of individual bodies join[s] forces with the *social good* of the body politic in ways that tacitly bracket the internal differentiation of the national body as such" (Athanasiou 2006: 239). Indeed, in the Greek context, where infertility is seen as a break with the future—both personally and nationally—assisted reproduction, or "the cure for infertility," is presented as the hope for both individual and collective futures, a way to sustain the "family" and the "nation."

The Changing Greek Family

The question remains: What actually constitutes a "family" in the Greek context? In many texts, the word "family" is not clearly defined. It is often described as a general term for domestic intimate relations. It is perceived as a form of organizing private life that remains firm and universal. Yet, the study of the history of the family shows that there are many types of families. Family types always exist as part of the structure of society. Sylvia Yanagisako argues,

> The units we label as families are undeniably about more than procreation and socialization. They are as much about production, exchange, power, inequality, and status. When we fully acknowledge that the family is as much an integral part of the political and economic structures of society as it is a reproductive unit we will finally free ourselves from an unwarranted preoccupation with its procreative functions and all the consequent notions embodied within such a stance. . . . Our usage of the terms "family" and "household" will then reflect an awareness that they are, like "marriage" and "kinship," merely "odd-job" words, which are useful in descriptive statements but unproductive as tools for analysis and comparison. (Yanagisako 1979: 200–201)

Changes in the modern Greek family are closely related to amendments of the Greek Family Law in 1983 that made divorce easier, guaranteed equality between spouses, ended official discrimination against illegitimate children, and introduced civil marriage (Law 1329 [1983]). Yet, discussing changes in the modern Greek family from 1974 to 1994, Evthymios Papataxiarchis (2013) claims that, in contrast to other European societies where cohabitation and single-parent households are recognized as strong alternatives, in Greece the model of the nuclear heterosexual family shows impressive persistence and an ability to reproduce in changing structural conditions. Sociologists Charis Simeonidou (2002) and Monica Carlos and Laura Maratou-Alibranti (2002) agree with this argument. Their research with Greek families at the turn of the millennium shows that recent changes in family and reproductive behaviors in southern Europe that affected the "traditional" family model (two married parents and their children)—such as an increase in divorce, the emergence of new forms of cohabitation, and a growing ambivalence toward the institution of the family—occur minimally in Greece. However, more recent demographic data present a different picture.

According to the most recent data available for the EU countries, 1.7 million marriages and an estimated 0.7 million divorces took place in the European Union in 2021 (Eurostat 2021b). These figures may be expressed as 3.9 marriages for every one thousand persons (crude marriage rate) and 1.7 divorces for every one thousand persons (crude divorce rate). Since 1964 (the first year for which data are available), the crude marriage rate in the European Union has declined by more than 50 percent. At the same time, the crude divorce rate has essentially doubled, increasing from 0.8 per thousand persons in 1964 to 1.7 in 2021. In Greece the crude marriage rate declined from 8.9 in 1964 to 3.8 in 2021, while the crude divorce rate increased from 0.8 in 1964 to 1.8 in 2017. It follows that Greece has moved from third place among European countries in terms of marriage in 1964 to the fifteenth place in 2021 (Eurostat 2021b). The rate of divorce has also increased. In terms of divorce among European countries, Greece moved from twenty-fifth place in 1964 to fifteenth in 2017 (Eurostat 2020a). Similar changes are also observed in the type of marriage that is being advanced in Greece. Civil marriage has outnumbered religious marriage in recent years, and cohabitation agreements have increased as well. In 2021, the proportion was 35.3 percent for religious marriages, 42.6 percent for civil marriages, and 22.1 percent for cohabitation agreements (Hellenic Statistic Authority 2022).

In reference to births, the fertility rate (live births per woman) in Greece is 1.43, which is significantly lower than the EU average of 1.53 (Eurostat 2021a). However, Greece has fewer births out of wedlock than other EU countries. In 2018, 42 percent of EU births were out of wedlock, which is 17 percent higher than in 2000. According to EU statistics, this number exemplifies the establishment of new family forms next to a more "traditional" model where children are born in the context of a marital relationship. In Greece, however, the percentage of out-of-wedlock births in 2018 amounted to only 11.1 percent of total births, in comparison to 4.3 percent in 2001 (Eurostat 2020b). Greece and Cyprus were deemed "traditional" EU countries in this regard.

Having said this, the decline in the marriage rate, the increase in cohabitation agreements, and the rise in the number of divorces represent the practices of a new cohort of Greeks who choose not to marry, not to have children, to divorce their spouses, and to raise children alone. Indeed, these trends suggest new ways of conceptualizing and understanding the Greek family. Furthermore, they suggest the escalating readiness of Greek society to keep up with "average" EU countries in terms of marriage and divorce options. Yet, the very low percentage of births out of wedlock in Greece also demonstrates something else—the deep entrenchment of the nuclear heterosexual family in Greece, a model that results in what I call "reproductive heterosexism."

Reproductive Heterosexism

Due to a complex amalgamation of medical perceptions, religious beliefs, legal regulations, and psychological and sociological prejudices, reproductive heterosexism persists in Greece. Parenthood is intrinsically related to the conjugal household, and little space is offered for single parenthood, let alone same-sex parenthood. According to the recent Europe Rainbow Map and Index (ILGA-Europe 2023), which charts the legal and policy human rights of lesbian, gay, bisexual, trans, and intersex people, in Greece same-sex rights do not include marriage equality, joint adoption, second-parent adoption, automatic coparent recognition, medically assisted reproduction for gay and lesbian couples, or the recognition of trans parenthood. Only registered partnership is recognized, although access to medically assisted donor insemination for single women is allowed.

Lesbian women in Greece were excluded from access to assisted reproduction with Law 3089 (2002). In 2002, the church put tremendous pressure on the government to exclude nonheterosexual couples and unmarried women from the law. While nonheterosexual couples were excluded, nonmarried, single women were included, but only because, as one of the exponents of the bill stated, "Women are natural-born mothers, this is a kind of information which is inscribed onto their DNA" (Kantsa 2006: 370).

Consequently, although a significant number of same-sex-desiring Greek women consider the possibility of having children by asking a friend, using a sperm donor, or adopting a child, only a small number of women become mothers through these means. Medically assisted insemination techniques and adoption are available to nonmarried people, but they are rarely used in practice. Insemination is a high-priced means of reproduction that is not always associated with success, and there are few chances for a single woman or a same-sex-desiring woman to adopt a child, because of the limited number of available children. Vasso Canaka was a thirty-six-year-old woman living in Athens and employed in the private sector. She had insemination performed in 2013 and underlines the significant financial demands: "Ok, it makes sense, you always know anyway that in case it succeeds, a child needs money. But it's another thing to have to cover some expenses every month, and quite another to have to shell out a few thousand for the procedure. It's not the same. So, yes, this is what stresses me the most. For the moment I can afford it, if it turns out that the attempts I have to make are too many for my budget, I'll see what I'll do" (Kantsa and Chalkidou-Chalkidis 2014: 94).

Similarly, very few single gay men or couples start families in Greece. In the Greek context, although surrogate motherhood was established by Law 3089 (2002), regulations exclude men. According to the existing legislation in Article 1458, "Judicial permission is granted upon application by the woman who wishes to have a child, as long as it is proven that she is medically unable to conceive and that the woman offering to conceive is, in view of her state of health, suitable for pregnancy" (Civil Code n.d.). Through this legislation, combined with the exclusion of gays and lesbians from adoption procedures, the state excludes gay men from the possibility of starting families. In his recent research on gay fatherhood in Greece, Savvas Triantafyllidis (2021) argues that, through their efforts to form families, gay men aspire to prove that they do not differ from heterosexuals and thus attempt to gain social recognition and full access to citizenship. Yet, it is the experience of existing homoparental families and their unequal treatment by the Greek state that underlines the stratified character of citizenship regarding family rights.

The absence of a legal framework for the recognition of same-sex-partner parental roles is crucial as it points out the interconnections of queer kinship, stratified reproduction, and reproductive citizenship (Smietana and Thompson 2018). This absence is not marked by a lack of framework; rather, it constitutes a specifically discriminatory framework that devalues the families of same-sex parents on the basis of sexuality. This practice is not so much an exclusion of same-sex families from social conditions as an inclusion in the social condition through the practice of exclusion. The regime of reproductive heterosexism in Greece excludes all but the recognized, permissible, intelligible, heterosexual forms of parenthood, relationality, and kinship.

It follows that, as Aspa-Pako Chalkidou-Chalkidis persuasively argues, "Parenthood in Greece gets established as a defined sexual category predicated on the exclusion of imagined deviance" (Chalkidou-Chalkidis 2022: 563). "Considering that in the Greek collective imaginary, the notion of family is inter-woven with the sexual fantasies of a heterosexually reproductive nation," Chalkidou-Chalkidis concludes that "institutional recognition entails legitimizing the presence of certain bodies (and not others) within the context of biopolitical democratic governance by configuring the terms of otherness" (Chalkidou-Chalkidis 2022: 570). Drawing on Sara Ahmed's argument that an institutional logic can be perceived as a logic of kinship—namely, as a way of relating to and reproducing social relations (Ahmed 2012: 38)—Chalkidou-Chalkidis suggests that an institutional logic of exclusion can also be understood as a logic of kinship, to the extent that it also proposes certain modes of relating to and producing social relationships that lead to exclusion (Chalkidou-Chalkidis 2022: 574).

In this context, the use of ARTs is understood as a way to make unimaginable family models and impermissible parenting roles intelligible. This is illustrated in the narrative of Katerina Stergiou, a forty-seven-year-old teacher who lives in Athens and underwent an insemination procedure in 2000. She comments on the use of ARTs by lesbians, who usually present themselves at clinics as single women: "In this case technology says 'gotcha.' The progress in science says 'gotcha.' I want to have a baby and not to go through what I have been told by everybody [meaning marriage], and especially in this case, technology is a kind of passe-partout; it takes you where they have not predicted. It's unpredictable; we went very quickly into something different, and I felt from the beginning that this change implies a huge social change" (Kantsa and Chalkidou-Chalkidis 2014: 97). Yet, in many cases of intentional single motherhood by means of assisted reproduction, the role of the natal household remains significant. Namely, most nonheterosexual women continue to be largely dependent upon their families of origin for practical and emotional support (Kantsa 2006). Due to the absence of a strong lesbian network in Greece or state policies that could act as substitutes for family relations, the family of origin preserves its role as the primary resource of emotional, practical, and financial support. Even in cases where nonheterosexual forms of reproduction and family formation are accepted and recognized, acceptance is strongly related to a kind of "protection" provided by the natal household. Protection takes practical and significant symbolic forms. The "proper environment" that a child needs in order to grow up "normally" is equated to the natal household of, in most cases, the biological mother. Thus, the ambiguities of nonheterosexual motherhood are absorbed by parental family members, who embrace their daughter for the "sake of their grandchild" and thus "legitimize" and "rationalize" their daughter's choices. However, it is through the same path that these choices are rendered invisible (Kantsa and Chalkidou-Chalkidis 2014: 98–99).

Family Making in the "Best Interests of the Child"

The best interests of the child is one of the four fundamental principles of the UN Convention on the Rights of the Child. Yet, its exact definition is often the object of litigation and negotiation across varying sociocultural contexts. Within the field of medically assisted reproduction, the idea of the child's welfare becomes the major argument for determining the acceptability of certain applications (Pennings 2011).

In the context of ARTs in Greece, the idea of the child's best interests has been used to argue both for and against donor anonymity and has been at the center of discussions concerning the principle of "socio-sentimental" kinship, age limits, the right of nonmarried women to have access to ARTs, and postmortem insemination (Galata 2018). In the same context, a concern "for the best interests of the child" excludes nonheterosexual couples and gay men from access to ARTs. It seems that, despite its denaturalization through new methods and technologies, kinship is still tied to "naturalized" notions of gender, age, and relationship that promote the heterosexual family and configure reproductive heterosexism.

As Kath Weston (1998) has successfully demonstrated, lesbian and gay families are not simple assimilations of dominant discourses as they do not build upon "prevailing beliefs about what makes a family"; but they transform these beliefs by focusing on the element of choice. However, Marilyn Strathern (1996: 48) argues that this particular detraditionalizing is also retraditionalizing in another guise, as "there always was a strong elective component to the enactment of family relationships, and those families that base themselves on choice (symbolized by 'friendship') claim traditional virtues in attending to the quality of interpersonal relations."

Thus, it is not surprising that reproduction in general and assisted reproduction in particular is still closely related to the heterosexual nuclear family in Greece, while the conjugal household is considered the proper "nurturing" environment for a child's upbringing. In an era when reproduction has been gradually disconnected from heterosexual sex due to the existence of ARTs, a connection between the "best interests of the child" and heterosexual conjugal families reinstates this norm, especially in a society imbued with the imperative of having children.

Conclusion

Reproduction is about more than just making children or making families. Reproduction is about technology and material, state policy and economic aspiration, and discrimination and exclusion. It can be used as a significant entry point to study how cultures are produced, contested, and transformed (Ginsburg and Rapp 1995), while assisted reproduction proves to be an exceptional reprolens into multiple domains of social life (Inhorn 2020). The ways in which a society regulates reproduction in general, and assisted reproduction in particular, are closely related to imaginations about its own future and aspirations for the next generations.

Recent demographic statistics suggest that Greek society is becoming increasingly open to marriage and divorce options, but these statistics also reflect greater resistance to the birth of children outside wedlock or the contestation of the nuclear heterosexual family model. It follows that, despite its pronatalist character, Greek society is ready to address infertility only under certain prerequisites, which assure that children will be placed within heterosexual conjugal households. Thus, although Greece has a highly permissive legislative framework allowing ARTs for heterosexual couples, it nonetheless denies access to same-sex individuals or couples. At the same time, the law does allow single women to access ARTs, drawing on a discourse about "natural maternity," which must be protected by the state, especially in the face of a dwindling population. But even when single women—same-sex-desiring or not—use this option, their default reality is to be subsumed within the "protective" environment of their natal household. This has the effect of "ghosting" their nonconjugal or nonheterosexual identities, choices, and families by "kinning" them to a more dominant overarching and essentially patriarchal household structure. The puzzle of the Greek case reveals the complexity of the relationship among gender, sexuality, and kinship relations in a society in which reproductive heterosexism persists amid a repronational commitment to family making.

REFERENCES

Ahmed, Sara. 2012. *On Being Included: Racism and Diversity in Institutional Life.* Durham, NC: Duke University Press.

Athanasiou, Athena, 2006. "Bloodlines: Performing the Body of the 'Demos': Reckoning the Time of the 'Ethnos.'" *Journal of Modern Greek Studies* 24: 229–56.

Calhaz-Jorge, Carlos, C. de Geyter, M. S. Kupka, J. de Mouzon, K. Erb, E. Mocanu, T. Motrenko, G. Scaravelli, C. Wyns, and V. Goossens. 2016. "Assisted Reproductive Technology in Europe 2012: Results Generated from European Registers by ESHRE." *Human Reproduction* 31(8): 1638–52.

Carlos, Monica, and Laura Maratou-Alibranti. 2002. "New Family Forms and Social Policies. The Cases of Greece and Portugal." In *Families and the Welfare State in Europe: Trends and Challenges in the 21ˢᵗ Century*, ed. Laura Maratou-Alibranti, 131–59. Athens: Gutenberg. [In Greek.]

Chalkidou-Chalkidis, Aspa-Pako. 2022. "Vanilla Democracy: Sexuality, Parenthood, and Kinship in Greece." *Sexualities* 25(5–6): 563–80.

Chatjouli, Aglaia. 2012. *Thalassemic Lives: Biological Difference, Normality, and Biosociality; An Anthropological Approach*. Athens: Patakis. [In Greek.]

Chatjouli, Aglaia, Ivi Daskalaki, and Venetia Kantsa. 2015. *Out of Body, Out of Home: Assisted Reproduction, Gender, and Family in Greece*. Athens: (In)FERCIT and Alexandria Publications.

Civil Code. N.d. https://www.ministryofjustice.gr. Accessed September 20, 2023. [In Greek.]

De Mouzon, Jacques, V. Goossens, S. Bhattacharya, J. A. Castilla, A. P. Ferraretti, V. Korsak, M. Kupka, K. G. Nygren, and A. Nyboe Andersen. 2010. "Assisted Reproductive Technology in Europe, 2006: Results Generated from European Registers by ESHRE." *Human Reproduction* 25(8): 1851–62.

Edwards, Jeanette. 2000. *Born and Bred: Idioms of Kinship and New Reproductive Technologies in England*. Oxford: Oxford University Press.

Edwards, Jeanette, Sarah Franklin, Eric Hirsch, France Price, and Marilyn Strathern. 1999 [1993]. *Technologies of Procreation: Kinship in the Age of Assisted Conception*. London: Routledge.

Edwards, Jeanette, and Carles Salazar, eds. 2009. *European Kinship in the Age of Biotechnology*. Oxford: Berghahn.

European Parliament. 2021. "Tackling the Major Demographic Problem Facing Greece." November 4. www.europarl.europa.eu.

Eurostat. 2020a. "EU Crude Divorce Rate on the Rise." July 10. https://ec.europa.eu.

———. 2020b. "42% of Births in the EU Are Outside Marriage." July 17. https://ec.europa.eu.

———. 2021a. "Fertility Statistics." https://ec.europa.eu.

———. 2021b. "Marriage and Divorce Statistics." https://ec.europa.eu.

Franklin, Sarah. 2013. *Biological Relatives: IVF, Stem Cells, and the Future of Kinship*. Durham, NC: Duke University Press.

Franklin, Sarah, and Helena Ragoné, eds. 1998. *Reproducing Reproduction: Kinship, Power, and Technological Innovation*. Philadelphia: University of Pennsylvania Press.

Galata, Martha. 2018. "The Interest of the Child in Medically Assisted Reproduction." MA thesis, Department of Public Administration, Panteion University, Athens, Greece.

Georges, Eugenia. 2008. *Bodies of Knowledge: The Medicalization of Reproduction in Greece*. Nashville, TN: Vanderbilt University Press.

Ginsburg, Faye D., and Rayna Rapp, eds. 1995. *Conceiving the New World Order: The Global Politics of Reproduction*. Berkeley: University of California Press.

Halkias, Alexandra. 2004. *The Empty Cradle of Democracy: Sex, Abortion, and Nationalism in Greece*. Durham, NC: Duke University Press.

Hellenic Statistic Authority. 2022. "Data on Vital Statistics: 2021." October 4. www.statistics.gr.

ILGA-Europe. 2023. "Rainbow Europe Map and Index." May 11. www.ilga-europe.org.

Inhorn, Marcia C. 2015. *Cosmopolitan Conceptions: IVF Sojourns in Global Dubai*. Durham, NC: Duke University Press.

——. 2020. "Where Has the Quest for Conception Taken Us? Lessons from Anthropology and Sociology." *Reproductive Biomedicine and Society Online* 10: 46–57.

Inhorn, Marcia C., and Daphna Birenbaum-Carmeli. 2008. "Assisted Reproductive Technologies and Culture Change." *Annual Review of Anthropology* 37: 177–96.

Kantsa, Venetia. 2006. "Family Matters: Motherhood and Same-Sex Relationships." In *Adventures of Alterity: The Production of Cultural Difference in Contemporary Greece*, ed. Evthymios Papataxiarchis, 355–81. Athens: Alexandria Publications. [In Greek.]

——, ed. 2013. *Motherhood at the Forefront: Recent Research in Greek Ethnography*. Athens: Alexandria Publications. [In Greek.]

——. 2014. "Presenting Hope: Body Technologies in Assisted Reproduction." In *The Body under Surveillance: Ethical and Political Dimensions of Medical Technology and Social Care*, ed. Aglaia Chatjouli, George Alexias, and Manolis Tzanakis, 180–206. Athens: Pedio. [In Greek.]

——, ed. 2015. *Changing Relations: Kinship and Medically Assisted Reproduction*. Athens: (In)FERCIT and Alexandria Publications. [In Greek.]

Kantsa, Venetia, and Aspa-Pako Chalkidou-Chalkidis. 2014. "Doing Family 'in the Space between the Laws': Notes on Lesbian Motherhood in Greece." *Lamda Nordica* 19(3–4): 86–108.

Kantsa, Venetia, Lina Papadopoulou, and Giulia Zanini, eds. 2015. *(In)Fertile Citizens: Anthropological and Legal Challenges of Assisted Reproduction Technologies*. Athens: (In)FERCIT and Alexandria Publications.

Kavakas, Dimitris. 2020. "Greece Fertility Destination 2021." Redia IVF, November 23. www.rediaivf.com.

Law 1329. 1983. "Implementation of the Constitutional Principle of Equality between Men and Women in the Civil Code, Its Introductory Law, Commercial Legislation, and the Code of Civil Procedure, as Well as Partial Modernization of the Provisions of the Civil Code concerning Family Law." Ministry of the Interior, www.ypes.gr. [In Greek.]

Law 3089. 2002. "Medical Assistance in Human Reproduction." Greek National Authority of Assisted Reproduction, https://eaiya.gov.gr. [In Greek.]

Law 3305. 2005. "Application of Methods of Medically Assisted Reproduction." Greek National Authority of Assisted Reproduction, https://eaiya.gov.gr. [In Greek.]

Law 4272. 2014. "Adaptation to National Law of Implementing Directive 2012/25/EU on the Establishment of Information Procedures on the Exchange between Member States of Human Organs Intended for Transplantation: Arrangements for Mental

Health and Medically Assisted Reproduction and Other Provisions." Greek National Authority of Assisted Reproduction, https://eaiya.gov.gr. [In Greek.]

Law 4958. 2022. "Reforms to Medically Assisted Reproduction and Other Emergency Adjustments." Greek National Authority of Assisted Reproduction, https://eaiya.gov.gr. [In Greek.]

Loizos, Peter, and Evthymios Papataxiarchis. 1991. *Contested Identities: Gender and Kinship in Modern Greece*. Princeton, NJ: Princeton University Press.

National Authority of Assisted Reproduction. 2018. "Presentation of Medically Assisted Reproduction Unit Statistics at ESHRE 2018." Greek National Authority of Assisted Reproduction, https://eaiya.gov.gr. [In Greek.]

———. 2023. "Licensed in Vitro Fertilization Units (IVFU) & Cryopreservation Banks (CB)." Greek National Authority of Assisted Reproduction, https://eaiya.gov.gr.

Papataxiarchis, Evthymios. 2013. "Shaping Modern Times in the Greek Family: A Comparative View of Gender and Kinship Transformations after 1974." In *State, Economy, Society: 19th–20th Centuries*, ed. Anna Dala and Niki Maroniti, 217–44. Athens: Metehmio.

Paraskou, Anastasia, and Babu P. George. 2017. "The Market for Reproductive Tourism: An Analysis with Special Reference to Greece." *Global Health Research and Policy* 2(16).

Paxson, Heather. 2004. *Making Modern Mothers: Ethics and Family Planning in Urban Greece*. Berkeley: University of California Press.

———. 2006. "Reproduction as Spiritual Kin Work: Orthodoxy, IVF, and the Moral Economy of Motherhood in Greece." *Culture, Medicine & Psychiatry* 30(4): 481–505.

Pennings, Guido. 2004. "Legal Harmonization and Reproductive Tourism in Europe." *Human Reproduction* 19(12): 2689–94.

———. 2011. "Evaluating the Welfare of the Child in Same-Sex Families." *Human Reproduction* 26(7): 1609–15.

Simeonidou, Charis. 2002. "Marriage-Divorce, Cohabitation-Breaking Up in Greece. Research Results EKKE." In *Families and the Welfare State in Europe: Trends and Challenges in the 21st Century*, ed. Laura Maratou-Alibranti, 115–30. Athens: Gutenberg.

Smietana, Marcin, and Charis Thompson, eds. 2018. "Making Families: Transnational Surrogacy, Queer Kinship, and Reproductive Justice." Special issue of *Reproductive BioMedicine and Society Online* 7: 1–160.

"Social Cohesion Ministry Will 'Strengthen' Family." 2023. *Ekathimerini*, June 27. www.ekathimerini.com.

Strathern, Marilyn. 1992. *Reproducing the Future: Essays on Anthropology, Kinship, and the New Reproductive Technologies*. New York: Routledge.

———. 1996. "Enabling Identity? Biology, Choice, and the New Reproductive Technologies." In *Questions of Cultural Identity*, ed. Stuart Hall and Paul du Gay, 37–52. London: Sage.

———. 2005. *Kinship, Law, and the Unexpected: Relatives Are Always a Surprise*. Cambridge: Cambridge University Press.

Trakas, Deanna. 2013. "Motherhood as a Midwifery Procedure." In *Motherhood at the Forefront: Recent Research in Greek Ethnography*, ed. Venetia Kantsa, 327–44. Athens: Alexandria. [In Greek.]

Triantafyllidis, Savvas. 2021. "Tracing Homosexual Fatherhood: Anthropological Approaches on Male Homosexual Relatedness in Modern Greece." PhD thesis, Department of Social Anthropology, Panteion University, Athens, Greece.

Weston, Kath. 1998. "Forever Is a Long Time: Romancing the Real in Gay Kinship Ideologies." In *Longslowburn: Sexuality and Social Science*, ed. Kath Weston, 84–93. New York: Routledge.

Wyns, C., C. De Geyter, C. Calhaz-Jorge, M. S. Kupka, T. Motrenko, J. Smeenk, C. Bergh, A. Tandler-Schneider, I. A. Rugescu, and V. Goossens. 2022. "Assisted Reproductive Technology in Europe, 2018: Results Generated from European Registers by ESHRE." *Human Reproduction* (3): 1–20.

Yanagisako, Sylvia. 1979. "Family and Household: The Analysis of Domestic Groups." *Annual Review of Anthropology* 8: 161–205.

4

Reproductive Imaginations

Process versus Outcome in Queer Family Making in Britain

ROBERT PRALAT

I do get asked quite a lot [whether I want to have children].
And inevitably, you know, the next question is, well, how?
And I'm sort of left going, I don't know! You're asking me as
if I should have an idea, but really? I mean, I'm vaguely aware
of different options, but . . . No. Realistically, I don't actually
know how I would go about it.
—Sally, thirty-one-year-old lesbian

For people who are unlikely to have children through sex, the prospect of
becoming a parent automatically raises the question of how to do so. Lesbians and gay men, as well as others who do not expect to reproduce in a
conventional way, must consider not only whether they want to become
parents but also—if they do desire to create a family with children—how
they would do it. As Sally explains in the opening quotation, a question
about parenting desire immediately prompts a question about possible
ways of fulfilling it, and responding to the latter question can be complicated. In fact, as I argue in this chapter, the difficulty of answering the
"how question" can make both questions difficult to answer.

In my research to date, I have explored how people who are not heterosexual think and talk about parenthood. The starting point for this
work was an observation that, in Britain (the geographical focus of
my research), lesbian motherhood and gay fatherhood achieved social
acceptance and legal recognition remarkably quickly. Not long ago, a
family headed by two people of the same sex was broadly perceived as
posing a major threat to children. Yet, just two years after the repeal in
2003 of Section 28, which banned the "promotion" of homosexuality as a

"pretended family relationship," same-sex couples in England and Wales were given not only the right to formalize their relationships through civil partnership but also the right to adopt. Coming into force in 2005, the two laws paved the way for other legal milestones that followed soon after, including antidiscrimination policies in fertility treatment and same-sex marriage.

In some way, it was in 2005 when my research on this topic began. That year, as a nineteen-year-old gay man, I moved to England from Poland, starting my adult life in a country that had just granted same-sex couples both partnering and parenting rights. I was keen to understand how my peers approached their adulthood in this new reality, with a much-altered relationship between sexuality and reproduction—and with multiple options for family making. The hitherto restricted options for lesbians and gay men to have children, which only acknowledged birth mothers (even if they had female partners) and single adoptive parents (even if they were not truly "single"), were expanded by an explicit validation of couple-based queer parenthood. It was now possible for same-sex couples not only to adopt jointly but also, thanks to civil partnership and then marriage, to pursue parenthood through assisted reproduction, with both partners recognized as parents and expected to be treated on a par with their heterosexual counterparts. This opened up several "pathways to parenthood": in addition to adoption, previously limited opportunities to have biological children through informal arrangements were supplemented by clinical donor conception for lesbians (with or without in vitro fertilization [IVF]) and surrogacy for gay men (the latter feasible on an "altruistic" basis in the United Kingdom, with possibilities of "commercial" surrogacy abroad; see Smietana, chapter 5).

Modest curiosity had turned into a full-time preoccupation as I embarked on studying for a PhD in 2011. Immersed in the academic literature on lesbian mothers and gay fathers, I noticed that scholarly understandings of queer reproduction relied almost exclusively on studies with people who have experienced parenthood—or at least attempted to achieve it. The growing visibility and variety of families headed by same-sex couples was documented in an expanding body of evidence demonstrating what it is like to form a family that departs from the norm by virtue of parents' sexual orientation. But this literature presented only part of a bigger picture. For there were many more people identifying as lesbian, gay, bisexual, or otherwise who did not have children but who were the potential beneficiaries of the socio-legal transformation in the family arena. I wanted to know what parenthood meant to them, and what kind of reflections the idea of it evoked.

In this chapter, I draw on interviews conducted between 2012 and 2015 in England and Wales with twenty-three lesbian, gay, and bisexual people in their twenties and thirties, who did not have children but who might have them in the future. Recruited mostly through a dedicated study website, a link to which was shared through LGBTQ organizations, staff networks, and Facebook, interviewees were predominantly white, middle-class lesbians and gay men residing in urban locations (for details about methodology and demographics, see Pralat 2018, 2020, 2021).

I focus on what I call the "how question"—that is, how to go about having children. By paying particular attention to the *process* of creating a family, I explore how nonheterosexual men and women envisage becoming parents. Navigating often-limited understandings of various parenthood possibilities facilitates what I refer to as *reproductive imaginations*—thoughts and ideas about what becoming a parent might involve. These imaginings, I find, can have very different effects. For some, the detail they uncover provides an impetus for ever more conscientious planning for parenthood. For others, the realized complexity of family making pushes the prospect of becoming a parent further away. A question remains about the extent to which the complicated nature of queer parenthood ultimately deters people from having children altogether. Whether or not it does, I argue, reproduction becoming more "imaginable" does not necessarily make it more likely to happen.

Researching Reproductive Imaginations

Social science research on lesbian mothers and gay fathers, as in the sociology and anthropology of reproduction more broadly, has traditionally centered on the "lived experience" of parenthood or the attempts to achieve it. Multiple studies document the everyday lives of families headed by two mothers, two fathers, and other parental alternatives to the straight-couple norm, shedding light, among other things, on how men and women navigate the complex realms of adoption and assisted reproduction in order to reach the goal of having children (e.g., Craven 2019; Gamson 2015; Hicks 2011; Lewin 2009; Ryan-Flood 2009). Undoubtedly, it is attending to the lived experience, with ethnographic precision and rich detail, that has allowed sociological and anthropological research on nonheterosexual reproduction to flourish, adding another perspective to primarily quantitative studies of lesbian mothers and gay fathers in psychology—not dissimilar to the way qualitative research on fertility and infertility has accompanied number-driven understandings of reproduction offered by demography.

Yet, as Carol Smart argues, scholars studying personal life "need to explore those families and relationships which exist in our imaginings" (Smart 2007: 4), not only those whose empirical reality is more easily perceptible. According to the late historian John Gillis (1997), over the past two hundred years, the meaning of family has expanded from a group of people one "lives with" in the here and now to an imagined entity one "lives by" through either a remembered past or an envisaged future. Arousing culturally constructed nostalgia and longings, the families we live by are anticipatory as well as memorial, as both the past and the future are increasingly drawn to the present. Just as most of the time we spend on family gatherings is in anticipation and remembering rather than in the actual current moment, so too should scholars pay more attention to how families are imagined. Here, I focus on one temporal dimension of family imaginings: the future.

All this is not to say that researchers of queer parenthood have not taken note of the imagination, or anticipation. Studies of lesbian mothers and gay fathers consider how people envisage their future families. For example, research on donor conception among lesbian couples asks questions about various aspects of family life that capture prospective parents' imagination: what kind of role sperm donors will play in the life they help to conceive (Dempsey 2010), what being conceived with sperm from different donors might mean for relationships between siblings (Nordqvist 2014), or what kind of "family story" donor-conceived children should be told (Donovan and Wilson 2008). Researchers have considered how same-sex couples imagine what it would be like to raise a child of a particular gender (Berkowitz and Ryan 2011; Goldberg 2009), while studies of gay fatherhood highlight the question of whether parenthood is imaginable at all for gay men (Goodfellow 2015; Murphy 2013; Smietana 2018).

Attending to the imagination reveals its central role in materializing the family and its various forms. For example, research on donor conception shows that what lesbian couples originally envisage when thinking about their future family is often revisited as women's circumstances change or as an initially anticipated relationship with a known sperm donor proves too difficult to negotiate (Donovan and Wilson 2008; Nordqvist 2014). Likewise, research on surrogacy sheds light on how, for gay male couples, decisions about paternity are shaped by imagined relationships with extended family members (Dempsey 2013). In the social studies of reproduction more broadly, focusing on the imagination provokes important questions about what it means to have "a child in mind" (Sandelowski 1993). For instance, Han (2013) and Roberts, Griffiths, and Verran (2017), in their studies of pregnant women's engagement with fetal ultrasound images, ask if sonograms replace the imagined fetus or act as prompts to imagining the new baby. Writing in the context of egg donation, Hudson (2020) observes that the use of assisted reproductive technologies involves a great deal of imaginative work as their users play out a range of possible future scenarios.

Research on parents and intended parents includes many insights about how people imagine their reproductive futures, even if these perspectives are often based on retrospective accounts. However, when studies of reproduction attend to the imagination, they tend to focus on children and families as imagined entities—as products or outcomes of whatever people go through when they become parents, whether it involves conception, pregnancy, adoption, surrogacy, gamete donation, or some combination thereof. What stood out to me instead, as I interviewed lesbians, gay men, and bisexual people without children, and with little to no experience of or knowledge about family making, is how the process of becoming a parent has the potential to capture people's imagination.

From the Outcome to the Process

> I like the idea of having kids, I like the idea of raising kids, I like the idea of having a family. . . . I think that's a very important aspect of how I

see happiness. But, what I have more mixed feelings about is the specific ways in which you can get kids as a gay man in this society. And I guess I didn't think about that process so much before, and now I think about that process. 'Cause now I think, hey, let's say in two years I decide to have kids—how am I going to go about doing it? And it doesn't seem that pleasant. (Louis, twenty-four-year-old gay man)

This quotation from my interview with Louis captures the disjuncture between the outcome and the process of becoming a parent—a discrepancy that underlines the importance of the "how question." The mixed feelings about specific ways of having children that Louis mentions were common among interviewees, especially if they had not yet decided whether they would ever try to pursue parenthood. While some expressed uncertainties and worries about various aspects of *being* a parent—such as caring for a child, protecting one's family from homophobia, changing one's lifestyle, or having the financial resources to raise children—many were unsure about parenthood primarily because of what *becoming* a parent would involve.

For Louis, the mental picture of a happy family contrasted starkly with the "unpleasant" vision of what was required to create this family in the first place. Pondering the possibilities of adoption and surrogacy, he continued further in our interview: "I don't know how I feel about the various methods that are available to us. And I'm more uncertain about those than I used to be, weirdly enough, even though the legal framework is now better than it was before." Explaining how his attitude toward having children had changed over time, Louis drew attention to a curious paradox: despite the fact that changes in law had clarified various family-making trajectories, so that queer families were no longer left in a legal vacuum, these changes had not necessarily made it easier for people like Louis to consider becoming a parent. The legal framework surrounding gay fatherhood may have become more defined and transparent, but the pathways to parenthood appear opaque—possibly, in part, because a greater awareness of them revealed their various complexities.

As I describe elsewhere (Pralat 2018), for lesbian, gay, and bisexual people, thinking about different ways of becoming a parent is often accompanied by moral discomfort, whichever means of creating a family is considered—whether it is adoption, surrogacy, donor conception, or friendship-based coparenting. This is the case because no single route to parenthood is evidently most "ethical." The available options can feel both "right" and "wrong," rendering the consideration of parenthood in its various forms an inherently ambivalent exercise. The ethically complex territory of pathways to parenthood contrasts with the seemingly ethically straightforward destination of having a family. Interviewees did voice some concerns about whether one would be a "good" parent or whether it would be "fair" to bring children into being, considering various forms of adversity they could face. But these concerns seemed secondary to the unease evoked by navigating the imagined trajectories for family making.

At times, the conceptual and procedural complexity of different methods of becoming a parent was sufficient to exclude them from the list of possibilities, simply because of being "too complicated." This was the case even for those who unquestionably wanted to have children in the future. Katie, a thirty-one-year-old lesbian who, along with her civil partner, was hoping to become a mother through donor insemination using sperm from a friend, felt uncomfortable with the envisaged over-reliance on clinical assistance in pursuing her parenting desire:

> KATIE: It just seems silly, when there's so many children that need homes, that some people go to such drastic medical extremes to create a new life.
>
> ROBERT: For example?
>
> KATIE: For example, um, women that spend six months injecting themselves with hormones and then . . . have—I think it's called inner-uterine . . . I can't remember—IUI, where they actually insert the sperm right into your uterus. Or test-tube babies where, you know, they create . . . gosh, I should know this terminology, shouldn't I? [laughs]—where they actually start the process with the fetus growing outside of the body and then insert it in. It just seems like a whole lot of trouble.

It is telling that Katie, somewhat apologetically, struggles to describe methods of assisted reproduction, which she seems to know enough about to reject them as potential options for having children.

The technicality of intrauterine insemination (IUI) or IVF (the latter being alluded to as "test-tube babies") makes these methods of achieving pregnancy seem like "drastic medical extremes" and "a whole lot of trouble." Clinically assisted reproduction may have become to a large extent normalized, as many chapters in this book demonstrate. But the medicalized process of conception does not sit easily with many of those whom it is intended to benefit, including lesbians who are reliant on some form of assistance anyway, even when they attempt to become parents without entering a clinic. This is exacerbated by the awareness of the "many children that need homes," which makes the use of medical interventions such as IVF seem somewhat unjustified.

The lack of fluency in talking about assisted reproduction, evident in Katie's effort to recall correct terminology, was common in my interviews. Even relatively nontechnical terms such as "surrogacy" did not seem to be part of everyday vocabulary. "I think to some extent girls, lesbian couples, have it easier than gay male couples in that you only need a sperm donor," said Gemma, a bisexual woman aged twenty-seven. "I think that's a much smaller ask than . . . I've forgotten the word—a much smaller ask than a tummy mummy." Beyond the interview context, it seemed much easier for people to talk about future children than about the ways of bringing the notional offspring into being. Interviewees were reluctant to discuss this with their own parents, possibly because the process is a temporal equivalent of having sex—a private act unlikely to be discussed openly with one's mother or father (Pralat 2016). The mechanics of assisted reproduction were uncomfortable to talk about not only between generations; it felt awkward to discuss them with straight peers, too (Pralat 2021). But just as detailed answers to the "how question" were best avoided in conversations with others, they also seemed easiest to ignore when thinking about the future—unless one was already committed to pursuing parenthood in a particular way.

Navigating Disorienting Imaginations

At the time [when I came out], I was kind of like . . . I do want to have a child of my own, I want to be pregnant and experience that—I guess that's . . . a woman thing, I don't know. But there's several ways of doing that. And obviously when there's two women in the relationship, are you both going to do that? Do you adopt? And if you don't adopt, if you do go down the insemination route, do you use a friend or a donor? How much does that matter? Yeah, quite a lot. And if it is a friend, then you'd have to involve the friend—how much? Then there's also the grandparents, so the parents of your friend that you've used, and the fact that they have a grandchild. And you gotta think about all these things! (Becky, twenty-five-year-old lesbian)

My interlocutors understood the possible pathways to parenthood to varying degrees. Those in relationships with partners who explicitly shared their parenting desires were likely to have considered different possibilities in greater detail. These interviewees' narratives indicate that answering the "how question" does not necessarily provide closure. Instead, it usually provokes a cascade of further, more specific questions, as shown by the extract from my interview with Becky, who recounted how her coming out as lesbian had affected the way she thought about future family life.

Becky's account sheds light on further questions that are likely to play a role in considering different ways of becoming a parent. Her narrative highlights the importance of being prepared for parenthood—something interviewees were universally aware of—but it also shows that there are no straightforward steps to follow in order to ensure that every decision made while creating a family is truly well informed and thought through. Although Becky had evidently considered these questions before, her listing of unknowns demonstrates that reproductive decision making in same-sex intimacy is not a progressive accumulation of satisfying responses requiring only further clarification; it is a constant vacillation. In other words, reproductive decision making is not only linear; it is also circular. Elsewhere in our interview, Becky admitted that she and her partner "feel a bit at sea" and that "it all feels like shrouded in fog." Her use of spatial imagery in describing what went through her mind reflected a profound feeling of disorientation.

Aligning same-sex desire with a desire to have a child can feel disorienting (Pralat 2021). For lesbians and gay men who entered adulthood at a time when queer parenthood had only just achieved (significant but still partial) socio-legal recognition, this feeling of disorientation results partly from a lack of clarity about one's life course: it may now be accepted for me to have a child, but am I actually expected to do that? Even though nonheterosexual reproduction has become more thinkable and "talkable," there are no established cultural scripts to follow when one wishes to have a child. This dearth becomes especially evident when an imagined method of creating a family relies on people other than intimate partners.

The inevitable need to negotiate relationships with "third" or "extra" parties was what many interviewees perceived as the biggest obstacle in becoming a parent. Some mentioned adoption agencies whose involvement in a couple's private life is an unavoidable part of pursuing adoptive parenthood. The prospect of being assessed on one's parenting capability—and a general awareness of this assessment as lengthy, intrusive, and undermining—did not encourage the pursuit of adoption. Even when interviewees were aware that discriminatory practices were illegal, some worried that their sexual orientation would be "an issue" for adoption workers. But it was the reliance on other people required to create a family based on biogenetic relatedness that men and, to a lesser extent, women referred to most often. Consider the following quotation from Stephen, a twenty-nine-year-old gay man in a relationship for two years: "I mean . . . that end of things [having a biological child], from a kind of—as an implementation problem, as it were [laughs]—is a bit of a nightmare. The whole . . . sort of fertility technology process of actually having a genetically related child as a nonheterosexual person is quite messy. I mean, you need to get the other half from somewhere and that's a negotiative nightmare. I can imagine just a whole world of very odd complexity there."

Stephen's account highlights how the idea of creating a biogenetic family is rife with potential complications. His framing of biological parenthood as an "implementation problem" suggests that creating relatedness is to some extent about logistics. But with no clear instructions to follow, "getting the other half from somewhere" can be "messy" and, indeed, terrifying—it can become a "negotiative nightmare." What seems to capture Stephen's imagination in the first place—and facilitate envisaging potential complications—also appears to inhibit imagining in greater detail. Unlike Becky, who was already invested in creating a family with her partner and seemed willing to engage in forecasting the complexity of donor conception, Stephen, without a similar commitment to parenthood and reliant on greater "assistance," appeared reluctant to proceed.

Amid the complicated mechanics of creating a new life (or bringing an existing life into one's world, as is the case in adoption), what appears most complex about navigating routes to parenthood is the awareness that any family-making project ultimately requires the involvement of an extra party. As Chris, a gay man aged twenty-eight, commented, "I think it's more straightforward for lesbian couples because one of them will typically be the incubator—not to try and make it sound too medicalized, but . . . yeah, having that extra party involved, really . . . murky waters for me." The unease about involvement of a third party can be explained by the centrality of the couple in people's thinking about parenthood—and it is a feeling that is highly gendered. Chris, like Gemma, quoted earlier, noted how it was generally easier for women than it was for men to have children "biologically." Lesbians, it seems, may find it easier than gay men to imagine having a biological child because for most female same-sex couples the process of reproduction takes place largely within the intimate bodily boundaries of two partners. For gay men, conception, gestation, and childbirth all need to occur outside of the couple's intimacy. Thus, although neither lesbian nor gay male couples can reproduce through sex, men need to depart more substantially from the norm of two individuals producing offspring through making love (Pralat 2020). This has implications for how people imagine their reproductive futures and how capable they are of incorporating the processual complexity of parenthood with more outcome-oriented visions of a future family.

Becoming More Imaginable

As shown in this chapter, for many lesbian, gay, and bisexual people, the question about whether they want to have children (yes or no?), when affirmed, instantly brings up the question about the means of creating a family (if yes, then how?). This is likely to prompt further questions about specific pathways to parenthood, which may, in turn, lead to revisiting the original question about parenting desire. The questioning seems both linear and circular: one question follows another, but answers to subsequent questions may require rethinking questions answered previously. The "how question" has cascading effects and, as the subsequent questions multiply, they turn the attention to the reproductive outcome (having children) or the reproductive process (becoming parents). When the object of the imagination shifts from the future family to the means of its creation, the unfolding intricacy leaves many with feelings of ambivalence and discomfort.

In a sense, what the narratives of imagining the possibility of having children reveal is not new. The cumulative complexity mirrors what we already know from studies of lesbian mothers and gay fathers recalling their rarely straightforward reproductive decision making. Accounts of queer parents reflect the multiplicity of considerations involved in the process of creating a family as a same-sex couple: be it deciding whether to adopt or use assisted reproduction (Goldberg, Downing, and Richardson 2009; Jennings et al. 2014); which female partner would carry the child (Geerts and Evertsson 2023; Hayman et al. 2015); which male partner would be the biological father (Dempsey 2013; Fantus and Newman 2019); whether to pursue clinical or self-arranged insemination (Mamo 2007; Nordqvist 2014); whether to pursue genetic or gestational surrogacy (Blake et al. 2017; Murphy 2013); whether to choose a known or an unknown sperm donor (Ryan-Flood 2009; Donovan and Wilson 2008); or whether to embrace or reject "racial matching" (Keaney 2021; Newman 2019). As existing research shows, the relative importance of various considerations depends on a variety of cultural, personal, relational, and socioeconomic circumstances.

Queer people pondering the prospect of becoming parents also echo to some extent the narratives of heterosexual couples undergoing infertility treatment. The spatial aspects of envisaging parenthood seem significant here. Having to navigate "murky waters" and feeling "at sea" or "shrouded in fog" (as observed by Chris and Becky) is not dissimilar to the obstacles (Franklin 1997) and disruptions (Becker 2000) facing straight people as they go through IVF. Reproductive decision making in same-sex intimacy feels disorienting, but these feelings need not be unique to the nonheterosexual experience. It seems that the awareness of the necessity for reproduction to take place outside of the intimacy of a loving couple is as significant as, if not more important than, nonnormative sexual orientation. As Sasha Roseneil and colleagues observe in multiple locations across Europe, the procreative norm is more tightly bound up with the couple norm than it is with the "hetero-norm" (Rose-neil et al. 2020). The validation of couple-based queer parenthood in countries such as Britain appears to confirm it.

What is it, then, that the perspectives of those who are not parents but who may consider parenthood in the future add to our understanding of reproduction, fertility, and infertility? I argue that by shedding light on reproductive imaginations grounded in limited knowledge about family making and varying levels of commitment to having children, these perspectives decenter the wholehearted dedication to parenthood that so often dominates the narratives of people who have "achieved" it (or are attempting to do so) in the context of obstruction, struggle, and effort. This decentering accommodates and illuminates instead mixed feelings about having children and the contingent nature of parenting desire.

Ambivalent responses to the "how question" illustrate why, despite socio-legal and medical advances, many lesbians, gay men, and bisexual people may not become parents after all. Reproductive imaginations that focus on process rather than outcome suggest that, even if families headed by lesbian mothers and gay fathers are now more imaginable (thanks to the greater awareness of the multiple ways to make a family), nonheterosexual parenthood will not necessarily become more prevalent. As Judith Stacey (2006) has argued, writing about gay men and fatherhood in the United States, the paradoxical consequences of the shift from closeted to open homosexuality are a concurrent rise in the visibility and legitimacy of gay paternity and a decline in its incidence. This is the case because the rising numbers of gay men pursuing fatherhood through adoption or assisted reproduction (as openly gay) are unlikely to compensate for the decreasing numbers of gay men becoming parents with female partners (while in the closet). It is difficult to determine how exactly the increase in societal acceptance of same-sex intimacy impacts the fertility of the general population. The rise in "intentional" queer parenthood is evident, as demonstrated, at least in the United Kingdom, by growing numbers of children adopted by same-sex couples, of women accessing fertility clinics with female partners, and of men applying for parental orders for surrogacy. But there is also consistent evidence, within a variety of national contexts, that lesbians as well as gay men are less likely to want to have children than their heterosexual counterparts (Baiocco and Laghi 2013; Kranz, Busch, and Niepel 2018; Leal, Gato, and Tasker 2019; Riskind and Tornello 2017). It may be that the complexity of becoming a parent as lesbian or gay acts as an important counterforce to parenting desire, otherwise facilitated by greater visibility and acceptance of queer-parent families. Having children outside heterosexuality has become more conceivable, but so have the intricacies of the family-making process.

Conclusion

I have aimed to show in this chapter that, prior to their material existence, families must be imagined, especially when their creation necessitates conscious decisions. However, there are different kinds of reproductive imaginations, and what exactly is imagined impacts how one feels about family making. If barriers to parenthood prove more effective at capturing the imagination than the appeal of having children, the imaginability of a future family may not be sufficient to facilitate its creation. This may be especially true for lesbians and gay men in Britain, where options to become parents for same-sex couples opened up and multiplied remarkably quickly in the 2000s. On one hand, public awareness that having children as lesbian or gay is possible has expanded. On the other, there has been little time for the development, within queer communities and beyond, of cultural literacy around what exactly various pathways to parenthood involve. The unease of envisaging the reproductive process, and how it contrasts with the comfort of imagining a future family as an outcome, may be less pronounced in other national contexts—such as my country of origin, where the unavailability of options to pursue parenthood as a same-sex couple limits the imaginability of queer family making (see Mizielińska 2022). At the same time, as the idea of nonheterosexual parenthood becomes more familiar, the ambivalence it evokes also resembles the mixed feelings about having children experienced by others. This includes straight people for whom parenting intention is increasingly called into question, whether due to concerns about austerity (Hall 2023), fears of the climate crisis (Dow 2016), or anxieties around reproductive uncertainties (Faircloth and Gürtin 2018). Paying greater attention to the way men and women envisage having children in the future, especially prior to their commitment to do so, reveals the important role that imagining can play in shaping fertility trends in the new reproductive order.

REFERENCES

Baiocco, Roberto, and Fiorenzo Laghi. 2013. "Sexual Orientation and the Desires and Intentions to Become Parents." *Journal of Family Studies* 19(1): 90–98.

Becker, Gaylene. 2000. *The Elusive Embryo: How Women and Men Approach the New Reproductive Technologies.* Berkeley: University of California Press.

Berkowitz, Dana, and Maura Ryan. 2011. "Bathrooms, Baseball, and Bra Shopping: Lesbian and Gay Parents Talk about Engendering Their Children." *Sociological Perspectives* 54(3): 329–50.

Blake, L., N. Carone, E. Raffanello, J. Slutsky, A. A. Ehrhardt, and S. Golombok. 2017. "Gay Fathers' Motivations for and Feelings about Surrogacy as a Path to Parenthood." *Human Reproduction* 32(4): 860–67.

Craven, Christa. 2019. *Reproductive Losses: Challenges to LGBTQ Family-Making.* New York: Routledge.

Dempsey, Deborah. 2010. "Conceiving and Negotiating Reproductive Relationships: Lesbians and Gay Men Forming Families with Children." *Sociology* 44(6): 1145–62.

———. 2013. "Surrogacy, Gay Male Couples, and the Significance of Biogenetic Paternity." *New Genetics and Society* 32(1): 37–53.

Donovan, Catherine, and Angelia R. Wilson. 2008. "Imagination and Integrity: Decision-Making among Lesbian Couples to Use Medically Provided Donor Insemination." *Culture, Health & Sexuality* 10(7): 649–65.

Dow, Katharine. 2016. *Making a Good Life: An Ethnography of Nature, Ethics, and Reproduction.* Princeton, NJ: Princeton University Press.

Faircloth, Charlotte, and Zeynep B. Gürtin. 2018. "Fertile Connections: Thinking across Assisted Reproductive Technologies and Parenting Culture Studies." *Sociology* 52(5): 983–1000.

Fantus, Sophia, and Peter A. Newman. 2019. "Motivations to Pursue Surrogacy for Gay Fathers in Canada: A Qualitative Investigation." *Journal of GLBT Family Studies* 15(4): 342–56.

Franklin, Sarah. 1997. *Embodied Progress: A Cultural Account of Assisted Conception.* London: Routledge.

Gamson, Joshua. 2015. *Modern Families: Stories of Extraordinary Journeys to Kinship.* New York: New York University Press.

Geerts, Allison, and Marie Evertsson. 2023. "Who Carries the Baby? How Lesbian Couples in the Netherlands Choose Birth Motherhood." *Family Relations* 72(1): 176–94.

Gillis, John. 1997. *A World of Their Own Making: Myth, Ritual, and the Quest for Family Values.* Cambridge, MA: Harvard University Press.

Goldberg, Abbie E. 2009. "Heterosexual, Lesbian, and Gay Preadoptive Parents' Preferences about Child Gender." *Sex Roles* 61(1–2): 55–71.

Goldberg, Abbie E., Jordan B. Downing, and Hannah B. Richardson. 2009. "The Transition from Infertility to Adoption: Perceptions of Lesbian and Heterosexual Couples." *Journal of Social and Personal Relationships* 26(6–7): 938–63.

Goodfellow, Aaron. 2015. *Gay Fathers, Their Children, and the Making of Kinship*. New York: Fordham University Press.

Hall, Sarah Marie. 2023. "A Pregnant Pause? Reproduction, Waiting, and Silences in the Relational Endurance of Austerity." *Geoforum* 142: 103755.

Han, Sallie. 2013. *Pregnancy in Practice: Expectation and Experience in the Contemporary US*. New York: Berghahn.

Hayman, Brenda, Leslie Wilkes, Elizabeth Halcomb, and Debra Jackson. 2015. "Lesbian Women Choosing Motherhood: The Journey to Conception." *Journal of GLBT Family Studies* 11(4): 395–409.

Hicks, Stephen. 2011. *Lesbian, Gay, and Queer Parenting: Families, Intimacies, Genealogies*. London: Palgrave Macmillan.

Hudson, Nicky. 2020. "Egg Donation Imaginaries: Embodiment, Ethics, and Future Family Formation." *Sociology* 54(2): 346–62.

Jennings, Sarah, Laura Mellish, Fiona Tasker, Michael Lamb, and Susan Golombok. 2014. "Why Adoption? Gay, Lesbian, and Heterosexual Adoptive Parents' Reproductive Experiences and Reasons for Adoption." *Adoption Quarterly* 17(3): 205–26.

Keaney, Jaya. 2021. "The Color of Kinship: Race, Biology, and Queer Reproduction." In *Long Term: Essays on Queer Commitment*, ed. Scott Herring and Lee Wallace, 175–98. Durham, NC: Duke University Press.

Kranz, Dirk, Holger Busch, and Christoph Niepel. 2018. "Desires and Intentions for Fatherhood: A Comparison of Childless Gay and Heterosexual Men in Germany." *Journal of Family Psychology* 32(8): 995–1004.

Leal, Daniela, Jorge Gato, and Fiona Tasker. 2019. "Prospective Parenting: Sexual Identity and Intercultural Trajectories." *Culture, Health & Sexuality* 21(7): 757–73.

Lewin, Ellen. 2009. *Gay Fatherhood: Narratives of Family and Citizenship in America*. Chicago: University of Chicago Press.

Mamo, Laura. 2007. *Queering Reproduction: Achieving Pregnancy in the Age of Technoscience*. Durham, NC: Duke University Press.

Mizielińska, Joanna. 2022. *Queer Kinship on the Edge? Families of Choice in Poland*. London: Routledge.

Murphy, Dean A. 2013. "The Desire for Parenthood: Gay Men Choosing to Become Parents through Surrogacy." *Journal of Family Issues* 34(8): 1104–24.

Newman, Alyssa M. 2019. "Mixing and Matching: Sperm Donor Selection for Interracial Lesbian Couples." *Medical Anthropology* 38(8): 710–24.

Nordqvist, Petra. 2014. "Bringing Kinship into Being: Connectedness, Donor Conception, and Lesbian Parenthood." *Sociology* 48(2): 268–83.

Pralat, Robert. 2016. "Between Future Families and Families of Origin: Talking about Gay Parenthood across Generations." In *Parenthood between Generations: Transforming Reproductive Cultures*, ed. Siân Pooley and Kaveri Qureshi, 43–64. New York: Berghahn.

———. 2018. "More Natural Does Not Equal More Normal: Lesbian, Gay, and Bisexual People's Views about Different Pathways to Parenthood." *Journal of Family Issues* 39(18): 4179–4203.

———. 2020. "Parenthood as Intended: Reproductive Responsibility, Moral Judgements, and Having Children 'by Accident.'" *Sociological Review* 68(1): 161–76.

———. 2021. "Sexual Identities and Reproductive Orientations: Coming Out as Wanting (or Not Wanting) to Have Children." *Sexualities* 24(1–2): 276–94.

Riskind, Rachel G., and Samantha L. Tornello. 2017. "Sexual Orientation and Future Parenthood in a 2011–2013 Nationally Representative United States Sample." *Journal of Family Psychology* 31(6): 792–98.

Roberts, Julie, Frances Griffiths, and Alice Verran. 2017. "Seeing the Baby, Doing Family: Commercial Ultrasound as Family Practice." *Sociology* 51(3): 527–42.

Roseneil, Sasha, Isabel Crowhurst, Tone Hellesund, Ana Cristina Santos, and Mariya Stoilova. 2020. *The Tenacity of the Couple-Norm: Intimate Citizenship Regimes in a Changing Europe*. London: UCL Press.

Ryan-Flood, Róisín. 2009. *Lesbian Motherhood: Gender, Families, and Sexual Citizenship*. London: Palgrave Macmillan.

Sandelowski, Margarete. 1993. *With Child in Mind: Studies of the Personal Encounter with Infertility*. Philadelphia: University of Pennsylvania Press.

Smart, Carol. 2007. *Personal Life: New Directions in Sociological Thinking*. London: Polity.

Smietana, Marcin. 2018. "Procreative Consciousness in a Global Market: Gay Men's Paths to Surrogacy in the US." *Reproductive BioMedicine and Society Online* 7: 101–11.

Stacey, Judith. 2006. "Gay Parenthood and the Decline of Paternity as We Knew It." *Sexualities* 9(1): 27–55.

5

Queer Calculations

Spreadsheet Fertility and British Gay Men's Reproductive Projects

MARCIN SMIETANA

This chapter introduces the concept of *spreadsheet fertility*, derived from almost two decades of research on gay-father families in the United Kingdom, Europe, and the United States (see e.g., Smietana 2017, 2019; Smietana and Twine 2022). While observing deliberate, intentional, and carefully planned strategies for family making among gay male couples, support groups, and communities, I became increasingly conscious of the central role of spreadsheets in calculating fertility costs and mapping out the various activities involved in creating babies. Particularly in the increasingly common context of baby making through surrogacy arrangements, the logistics, as well as the finances, are daunting. Initially, I used the concept of "spreadsheet fertility" to capture the complexity of the fertility journey for gay men using surrogates and also the complex labor of fertility planning and deliberation this involved. However, I quickly began to appreciate that the spreadsheet entries detailed more than financial or logistical matters. These spreadsheet entries, and the many deliberations they condensed into a single document, were also personal, philosophical, political, and intimately conjugal maps of identity, kinship, desire, and belonging. In addition to revealing the complex "fertinomics" (Franklin 2021) of family making in the current age, the spreadsheets act as condensed signifiers of an important form of fertility change, a shift toward deliberate, proactive, and calculated approaches to achieving desired fertility goals, characterized by Sarah Franklin (2022 [1997]) as "iFertility." Initially a descriptive and handy summary of gay-father family making, spreadsheet fertility gradually came to acquire even more significance in the context of the Changing (In)Fertilities Project (Franklin and Inhorn 2018; see also Franklin and

Inhorn, Introduction), which depicted many examples of complex fertility planning, calculation, and almost artisanal crafting of families.

When I first began my research on gay-father families in 2005, it was widely assumed that one of the most important distinctive features of the gay male couple was the inability to have a baby without assistance—be it through adoption, informal coparenting arrangements with lesbian couples, surrogacy, or the formation of blended and stepfamilies. Today, the situation of needing to use a spreadsheet to plan one's baby increasingly characterizes many heterosexual couples and singles as well, and might even be described as a new norm of the "IVF era" (Franklin and Inhorn 2018).

If so, could it even be claimed that the IVF-ification of fertility (Franklin 2022 [1997]), defined by a new reproductive order in which fertility is less taken for granted by an increasing number of people, even young, presumed-to-be-fertile, straight cis couples and women (Inhorn 2023), has made fertility queerer? This argument would follow Franklin's (2014) observation that the meaning of biology has changed; it has increasingly become malleable, relative, and "queer."

Although this chapter does not answer this provocative question definitively, it does suggest that "spreadsheet fertility" is a concept we can use to explore how changing perceptions of fertility are changing the fertility behaviors, intentions, and actions of both gay and straight would-be parents in ways that are strikingly similar. It is a concept that helps us map the increasingly not-just-gay awareness that fertility needs to be managed, pushed, and driven to be realized. Fertility in this view, and in the new reproductive order this volume attempts to characterize, is not just a natural biological given, an almost automatic assumption, or simply a biological fact: it is instead a choice that requires deliberate and strategic planning. Indeed, the carefully calculated means of conception encountered both in the heterosexual world of in vitro fertilization (IVF) and in the gay-father surrogate family are most similar in the sense that they are at once fervently desired and strategically crafted. For babies to be brought into being in either context, fertility needs to be brought into being, and this requires an explicitly managerial mindset as well as intense and sustained determination. As one of the interviewees put it succinctly, you need to "kind of hammer it through, make it happen."

The concept of spreadsheet fertility is especially useful, too, because it illustrates, in whatever context it is used, how many nonmonetized considerations also enter the spreadsheet columns. As intended fathers calibrate the cost of a future child, they also integrate their employment, home, mortgage, surrogacy arrangements and the kinds of children they want to have. These calculations inevitably include considerations of how they will be positioned in the social system, such as the degrees of potential stigmatization they might suffer as gay-father families, and the burden this might place on their children. But they extend still further too, for example, in terms of national, racial, religious, and cultural considerations, which are, of course, also questions linked to forms of economic, racial, and social inequality.

The first part of this chapter looks at what spreadsheet fertility means where I first encountered it—in interviews with gay men who were either considering or undergoing surrogacy journeys. I focus on the latest set of qualitative interviews I conducted between 2020 and 2022 with thirty families of gay men created through surrogacy in the United Kingdom or overseas. Of the thirty families, twenty-eight were couples and two were singles. The men, aged twenty-four to fifty-two, were in the process of surrogacy or had young children. They were UK residents with twenty-two different national identifications. Twenty-three families identified as White, and seven were multiethnic couples, where one partner identified as Latin American, Filipino, South Asian, British South Asian, Black British Caribbean, Ghanaian, or British Nigerian. Most were university-educated professionals. In this chapter, all interviewees' names are pseudonyms. The second part of the chapter then turns to wider questions of changing in-fertilities—that is, changing reproductive perceptions and behaviors—and the meaning of spreadsheet fertility for the new reproductive order.

A Gay Couple and Straight Surrogacy

"We'd been together for six, seven years, we were both in good jobs, and we were saving with a view to having a child," said Harvey in answer to my question about how he was able to cover surrogacy expenses. Indeed, Harvey and his husband, Oliver, needed almost £13,000 (approximately $16,400) to pay for their surrogacy arrangement in the United Kingdom.

With their annual household income situated in the bracket of £30,000–50,000 ($37,700–62,900), this required careful planning. Indeed, their income—just above the annual UK average of £32,300 ($40,640) in 2022 (Office for National Statistics 2022)—was one of the lowest among the families interviewed in this study. Harvey ran a food tour company and Oliver was a medical doctor, and they were both thirty-two years old at the time of their first surrogacy arrangement. They met in 2005, entered a civil union in 2006, and got married in 2013. From the start of their relationship, they both wanted children. They began networking via the group Surrogacy UK, one of the main surrogacy organizations in the United Kingdom (Department of Health & Social Care 2023). They were introduced to their surrogate, Debbie, via another surrogate. After they developed a friendly relationship with Debbie and her children, which involved traveling across the country to see and get to know each other, she offered to be their surrogate, ultimately giving birth to their two children. Harvey was father to their first child, using at-home artificial insemination, while Oliver became father to their second child with the help of a fertility clinic. At the time of the interview, their son was seven years old, and their daughter was three.

In both cases, Harvey and Oliver opted for "traditional surrogacy," which in the United Kingdom is commonly called "straight surrogacy," with Debbie acting as both egg donor and surrogate. Their surrogacy arrangement was also altruistic, given that in the United Kingdom only "altruistic surrogacy" is legal, whereby the surrogate can be reimbursed for related expenses but cannot receive additional compensation. Among the thirty families in this study, eight pursued traditional surrogacy, just like Harvey and Oliver. The remaining twenty-two families used "gestational surrogacy," which involves two women: one as an egg donor and the other as a surrogate. Among those twenty-two families, fourteen carried out their gestational surrogacy arrangements in the United Kingdom, and eight traveled overseas to the United States and Canada.

Those who went for surrogacy abroad paid for it on a commercial basis, whereas surrogacy arrangements in the United Kingdom were altruistic. However, the "altruistic" nature refers to the surrogate's labor, but not to egg donation and IVF. In the United Kingdom, commercial fertility clinics exist alongside the public healthcare system, the National Health Service (NHS), thus forming a hybrid public-private healthcare system (Hamper and Perrotta 2023). Egg donation and IVF are provided within the NHS based on a medical definition of infertility, which does not usually apply to LGBTQ+ intended parents. For this reason, all fourteen families in this study that pursued gestational surrogacy in the United Kingdom used a hybrid model: while they dealt with surrogates on the altruistic basis, they resorted to private commercial clinics for egg donation and IVF. This raised their surrogacy costs up to as much as four times higher than the initial sum of £13,000 (approximately $16,400) that Harvey and Oliver paid for their traditional surrogacy arrangement.

Harvey and Oliver's surrogacy expenses were itemized on a spreadsheet (see figure 5.1), not only because it was required for the final transfer of parentage. The spreadsheet was also helpful for Harvey and Oliver to plan for the expenses they needed to incur to become parents. During our research interview, Harvey commented on the expenses included in the spreadsheet: "Things like maternity clothes, or compensation for lost earnings if Debbie was at home or indeed in hospital for a number of weeks. . . . Twenty pounds [twenty-five dollars] to be able to buy a takeaway pizza at the end of the pregnancy because she was too tired to cook for her kids, a taxi . . . You know, genuine things that were taking place as a direct result of being pregnant with our child."

What is more, the expenses itemized on Harvey and Oliver's spreadsheet had to be synchronized in time. Initial surrogacy meet-ups and socials were organized all around the United Kingdom, and it was there that the men could meet potential surrogates. This often involved "two train tickets at full price, often at short notice," which "over the course of many months, ran into several hundred, if not a couple of thousand pounds," as Harvey explained. However, travel expenses had to be carefully synchronized in time, in particular at a later stage, when, in Surrogacy UK's language, "the team" (that is, the intended parents and the surrogate) were doing "insems" (that is, home inseminations). This involved, as Harvey explained, "having to respond at short notice to Debbie saying 'I'm ovulating, you need to get up here within the next forty-eight hours to produce three samples over three days!' And then the cost associated with traveling up there."

Type of Expense	Amount	No of Weeks	Total Amount
Vitamins	40	5	200
Extra food + healthy options	30	40	1200
Convenience food (sickness)	40	40	1600
Loss of earnings (months 1-7) 9 days	100	40	300
Loss of earnings (months 8-11) 30 days	100	40	1000
Maternity clothes (approx 16 items)	800		800
Interim clothing (after birth)	200		200
Pregnancy underwear	60		60
Holiday after birth	1000		1000
Hospital kit	80		80
Chiropractor	10	40	400
Hospital parking	5	8	40
After pregnancy toiletries	40		40
Physio (months 8-11)	30	10	300
Childcare 2 days per month months 1-10	100	10	1000
Childcare after birth 2 weeks	250	2	500
Taxi (for school) 2 days per month - months 1-10	30	20	600
Taxi (for school) after birth 2 weeks	30	10	300
Surrogate's husband's loss of earnings (2 days)	240		240
Mileage to midwife x 10 appointments	48		48
Mileage to hospital x 8 appointments	40		40
Get togethers 4 x hotel	200		200
Get togethers 4 x 150 mileage	240		240
Get togethers 4 x food and incidentals	400		400
Help with cleaning 5 hrs per week for 12 weeks	35	12	420
Personal appointments at end of pregnancy	30	6	180
Activities with children 2 per month	50	20	1000
Help with ironing for 8 weeks	30	8	240
Swimmng	5	40	200
Aqua natal	6	20	120
Total not including unforeseen items			12948

Figure 5.1. Harvey and Oliver's Surrogacy Expense Spreadsheet: Altruistic and Traditional ("Straight") Surrogacy in the United Kingdom (Arrangement 1)

Yet Harvey and Oliver's surrogacy planning also included nonmonetized calculations, some of which were taken for granted and thus not listed explicitly on the spreadsheet. They involved physical resemblance between Harvey's male partner (Oliver) and the woman who donated her eggs. As also shown by other interviews in this study (see Smietana and Twine 2022), physical resemblance was racialized, given that the egg donors the men picked usually resembled the nongenetic father in racialized terms. This kind of resemblance was prioritized by the men not only as an expression of kinship they sought to establish with the children but also as a means to counter potential questions or stigmatization from people around them. Most of the men sought egg donors who would, in their view, help them produce children who would resemble both fathers' skin color, regardless of how they identified. Following this logic, Harvey and Oliver desired a White European egg donor, as they both identified as White European. This process of "strategic racialization" (Smietana and Twine 2022) characterized almost all of the thirty interviewed families: regardless of their racial identification, the intended fathers sought to match the egg donor's skin color to their own. Harvey noted,

> I actually really wanted our child to have a genetic link to my partner. You know, I think, for me, when you're attracted to someone, you're attracted to all aspects of that person, their personality, their skills, their interests, but also, you know, how they look and how they move. And so, for me, it feels quite natural to want to take elements of someone that you are in love with, and have that come through your child, and again, that can come through in a myriad of ways, not just physically. But for me, that physical element was something that was of interest.

With all of these criteria in mind, Harvey and Oliver also sought a friendly, interpersonal relationship with the woman who acted as a surrogate and an egg donor. When discussing his relationship with Debbie, Harvey said, "I don't even like calling her our surrogate. This is kind of a really loaded term that makes me feel like I'm using someone. And that isn't really the nature of our relationship."

Spreadsheet Fertility

Yet ticking all these boxes required a particular mindset: pursuing one's plan with clarity, determination, and skill. The use of surrogacy, and the costs involved, require a significant amount of planning. Harvey and Oliver saved for approximately seven years due to the costs involved. This achievement required determination as well as managerial and entrepreneurial skills on their part—or, in other words, spreadsheet fertility, through which fertility was created and implemented. Spreadsheet fertility is a result of perceptions and intentions. It needs to be created, organized, and moved forward. In Harvey and Oliver's first surrogacy arrangement, for example, they were able to keep the costs relatively low as they were able to pursue surrogacy on an altruistic and traditional basis. However, in their second arrangement, they needed to resort to IVF with the help of a fertility clinic, given that they were unable to

IVF Expenses		
Date	Item	Cost
11/01/2016		1095
13/01/2016	Semen analysis and test freeze	200
13/01/2016	Known donor screening package (stage 1)	1000
15/01/2016	Embryo/gamete freezing	325
15/01/2016	Embryo/gamete storage	500
27/01/2016	DNA profile and thalassaemia	400
27/01/2016	Haemoglobin electrophoris	70
16/02/2016	Post-quarantine screening (inc NAT testing)	700
01/03/2016	(Bloods (LWD6) - returning egg donors	220
07/03/2016	Thalassaemia	55
12/03/2016	Cyclogest 400mg pessary 1 Box	240
12/03/2016	Progynova 2mg (strip of 28)	24
14/03/2016	HFEA FEE (IVF/FET/surrogacy/egg donation/egg recipient)	75
14/03/2016	IVF surrogacy (using surrogate/commissioning mother eggs)	7850
30/03/2016	Embryo/gamete freezing	325
30/03/2016	Embryo/gamete storage (2 years)	500
	Total	13579

Figure 5.2. Harvey and Oliver's IVF Expense Spreadsheet: Commercial IVF in the United Kingdom (Arrangement 2)

get pregnant with home inseminations. This more than doubled the costs: in contrast to the £13,000 ($16,400) they had used for their first surrogacy arrangement, this time they needed to spend approximately £30,000 ($37,700). The IVF expenses alone amounted to almost £13,600 ($17,100) (see figure 5.2), to which another almost £11,600 ($14,600) of more standard surrogacy expenses needed to be added (see figure 5.3). The latter included visiting Debbie (the surrogate) on short notice when she was ovulating, paying for maternity clothes, compensating for Debbie's lost earnings, and paying for care for her children who were affected by the pregnancy. This expense structure reported by Harvey and Oliver was common among the men in this research. The IVF expenses (see figure 5.2) were coupled with the altruistic surrogacy expenses in the United Kingdom (see figure 5.3).

Spreadsheet fertility also reveals the impact of social class on fertility. A striking finding from this study is that none of the thirty families I talked to received any public funding for IVF during surrogacy

Surrogacy Expenses			
Type of Expense	Amount	No of Weeks	Total Amount
Vitamins	40	5	200
Extra food + healthy options	30	40	1200
Convenience food (sickness)	25	40	1000
Loss of earnings (months 1-7) 14 days	120	7	840
Loss of earnings (months 8-11) 12 days	120	6	720
Maternity clothes (approx 16 items)	800	1	800
Interim clothing (after birth)	200	1	200
Pregnancy underwear	60	1	60
Holiday after birth	1000	1	1000
Hospital kit	80	1	80
			0
Hospital parking	5	8	40
After pregnancy toiletries	40	1	40
			0
Childcare 2 days per month - months 1-10 (£50 per day)	100	10	1000
Childcare after birth 2 weeks	250	2	500
Childcare during birth	200	1	200
		10	0
			0
Mileage to midwife x 10 appointments	48	1	48
Mileage to hospital x 8 appointments	40	1	40
Get togethers 4 x hotel	200	1	200
Get togethers 4 x 150 mileage	240	1	240
Get togethers 4 x food and incidentals	400	1	400
Help with cleaning 5 hrs per week for 12 weeks	35	12	420
Personal appointments at end of pregnancy	30	6	180
Activities with children 2 per month	80	20	1600
Help with ironing for 8 weeks	30	8	240
Swimming	5	40	200
Aqua natal	6	20	120
Total not including unforeseen items			11568
Unforseen items will include the following in the event of a hospital stay - loss of earnings, childcare, taxis, hospital costs etc.			
Payment of expenses should be as follows:			
	INSTALLMENT	INSURANCE	PAYMENT
Payment 1 (upon positive pregnancy test @ 2 weeks)	1056.8	19	1075.8
Payment 2 (4 weeks later)	1056.8	19	1075.8
Payment 3 (8 weeks later)	1056.8	19	1075.8
Payment 4 (12 weeks later)	1056.8	19	1075.8
Payment 5 (16 weeks later)	1056.8	19	1075.8
Payment 6 (20 weeks later)	1056.8	19	1075.8
Payment 7 (24 weeks later)	1056.8	19	1075.8
Payment 8 (30 weeks later)	1056.8	19	1075.8
Payment 9 (34 weeks later)	1056.8	19	1075.8
Payment 10 (38 weeks later)	1056.8	19	1075.8
Payment 11 (upon birth - expenses for holiday)	1000		1000
Total			11758

Figure 5.3. Harvey and Oliver's Surrogacy Expense Spreadsheet: Altruistic and Traditional ("Straight") Surrogacy in the United Kingdom (Arrangement 2)

from the National Health Service (NHS). So far, there has been only one known case of a gay couple receiving such funding in the United Kingdom, namely, from the NHS Scotland (Laycock 2020). In contrast, heterosexual couples have a right to receive NHS funding for IVF, even if its actual application and the number of cycles (often two or three) vary depending on the area where patients live. I suggest that the difference in access to IVF funding for gay versus heterosexual couples is due to heteronormativity, as it is based on the medical definition of infertility: it is only after "trying to get pregnant through regular unprotected sex for two years" (National Health Service 2021) that women under forty years of age can be deemed medically infertile and authorized to use public IVF funding in the United Kingdom. This also excludes most lesbians from publicly funded IVF (Schorscher-Pecu 2021). Applying the medical definition of infertility as a criterion for receiving IVF funding for LGBTQ+ people can be viewed as discriminatory both in public healthcare systems such as that of the United Kingdom and in private health insurance systems such as the one in the United States. Denying IVF funding to gay people undergoing surrogacy arrangements also increases the highly intentional character of their spreadsheet fertility. In this case, fertility becomes available only to those who can afford crafting it. In other words, it is social class that determines access to parenthood.

Spiraling Spreadsheets

In the United Kingdom, fertility becomes even more exclusive for those who cannot achieve it, such as Alex and Mateo, a London-based couple in their early forties. Alex, who worked in the translation and interpreting industry, and Mateo, who was a self-employed physiotherapist, had been together for six years at the time of the interview. When I first met Alex on a Zoom video call, the couple had just had twins through surrogacy in Canada. Alex had immigrated to the United Kingdom from a European country and Mateo, from South America. At the time of the interview, they were already British citizens. Despite having citizenship, however, they did not have a right to access surrogacy in the country, due to their HIV+ status. Until May 2024, the Human Fertilization and Embryology Authority (HFEA) legally treated men providing sperm for surrogacy as sperm donors, and the latter could not be HIV positive according to the UK legislation (Department of Health & Social Care 2024; National AIDS Trust 2022). Needless to say, the couple's HIV status translated into a particularly complicated expense spreadsheet for international surrogacy in Canada, where sperm treatment techniques ensured the safety of the surrogate without the risk of HIV transmission. As Alex explained,

> We are both HIV positive. And when we researched surrogacy in the United Kingdom for a good year, we then eventually hit a brick wall. . . . After all this work and establishing connections and talking to people, and you know, reading and researching, we then eventually got this email from this medical director at one of the clinics in London, who basically said, "I'm afraid you won't be able to do surrogacy in the United Kingdom." And that was, you know, quite heart-breaking . . . and then we looked at Canada while we explored the United States again, but the United States is just, you know, a lot more expensive, it's a lot more commercialized . . . whereas in Canada, I mean, everything is so different in Canada. You know, from in terms of regulation, in terms of perception, people are so much more relaxed about HIV, you know, it was no issue finding an agency, finding a clinic, and finding a surrogate who had any issues with the HIV.

Luckily, Alex and Oliver were able to afford the £100,000 ($125,800) they needed for overseas surrogacy in Canada. (Other interviewees' total expenses for surrogacy in Canada were slightly lower, approximately £65,000, or $82,000.) Yet even with their annual household income of almost £150,000 ($188,700), the process required a lot of work and the managerial mindset characterized by spreadsheet fertility. This mindset could be seen in the expressions that Alex used to talk about his surrogacy experience: "You think about it and you *make it work*"; "I started my *research* a long time ago"; "I was the one *driving it* and *doing all the research*"; "When we started signing up with the agency and we met the surrogate etc., that's when he really *put effort in the topic*"; "It's *hard work* and the journey is a *long* journey, it's *expensive*"; "Finding an egg donor was such *a long and hard process* for us because we had these certain criteria in mind" (emphasis added). Statements of this kind were common among the interviewees.

Alongside Alex and Mateo, seven other families in this study, out of the thirty interviewed, resorted to overseas surrogacy. Apart from the HIV+ status in the case of Alex and Mateo, several other considerations convinced them to seek parenthood overseas: relatively long waiting times in the United Kingdom; social and cultural skills required for networking within the UK surrogacy community; and, perhaps most importantly, calculating risks linked to the fact that in surrogacy in the country, parental orders for intended parents are granted only after the child's birth (Law Commission 2023).[1]

Among those who sought surrogacy overseas was Paul, a Black Caribbean-British thirty-seven-year-old marketing professional, married to Federico, a forty-two-year-old White Italian real estate professional. The couple met nine years before I interviewed them and had gotten married six years earlier. They lived in London. When I met Paul for the first time in autumn 2021, they had a young son through surrogacy in the United States, and they were in the process of their second transatlantic surrogacy arrangement. Both Paul and Federico said they had always wanted to have children. They opted for international surrogacy in the United States given the legal uncertainty and long waiting times in the United Kingdom. They used an anonymous mixed-race egg donor, to reflect their own multiethnic family composition, and they took turns becoming genetic fathers. Paul emphasized the friendship they established with their surrogate, her husband, their children, and their extended family, which involved mutual transatlantic visits.

For their first surrogacy arrangement, they spent approximately £94,000 ($118,300) (see figure 5.4). By far their highest expense was IVF, followed by agency fees and legal fees, as well as gestational fees for the surrogate. In order to be able to afford the surrogacy arrangement, Paul and Federico had to use all their savings, as well as refinance their house payment and take a mortgage loan. They were able to afford surrogacy in the United States thanks to their status as homeowners, even if it was based on a mortgage and required refinancing. It was also possible thanks to their middle-class annual household income of £150,000–£200,000 ($188,700–$251,600). The surrogacy arrangement required thinking in economic terms. As Paul explained, "We had a budget. And we had to stick to that. So everything that we did, we were conscious of,

CATEGORY	DATE	DESCRIPTION	TOTAL USD	TOTAL GBP (APPROX)
COORDINATION	09-Apr-17	Agency fee - paid upon commencement	$8,500.00	£6,545.00
COORDINATION	13-Jun-17	Agency fee - paid upon surrogate match	$8,500.00	£6,771.00
IVF/MEDICAL	22-Jun-17	Center for reproductive medicine - IVF installment	$10,000.00	£7,977.00
IVF/MEDICAL	05-Jul-17	Center for reproductive medicine - IVF installment	$10,000.00	£7,790.00
IVF/MEDICAL	18-Jul-17	Center for reproductive medicine - IVF installment	$10,000.00	£7,727.00
IVF/MEDICAL	31-Jul-17	Center for reproductive medicine - IVF installment	$10,000.00	£7,643.00
SURROGATE	01-Aug-17	Surrogate travel - for medical tests	$273.60	£210.00
IVF/MEDICAL	01-Sep-17	Center for reproductive medicine - IVF installment	$9,700.00	£7,550.00
SURROGATE	11-Sep-17	Surrogate travel - for medical tests	$189.28	£145.00
SURROGATE	02-Oct-17	Psychological consultation for surrogate	$400.00	£308.00
LEGAL	05-Oct-17	Legal fees - for surrogate contract creation	$1,400.00	£1,078.00
LEGAL	05-Oct-17	Legal fees - for escrow account management	$1,025.00	£789.25
COORDINATION	10-Oct-17	Agency fee - paid upon legal clearance	$8,500.00	£6,572.00
SURROGATE	11-Oct-17	Monthly disbursment	$100.00	£77.00
SURROGATE	12-Oct-17	Monthy disbursment	$100.00	£77.00
LEGAL	12-Oct-17	Surrogate's legal fee - for surrogate contract creation	$650.00	£500.50
SURROGATE	30-Oct-17	Surrogate travel - for transfer	$703.34	£541.57
SURROGATE	31-Oct-17	Monthly disbursment	$100.00	£77.00
SURROGATE	06-Nov-17	Life insurance for surrogate	$698.70	£538.00
IVF/MEDICAL	15-Nov-17	Surrogate - ultrasound (lining check)	$395.00	£304.15
SURROGATE	30-Nov-17	Monthy disbursment	$100.00	£77.00
SURROGATE	01-Dec-17	Transfer fee	$1,000.00	£770.00
IVF/MEDICAL	04-Dec-17	Reproductive medicine center - medications and ultrasound	$495.00	£381.15
IVF/MEDICAL	11-Dec-17	Reproductive medicine center - medications	$175.00	£134.75
SURROGATE	12-Dec-17	Surrogate car hire - for transfer appointment	$147.09	£113.26
IVF/MEDICAL	13-Dec-17	Pharmacy - medications	$709.44	£546.27
COORDINATION	13-Dec-17	Agency fee - paid upon positive BETA test	$4,500.00	£3,408.00
IVF/MEDICAL	21-Dec-17	Reproductive medicine center - medications	$175.00	£134.75
SURROGATE	22-Dec-17	Gestational fee - upon Beta confirmation	$575.00	£442.75
SURROGATE	28-Dec-17	Monthy disbursment	$100.00	£77.00
IVF/MEDICAL	02-Jan-18	Reproductive medicine center - HcG pregnancy test	$235.00	£180.95
SURROGATE	08-Jan-18	Gestational fee	$2,380.00	£1,832.60
IVF/MEDICAL	11-Jan-18	Reproductive medicine center - surrogate ultrasound	$220.00	£169.40
IVF/MEDICAL	18-Jan-18	Pharmacy - medications	$464.45	£357.63
SURROGATE	31-Jan-18	Monthly disbursment	$100.00	£77.00
SURROGATE	05-Feb-18	Gestational fee	$2,380.00	£1,832.60
SURROGATE	28-Feb-18	Monthly disbursment	$100.00	£77.00
SURROGATE	05-Mar-18	Gestational fee	$2,380.00	£1,832.60
SURROGATE	05-Mar-18	Maternity clothing allowance	$500.00	£385.00
SURROGATE	29-Mar-18	Monthy disbursment	$100.00	£77.00
SURROGATE	02-Apr-18	Gestational fee	$2,380.00	£1,832.60
SURROGATE	30-Apr-18	Monthy disbursment	$100.00	£77.00
SURROGATE	01-May-18	Gestational fee	$2,380.00	£1,832.60
SURROGATE	29-May-18	Gestational fee	$2,380.00	£1,832.60
SURROGATE	31-May-18	Monthy disbursment	$100.00	£77.00
SURROGATE	19-Jun-18	4D ultrasound and souvenir DVD	$189.74	£146.10
SURROGATE	25-Jun-18	Gestational fee	$2,380.00	£1,832.60
SURROGATE	28-Jun-18	Monthy disbursment	$100.00	£77.00
SURROGATE	23-Jul-18	Gestational fee	$2,380.00	£1,832.60
SURROGATE	31-Jul-18	Monthy disbursment	$100.00	£77.00
SURROGATE	06-Aug-18	Gestational fee	$2,385.00	£1,836.45
LEGAL	13-Aug-18	US parentage processing fee - birth certificare, parental order	$3,104.00	£2,390.08
SURROGATE	20-Aug-18	Surrogate - post-partum wages	$977.58	£752.74
IVF/MEDICAL	23-Aug-18	Hopsital and delivery costs	$2,180.93	£1,679.32
LEGAL	27-Aug-18	US passport application - expedited service	$445.00	£342.65
SURROGATE	04-Sep-18	Surrogate - post-partum wages	$977.58	£752.74
IVF/MEDICAL	13-Sep-18	Hospital and delivery costs	$175.00	£134.75
SURROGATE	19-Sep-18	Surrogate - post-partum wages	$977.58	£752.74
TOTAL			$121,636.22	£94,385.73

Figure 5.4. Paul and Federico's Expense Spreadsheet: Overseas Commercial Gestational Surrogacy in the United States

you know, retainer fees, and variable fees, and all these kind of things of . . . how that would impact our overall budget."

Just as in the cases of the families discussed earlier in this chapter—Harvey and Oliver, and Alex and Mateo—Paul also referred to the managerial mindset required for surrogacy to happen. Throughout the interview, he compared the mindset required to undertake surrogacy with the mindset he needed for his job in marketing. His path to parenthood required substantial planning, determination, and entrepreneurship: "I think in these kinds of situations, someone needs to *drive it and take charge*, because otherwise things will drop. So that turned out to be me. I think it's also my personality, because you know, in my line of work, and everything, I *need to be really organized*. And you know, I'm very Type A personality. So it made sense that I would *drive it and push things forward*, which I did and it worked quite well" (emphasis added).

The labor of organization, planning, and calculation characterized the entire surrogacy journey. One example of this was the final transfer of parentage after the child's birth, upon return to the United Kingdom. As Paul described it, "It's just a lot of paperwork, and a lot of it is very procedural, so you have to do certain things at certain times." To deal with preparing and sending the necessary documents on time, the couple hired a lawyer. This alleviated the labor that Paul would otherwise have had to do by himself: "But I had pretty much underestimated how tired I was going to be and how frazzled my brain was, and I couldn't, there was no way I could do that myself. So they did a lot of the paperwork for us."

Multiple considerations would populate the literal or metaphorical spreadsheet columns in the choice of the egg donor as well. In the case of Paul and Federico, this included her medical records, talents, intelligence/education ("She was a ballet dancer and a chemical engineer"), and motivations ("She also had really good reasons for being an egg donor. . . . She wants to do everything that she can to help someone else"). Another important criterion was the egg donor's racial identification, which Paul and Federico sought to match to their own. They therefore both used the same mixed-race egg donor, who was half African American and half Italian.

Conclusion

Gay parents' reproductive thinking in terms of spreadsheets evidences the particularly intentional character of gay fertility and parenthood (see also Stacey 2006; Smietana 2019; Pralat 2020). In the new reproductive order, many people experience fertility as not given and not obvious; rather, it has to be created. For babies to be brought into being, fertility needs to be brought into being: fertility needs to be managed, pushed, driven, crafted; it is a product of calculation, not automation; it is something deliberate and strategic. Creating fertility involves planning for money, time, travel, housing, relationships, and more. It is mediated through spreadsheets with both monetized and nonmonetized calculations.

Spreadsheet fertility is a new phenomenon. Even if LGBTQ+ parenthood has been characterized by particular intentionality for a few decades now, spreadsheets were not commonly used in building personal DIY reproductive arrangements between gay men and lesbian women in the early days of queer reproduction, such as the 1980s in the United States (Weston 1991). They may not be common either today in some places, such as Central and Eastern Europe (Mizielińska 2022). Yet spreadsheet fertility appears to be emerging in several contexts now, including different kinds of surrogacy arrangements as well as international reproductive travel in contexts as distinct as the United States (Smietana 2017), the United Kingdom, several other European countries, such as Norway (Stuvøy 2018), and Taiwan (Chen 2023).

In the United Kingdom, with increasing social support as well as favorable social and legal structures, the number of surrogacy cases has been steadily increasing, "with clear evidence that the proportion of same-sex male couples accessing surrogacy is a major contributor to this growth" (Horsey et al. 2022: 1). This shift may be at least partly due to the recent emergence of the "imaginability" (Pralat 2016; see also Pralat, chapter 4) and "thinkability" (Smietana 2019) of gay parenthood. The latter also exemplifies one of the tenets of this volume: that people's perceptions of fertility—such as the new thinkability of gay parenthood— are driving new reproductive behaviors, identities, and even activisms (see Franklin and Inhorn, Introduction).

Spreadsheet fertility represents the new reproductive order that the current volume characterizes, whereby fertility is subject to IVF-ication. It maps onto previous ways of bureaucratization and family planning, as well as, more recently, datafication of reproduction. It is also linked to processes such as biomedicalization (Mamo 2007) and the biomedical mode of reproduction (Thompson 2005), the globalization of IVF (Inhorn 2015), the industrialization of IVF (Franklin 2013) and of surrogacy (Rudrappa 2015), the routinization of IVF (Wahlberg

2018), and the financialization of reproductive technologies (Stuvøy 2018; Van de Wiel 2020).

Yet such a highly intentional and calculative approach to reproduction increasingly characterizes not only LGBTQ+ family making but also contemporary reproduction at large (Franklin 2022 [1997]). Indeed, spreadsheet fertility appears not to be limited to the LGBTQ+ community, as recent literature on heterosexual reproduction shows, too: for many people, reproduction is increasingly becoming a product of calculations and transactions. Scholars of reproduction have demonstrated that fertility is becoming ever more intentional also for heterosexual women contemplating and undergoing egg freezing (Inhorn 2023; Van de Wiel 2020), couples undergoing IVF (Franklin (2022 [1997]); Inhorn 2015), and even those trying to conceive "naturally" (Faircloth and Gürtin 2018). The onset of thinking about one's reproductive life in terms of calculations and planning is also part of a broader "intensive parenting" culture (Faircloth and Gürtin 2018: 986), characterized by the "expansion of 'parenting' into an expertise-saturated, policy-focused, and commercially fuelled area of social life." Therefore, the spreadsheet fertility that I found in the study of gay parents' reproductive projects increasingly refers to heterosexual reproduction, too. Reproduction at large is characterized today by what Sarah Franklin (2022 [1997]: 10) called "iFertility": "a new, technologically mediated fertility formation" that "is not given, 'natural' or 'automatic': it is planned, resourced, calculated, monitored, assisted and achieved."

Thus, fertility—just like biology (Franklin 2014)—is becoming ever more queer: its meaning changes, it is malleable, uncertain, and relative, it cannot be taken for granted, and it therefore requires careful calculation and planning. As Franklin (2022 [1997]: 214] notes, "LGBTQ+ people have often taken fewer conjugal and procreative liberties for granted" and "an important overarching trend that is likely to become more prominent is that the LGBTQ+ model of more deliberate fertility and family planning could in some ways be seen to be the 'new normal' for many heterosexual couples too" (see also Inhorn 2023). Likewise, a characteristic of spreadsheet fertility is a paradoxical destabilization of the previous reproductive norms: while it is now more common for LGBTQ+ people to have children in queer reproductive arrangements, it is also less common for heterosexual people to take their reproduction for granted (see Franklin 2022 [1997]: 214). Spreadsheet fertility may therefore be making reproduction queerer: less normative (Twine and Smietana 2021), less predictable, and more precarious. As Laura Mamo (2007: 6) argued in her study of lesbian mothers in the United States, "queering reproduction" entails "processes by which lesbian reproductive practices simultaneously alter and maintain dominant assumptions and institutions."

Spreadsheet fertility is part of the new reproductive order. One distinct feature of this order is the paradoxical way that the marketing and management of fertility increases its precarity, due to lack of money, time, knowledge, and other resources (see Franklin 2022 [1997]: 24; Franklin and Inhorn, Introduction). In other words, the more complex the spreadsheet, the more difficult it is for prospective parents to tick the boxes and achieve parenthood. This also shows that fertility is a matter of social justice and that queer fertility requires "queer reproductive justice" (Mamo 2018; Smietana, Thompson, and Twine 2018). We must therefore be wary of social inequalities that spreadsheet fertility may be reproducing. It often goes in tandem with middle-class positionalities and may thus exclude people of lower socioeconomic status from parenting options (see also Jacobson 2018). Among the thirty families I spoke to in this United Kingdom study, I was not able to recruit any family whose average annual household income fell below the UK average of £32,300 ($40,640). In addition, spreadsheet fertility may contribute to economic and other inequalities between parents and people who help them have children, such as surrogates and donors. This prompts a search for alternatives: public or insurance funding for IVF in gay surrogacy; traditional surrogacy arrangements without the involvement of egg donors and fertility clinics where possible and desired; and the recognition and equal valorization of multiple queer family forms, including different kinds of surrogacy. In the end, we must ask, if spreadsheet fertility is here to stay, can we do anything to mitigate its paradoxical effects?

Acknowledgments

The research was funded by the Wellcome Trust, UK (Grant no. 209829/Z/17/Z). The paper was written with further support from the Spanish Ministry of Science and Innovation (Grant

PID2020–112692RB-C21/AEI/10.13039/501100011033). I owe my gratitude for inspiration, guidance, and support in writing this chapter to Professors Sarah Franklin and Marcia C. Inhorn, to the Changing (In) Fertilities network, and to Bonnie Rose Schulman, Alessandro Biagini, Dr. Manuela Perrotta, and the gay fathers I spoke to within this research.

NOTE

1 The new surrogacy law reform, proposed by the Law Commission of England and Wales and the Scottish Law Commission for the UK government to consider, includes the option of intended parents becoming the child's parents from birth (Law Commission 2023).

REFERENCES

Chen, Jung. 2023. "Queering Reproductive Justice: Framing Reproduction of Gay Men from a Transnational Perspective; Taiwan as a Case." *Sociology Compass* 17(12): e13139.

Department of Health & Social Care. 2023. "Guidance: The Surrogacy Pathway; Surrogacy and the Legal Process for Intended Parents and Surrogates in England and Wales." www.gov.uk.

———. 2024. "People with HIV Can Now Donate Eggs or Sperm to Start a Family." May 15. www.gov.uk.

Faircloth, Charlotte, and Zeynep Gürtin. 2018. "Fertile Connections: Thinking across Assisted Reproductive Technologies and Parenting Culture Studies." *Sociology* 52(5): 983–1000.

Franklin, Sarah. 2013. *Biological Relatives: IVF, Stem Cells, and the Future of Kinship.* Durham, NC: Duke University Press.

———. 2014. "Queer Biology." *Lambda Nordica* 19(3–4): 173–80.

———. 2021. "Fertinomics: What Is the Relationship of Reproduction to Political Economy?" Lecture at Freie Universität Berlin. October 14.

———. 2022 [1997]. *Embodied Progress: A Cultural Account of Assisted Conception*, 2nd ed. London: Routledge.

Franklin, Sarah, and Marcia C. Inhorn. 2018. Changing (In)Fertilities Project (2018–2022). Funded by the Wellcome Trust, UK (Grant no. 209829/Z/17/Z). University of Cambridge and Yale University. www.cifp.sociology.cam.ac.uk/.

Hamper, Josie, and Manuela Perrotta. 2023. "Blurring the Divide: Navigating the Public/Private Landscape of Fertility Treatment in the UK." *Health & Place* 80 (March).

Horsey, Kirsty, Grace Gibson, Giuseppina Lamanna, Helen Priddle, Elena Linara-Demakakou, Shailaja Nair, Mimi Arian-Schad, Hemlata Thackare, Michael Rimington, Nicholas Macklon, and Kamal Ahuja. 2022. "First Clinical Report of 179 Surrogacy Cases in the UK: Implications for Policy and Practice." *Reproductive BioMedicine Online* 45(4): 831–38.

Inhorn, Marcia C. 2015. *Cosmopolitan Conceptions: IVF Sojourns in Global Dubai.* Durham, NC: Duke University Press.

———. 2023. *Motherhood on Ice: The Mating Gap and Why Women Freeze Their Eggs.* New York: New York University Press.

Jacobson, Heather. 2018. "A Limited Market: The Recruitment of Gay Men as Surrogacy Clients by the Infertility Industry in the USA." *Reproductive BioMedicine and Society Online* 7: 14–23.

Law Commission. 2023. "Surrogacy Laws to Be Overhauled under New Reforms: Benefitting the Child, Surrogate, and Intended Parents." March 29. www.lawcom.gov.uk.

Laycock, Emma. 2020. "Male Couple Expecting Baby after NHS IVF." *BioNews*, May 11.

Mamo, Laura. 2007. *Queering Reproduction: Achieving Pregnancy in the Age of Technoscience.* Durham, NC: Duke University Press.

———. 2018. "Queering Reproduction in Transnational Bioeconomies." *Reproductive BioMedicine and Society Online* 7: 24–32.

Mizielińska, Joanna. 2022. *Queer Kinship on the Edge? Families of Choice in Poland.* London: Routledge.

National AIDS Trust. 2022. "Government Challenged over 'Cruel' Ban on People Living with HIV Using Fertility Treatment." August 7. www.nat.org.uk.

National Health Service. 2021. "IVF: Availability, 11 October 2021." www.nhs.uk.

Office for National Statistics. 2022. "Average Household Income, UK: Financial Year Ending 2022." www.ons.gov.uk.

Pralat, Robert. 2016. "Between Future Families and Families of Origin: Talking about Gay Parenthood across Generations." In *Parenthood between Generations: Transforming Reproductive Cultures*, ed. Siân Pooley and Kaveri Qureshi, 43–64. Oxford: Berghahn.

———. 2020. "Parenthood as Intended: Reproductive Responsibility, Moral Judgements, and Having Children 'by Accident.'" *Sociological Review* 68(1): 161–76.

Rudrappa, Sharmila. 2015. *Discounted Life: The Price of Global Surrogacy in India.* New York: New York University Press.

Schorscher-Pecu, Ana. 2021. "Lesbian Couple Takes CCG to Court over IVF Discrimination." *BioNews*, November 15. www.progress.org.uk.

Smietana, Marcin. 2017. "Affective De-commodifying, Economic De-kinning: Surrogates' and Gay Fathers' Narratives in U.S. Surrogacy." *Sociological Research Online* 22(2): 2.

———. 2019. "Procreative Consciousness in a Global Market: Gay Men's Paths to Surrogacy in the USA." *Reproductive BioMedicine and Society Online* 7(November): 101–11.

Smietana, Marcin, Charis Thompson, and France Winddance Twine. 2018. "Making and Breaking Families: Reading Queer Reproductions, Stratified Reproduction, and Reproductive Justice Together." *Reproductive BioMedicine and Society Online* 7(November): 112–20.

Smietana, Marcin, and France Winddance Twine. 2022. "Queer Decisions: Racial Matching and Stigma Management among Gay Male Intended Parents." *International Journal of Comparative Sociology* 63(5–6): 324–44.

Stacey, Judith. 2006. "Gay Parenthood and the Decline of Paternity as We Knew It." *Sexualities* 9(1): 27–55.

Stuvøy, Ingvill. 2018. "Accounting for the Money-Made Parenthood of Transnational Surrogacy." *Anthropology & Medicine* 25(3): 280–95.

Thompson, Charis. 2005. *Making Parents: The Ontological Choreography of Reproductive Technologies*. Cambridge, MA: MIT Press.

Twine, France Winddance, and Marcin Smietana. 2021. "The Racial Contours of Queer Reproduction." In *The Routledge Handbook of Anthropology and Reproduction*, ed. Sallie Han and Cecília Tomori, 285–304. New York: Routledge.

Van de Wiel, Lucy. 2020. *Freezing Fertility: Oocyte Cryopreservation and the Gender Politics of Aging*. New York: New York University Press.

Wahlberg, Ayo. 2018. *Good Quality: The Routinization of Sperm Banking in China*. Oakland: University of California Press.

Weston, Kath. 1991. *Families We Choose: Lesbians, Gays, Kinship*. New York: Columbia University Press.

PART II

In-Fertile Nations

In-fertility has always been a national concern, with population reduction being one of the leading mantras of the twentieth century. However, in the twenty-first-century new reproductive order, that mantra has come into question for a number of reasons. First, some societies in which population reduction was most vigorously pursued have been forced to reassess the wisdom of their actions in the face of plummeting birth rates. Second, efforts to manage fertility on a national level have proven difficult in many cases, given the human values, perceptions, and practices that ultimately fuel or resist fertility change. Third, government investments in national in-fertility welfare increasingly include a commitment to ARTs as a symbol of national values. Indeed, for many twenty-first-century governments, *repronationalism* entails a mandate to make ARTs available to the public, through either state-sponsored programs or the development of robust private ART markets.

Nowhere are these issues more evident than in China, the nation whose "one-child" policy has finally been relaxed and ART treatments encouraged in the nation's five-hundred-plus IVF clinics. However, the Chinese government has refused to accept responsibility for the nation's falling fertility rate, instead shifting the blame onto three "fertility figures"—namely, "leftover women," "bare branches," and "DINKs" (i.e., dual income, no kids) (chapter 6). Israel offers the counterexample to China. The Israeli state has never encouraged or enforced birth control and has instead offered the most generous state-subsidized ART regime in the world, leading to continued high fertility rates and strong child desires among a population characterized by its "resilient pronatalism" (chapter 7). Unlike China or Israel, Mexico has undergone a century of "shifting reproductive agendas" forwarded by the varying governments in power. Yet, today, the Mexican government has lost control of its largely private and unregulated "hyper-market" of in-fertility products and services (chapter 8). As in Mexico, in Iran, historic anxieties about the rise and fall of fertility levels have led to shifting state-sponsored "fertility regimes" and the growth of a high-tech ART sector. Yet, the current government's pronatalist regime and encouragement of ARTs is being met with "reproductive rebellion" among a new generation of reproductive-aged Iranians, who are questioning the very meaning of childbearing (chapter 9). As seen in these examples, demography has been the reigning conceptual framework upon which nation-states have come to rely in making their population projections. Yet, with its narrow focus on the "proximate determinants of fertility," which are individual, biological, and choice dependent, demography has often failed to capture the complex social, cultural, political, and economic factors driving in-fertility change in particular national settings (chapter 10). As each of these chapters demonstrates, the consequences of widespread changes to previous logics of reproductive cause and effect are as evident in national policies as they are in individuals' family making. Together, the chapters in this section offer further evidence that in-fertility has itself become a key contested signifier in the relations between people and their governments.

6

Fertility Figures

The Reconfiguring of "One-Child" China

AYO WAHLBERG

In one of the many harrowing scenes in Xu Huijing's documentary film *Mothers* (Xu 2013), local family-planning officials in a village in northern China hound Rong Rong, a young mother of two, threatening her (and her family) with hefty fines if she does not succumb to sterilization. Such confrontations were common, especially in rural China, throughout the long reign of China's one-child policy beginning in the early 1980s. It was Chairman Mao Zedong's successor, Deng Xiaoping, who implemented these notoriously strict family-planning measures in 1979, insisting that "while there are advantages to having a large population, there are disadvantages as well . . . [as it] poses serious problems with regard to food, education and employment" (Deng 1984 [1979]: 171). Hence, the one-child policy was from its very beginnings seen as an instrument of socioeconomic development. In the words of Wu Cangping, demographer and government adviser at the Population Institute in Beijing at the time, "If we make energetic efforts to develop production and at the same time effectively control population growth . . . it is entirely possible to transform [China] from a *backward* country into an advanced one" (Wu 1980 cited in Greenhalgh 2008: 120, emphasis added).

Indeed, this developmental trope of "backwardness" is ubiquitous, used by demographers, economists, international organizations, and governments alike to justify state-led programs of modernization and industrialization in China and beyond (Escobar 1995). With thinly veiled reference to evolutionary and racist descriptions of "uncultivated," "immature," and "uncivilized" peoples, the notion of backwardness underpinned countless twentieth-century figurations in a relentlessly stratified and modernizing world. In China, as Greenhalgh and Winckler show, it was predominantly the figure of the "backward" peasant with "out-moded reproductive beliefs" that came to be "demonized as 'backward elements' whose excess childbearing and low quality were preventing the whole nation from attaining its place of glory in the world" (Green-halgh and Winckler 2005: 250). And so, in the technoscientific making of China's one-child policy, it was these kinds of depictions that explic-itly sanctioned state-led corporeal interventions into women's bodies in the form of contraception, sterilization, and abortion.

In the period from 1980 to 2015, this reproductive complex coalesced around dual objectives of controlling population growth and improving population quality (*kòngzhì rénkǒu shùliàng, tígāo rénkǒu sùzhì*; 控制人口数量，提高人口素质), comprising a total set of laws, family planning institutions, birth quotas, awareness campaigns, hospitals, clinics, phar-maceuticals, premarital counseling sessions, prenatal screening services, and more. Medical procedures and techniques related to birth control (population quantity) included contraception, sterilization, and abor-tion, as well as assisted reproductive technologies (ARTs), while those related to the health of newborns (population quality) included genetic counseling, fetal education, prenatal screening, abortion, and selective reproductive technologies (SRTs) (see Wahlberg 2018; Wahlberg and Gammeltoft 2018; Zhu and Dong 2018).

Today, following four decades of unyielding efforts to prevent birth in the name of economic and social development, the tables have turned. An opposite fear has emerged among the political elite wherein *a lack of births* is now viewed as a potential cause of economic stagnation and social crisis (Whittaker 2022: 117; De Zordo, Marre, and Smietana 2022). This reversal in demo-economic reasoning is a foundational feature of China's new reproductive order. Having suffered the consequences of the one-child policy on their own bodies, millions of women like Rong Rong are now witnessing a profound reconfiguration of the organizing logics of China's reproductive complex. In 2015, the government made the first in a series of adjustments to its family-planning policies by per-mitting couples to have two children (Huang 2022). The Office for Na-tional Statistics had estimated that such an adjustment would lead to an increase in annual births from sixteen million in 2014 to twenty million in the following years (see figure 6.1). In reality, this number fell to 9.56 million in 2022, despite a further adjustment of family-planning policies

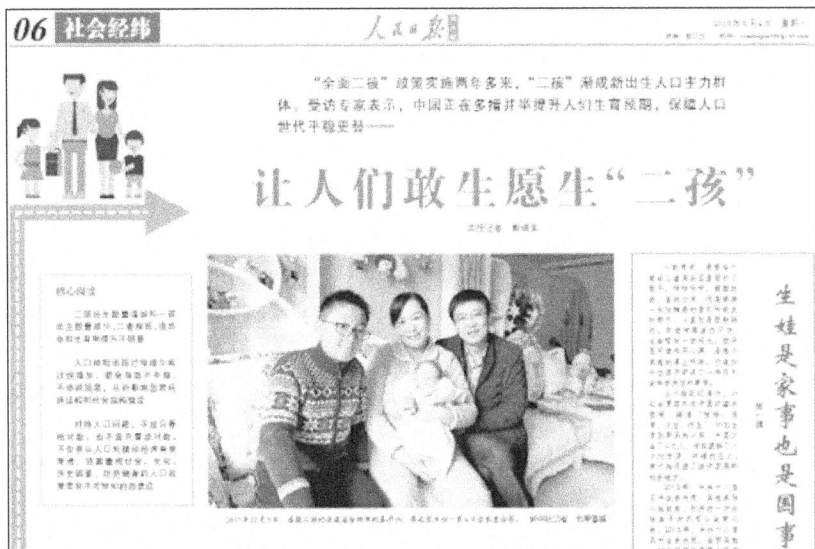

Figure 6.1. "Let People Dare to Give Birth to 'Two Children.'" Credit: *People's Daily* (2018)

in August 2021 into China's current "three-child policy." In October 2022, President Xi Jinping cemented this transformation when proclaiming in his speech to the Twentieth National Congress of the Communist Party, "We will improve the population development strategy, establish a policy system to boost birth rates, and bring down the costs of pregnancy and childbirth, child rearing, and schooling" (Xi 2022).

In this chapter, I show how novel *fertility figures* have emerged in the wake of newfound political concerns about the potential social and economic consequences of falling fertility in China. Gone are the so-called backward peasants who were so foundational in the making of the one-child policy. Instead, a cluster of novel fertility figures— "leftover women" (*sheng nu*; 剩女), "bare branches" (*guang gun*; 光棍), and "DINKs" (*dīngkè yìzú*; 丁克一族)—emerged as sociocultural culprits in discussions about what might be causing China's falling fertility rates, despite a relaxing of family-planning policies. The chapter builds on my decades-long, episodic ethnographic research in China, where I have focused on the development and routinization of ARTs (Wahlberg 2016, 2018). It was exactly at the moment when my fieldwork in Changsha (the capital of Hunan province) was coming to a close in 2018 that the government announced that it would be loosening its strict family-planning policies. As the COVID-19 pandemic complicated the regularity of my fieldwork visits, I began tracking changes to family-planning policies online, paying particular attention to governmental announcements and speeches by key political figures while also following media reports and popular discussions that were playing out through blog posts and social media commentary, as well as movies and literature. It is this collection of written documents, social media postings, and audiovisual materials that forms the basis of the analysis that follows. Far from being exhaustive, these materials are indicative of the ways in which reproductive futures are discussed and debated as China's new reproductive order continues to take shape.

Figurations of Fertility

"'To figure,'" writes Donna Haraway, "means to count or calculate and also to be in a story, to have a role" (Haraway 1996: 11). Indeed, if we are to understand processes of "worldmaking" in the sense proposed by Haraway (2016), we must pay close attention to material-semiotic processes of figuration, as they incorporate a double force of constitutive effect and generative circulation. Representations are material in the ways that they constitute social life, with imagery and depiction generating dominant frames of reference that make the world both graspable and intervenable while at the same time providing legitimations and justifications for particular social worlds.

Fertility figures play central roles in stories of looming crises, whether construed in terms of unsustainable "population bombs" or demographic "collapse." Much as "designer babies" became a kind of "condensed signifier" of broader anxieties about the risks and dilemmas posed by new genetic technologies (Franklin and Roberts 2006), fertility figures here emerge as troubling quantified demographic projections that come to be personified and stereotyped in speculations about the future. These portrayals circulate through journal articles, parliamentary hearings, news media, social media, art, scholarship, and more. For example, against a twentieth-century backdrop of figurations of "backward" women peasants, Jade Sasser shows how, in the twenty-first-century remaking of global family-planning policy through international organizations such as the United Nations Population Fund and World Health Organization in a time of anthropogenic climate crisis, "an idealized model of a woman . . . as a sexual steward" has taken form, "framed within the logics of private, individual decision-making and choice, who adopts a modicum of embodied environmental responsibility in the service of global development goals" (Sasser 2018: 4). Likewise, Birgit Kvernflaten and colleagues have argued that, amid concerns about falling fertility rates, politicians and policymakers have emphasized Norwegian "women's role as reproducers of the nation" (Kvernflaten, Fedorcsák, and Solbrække 2023: 278; see also Homanen and Meskus 2023). In her analysis of the rise of egg-freezing technologies in the United States, Marcia C. Inhorn shows how "stereotypical images of the kind of women who might turn to egg freezing were beginning to form in the media" in the late 2010s, "often referred to as 'career women'" (Inhorn 2023: 7). It can therefore be helpful to examine empirically the material-semiotic processes of figuration that constitute these fertility figures. In this way, scholars can unpack the domains of practice and significance that are built into each figure as essential constituents of national reproductive biopolitics.

In the time leading up to the ongoing reconfiguration of China's reproductive complex, demographers and economists began highlighting a series of (unintended) effects of the country's one-child policy. Through illustrative diagrams and graphs, scholars and policymakers showed how a mandated decrease in family size had led to a substantial skewing of sex ratios as female fetuses came to be aborted, abandoned, or given up for adoption in a cultural context of "son preference" (Nie 2011). Moreover, with smaller birth cohorts coming through, China's population pyramid was inverting at an unprecedented rate, predicting an aging population that would ultimately shrink the country's labor force while increasing its care burden (Keimig 2021; Chen and Liu 2009). And so, with fewer young people to look after aging parents and a healthcare system struggling to keep up with growing numbers of chronically ill, a new sense of urgency has permeated the political establishment. Hence, not only did Xi Jinping pledge to boost birth rates in his 2022 speech to the National Congress of the Communist Party; he also proposed a proactive national strategy in response to population aging, including improved "elderly care programs and services" and strengthened "health management for major chronic diseases" (Xi 2022). In demographer Wang Feng's assessment, "In the long run, we are going to see a China the world has never seen. It will no longer be the young, vibrant, growing population." Rather, "We will start to appreciate China . . . as an old and shrinking population" (Stevenson and Wang 2023).

It is amid this renewed set of anxious demographic projections and policy responses that we can discern the outlines of novel fertility figures in China. Demographic calculations of "marriage squeezes," "age at first marriage," "reproductive deferral," and "age at first birth" have come to be intertwined with moral characterizations of certain subgroups that are portrayed as obstacles to China's newfound biopolitical objective of increasing annual births. Such figurations, as Rosi Braidotti has argued, "are not figurative ways of thinking, but rather more materialistic mappings of situated, embedded, and embodied positions . . . highly specific geo-political and historical locations: history tattooed on your body" (Braidotti 2014: 13). In this sense, the fertility figures that emerge out of sociodemographic figuration processes are inextricably bound up in the shaping of national reproductive biopolitics with stigmatizing and stratifying consequences (Winndance Twine 2017; Homanen and Meskus 2023). In tracing these processes, this chapter contributes to the social study of what Greenhalgh has called the "demographic subjects" of situated fertility transitions, as "to situate fertility . . . is to show how it makes sense given the sociocultural and political economic context in which it is embedded" (Greenhalgh 1995: 13).

Fertility Figures in Three-Child-Policy China

In May 2022, as tempers flared during Shanghai's three-month COVID-19 lockdown, a viral video showed a health official threatening a family and three generations with repercussions if they refused to accept being taken into quarantine. The young man being yelled at in the video coolly responded, "We are the last generation, thank you" (Gan 2022). The episode led to vigorous online discussions about the merits and pitfalls of raising children in China at a time when the cost of childcare was soaring, competition for university places and subsequently for good jobs was intensifying, and more generally, concerns about economic, social, and environmental security were rife. Amid these everyday worries, in recent years, we can see how particular demographic subgroups have come to be singled out for their childlessness, in novels, movies, social commentaries, news reports, and more. In this section, I show how three groups in particular have emerged as prominent fertility figures in three-child-policy China.

Leftover Women

In Inhorn's (2023) book *Motherhood on Ice: The Mating Gap and Why Women Freeze Their Eggs*, we learn how a "mating gap" has emerged in the United States for those women who have turned to egg-freezing technology as a "reproductive suspension bridge." Inhorn writes that "a lack of stable reproductive relationships is the bane of women's existence, with significant deleterious consequences for women's reproductive lives" (2023: 21). A similar mating gap exists in China, as increasing numbers of women obtain university degrees and seek better-paid jobs in China's many urban centers. As a direct consequence, sociologists Jing Song and Yingchun Ji argue, "There has been a tension between growing opportunities for women outside the family and limited change in expectations and obligations within the family. Such a mismatch . . . will make the 'package' of marriage and family less attractive to women. The conflict between traditional expectations and economic opportunities, rather than individualism itself, leads to people's new marital and intimacy practices, such as delayed marriage and rising singlehood" (Song and Ji 2020: 6).

At the same time, in China, this mating gap is further compounded in a country where birth cohorts that are currently in their thirties have some of the most skewed gender ratios ever seen (Guilmoto 2012). Born during the one-child policy of the 1980s and 1990s, these singletons have now reached their late twenties and early thirties, a demographically significant period that has historically been linked to finding a partner, getting married, and having a first child. Yet on all three fronts, "expected behaviors" are changing as annual numbers of marriages and births continue to fall and living alone increases (Yeung, Desai, and Jones 2018).

One group that has been singled out for exacerbating an already skewed mating gap are those women who are approaching or have surpassed the age of thirty without having married. This group has come to be derogatively labeled as "leftover women" (*sheng nu*; 剩女), judged for not finding partners because of personal deficiencies. For example, in a 2019 blog post entitled "Looking forward to love and preparing to spend a lifetime alone," a young woman from Guangxi province explains how hometown visits during the Chinese lunar new year holiday can be experienced as distressing for many unmarried young women: "Our hometown is in a small county in Guilin, Guangxi, surrounded by mountains and traffic jams. Most of the people who stayed behind in the country married early, especially women. If they are not married after twenty-five, they will inevitably be pointed at and labeled as 'leftover women.' I am twenty-three years old and have just graduated from university. After [I returned] home, my relatives started discussing my relationship problems at the dinner table and urging me to find a boyfriend" (Zhou 2019).

Given the pressures that so-called *sheng nu* can face, it is not surprising that an advertising campaign devised by a skin care company with a short video entitled *Marriage Market Takeover* was shared widely on social media when it came out (SK-II 2016). The video opens with a collage of flashing photographs of young women overlaid with sound bites of stern parental voices stating, "You're not a kid anymore"; "I won't die in peace unless you're married"; "You're too picky"; and "You are a leftover woman" (see figure 6.2). The video revolves around the stories of four unnamed young single women who describe the many unpleasant societal and familial pressures they face, interlaced with comments from their disapproving parents. One mother, seated on a sofa, matter-of-factly states, "She's just average looking. Not too pretty. That's why she's leftover," as her daughter listens tearfully beside her. The video uses Shanghai's well-known marriage market, where parents bring pictures and descriptions of their sons and daughters in the hopes of finding a match for their child, as the setting for an empowering plot that culminates with the four young women bringing their parents to the marriage market only to find beautifully stylized photos of their daughters hanging up accompanied by messages directed at their parents such as, "I don't want to get married just for the sake of marriage; I won't live happily that way" and "Even if I am alone, I will be happy, confident, and

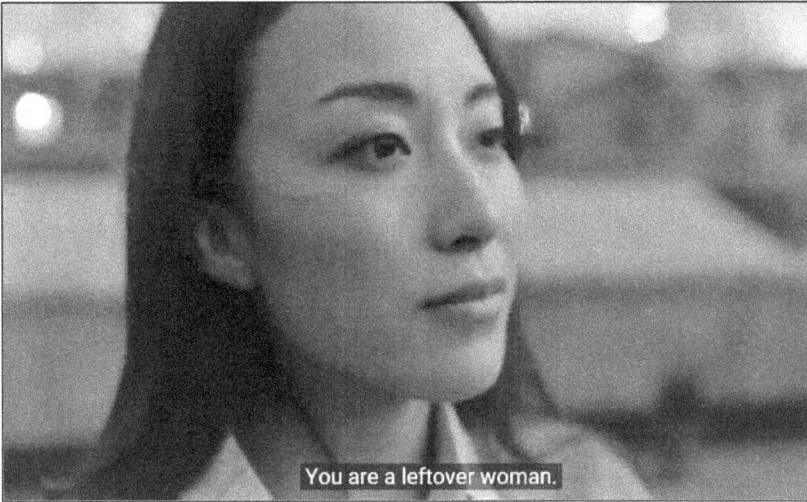

Figure 6.2. Still Image from *The Marriage Market Takeover*. Credit SK-II (2016)

have a good life." With careful emotional choreography, the video ends with one of the mothers proclaiming "*Sheng nu* should be proud" as she looks up beamingly at a photograph of her daughter.

While the message of empowerment for young professional women in China serves as a brand-booster for the cosmetic skin care company behind the video, such culturally circulating clips and blog posts are at the same time effective material-semiotic conduits in the kinds of sociodemographic figuration processes I suggest are so crucial in the shaping of national reproductive biopolitics. Such videos may challenge the stigma associated with the so-called *sheng nu*, yet they also play their part in socioculturally cementing this fertility figure. This is one of the reasons why, as Tianhan Gui has argued, in China today, "Women who are considered as too intelligent and successful in their career might no longer be regarded as 'women'" (Gui 2020: 1957). Given these forms of stigmatization that successful, educated women have faced, it is perhaps not surprising that in July 2022 Xu Zaozao lost her high-profile legal challenge to allow her to freeze her eggs for later use as a single woman. This assisted reproductive technology is currently only available by law to married women undergoing fertility treatment in China (Wang 2023).

Bare Branches

As already noted, this moral disapproval of young, unmarried women in China today is compounded by the "missing women" that demographers have identified as an adverse outcome of China's one-child policy. However, whereas single, unmarried women are more often met with censure, a growing group of young men who are seen as unable to find marriage partners, establish families, and thereby continue their family lineages, have come to be known as "bare branches" (*guang gun*; 光棍) (Greenhalgh 2014). Contrary to "leftover women," this group is often depicted as having been "left behind" by China's rapid modernization and industrialization, either in a literal sense as they have remained in China's rural villages or in a socioeconomic sense as they become a part of China's so-called floating population who move to cities in search of employment. While the group is in many ways stigmatized because of a perceived lack of formal education, it is to some extent also pitied for its predicament of belonging to a generation marked by a significantly skewed sex ratio: "With no support from a spouse or children, and no emotional communication with family members, old bare branches will be trapped in both material and psychological poverty" (Jiang et al. 2013: 10; see also Blair, Madigan, and Fang 2022). Indeed, as Greenhalgh argues, to understand how *guanggun* as a fertility figure has taken on a renewed meaning in China today, we must look to the pre-Communist era when "poor and ill-educated, village men who had no wife, no children, and no way to fulfill their filial duties had no place in the social order . . . [as] one of the most pitiable figures on the social landscape" (Greenhalgh 2014: 368).

In Jie Hao's (2010) comedy film *Single Man* (*guanggun er*; 光棍儿), we follow the sexual and daily life frustrations of four elderly single men—Bighead Liang, Gu Lin, Liuruan, and Old Yang—with flashbacks to their different routes to singlehood in the rural village of Gujiagou, north of Beijing. The title of the film plays on the double meaning of the Chinese word for both "bachelor" and "ruffian," as it portrays the difficulties of rural life, whether in trying to get a decent price for a batch of watermelons or dealing with human traffickers who aim to profit from China's "missing women" (see figure 6.3). While Hao's film emphasizes the

Figure 6.3. Bighead Liang, Gu Lin, Liuruan, and Old Yang in Jie Hao's *Single Man Watch as the Sun Sets*. Credit: Hao (2010)

creative and pragmatic ways that daily life is made to work under often harsh conditions, the film also stands as commentary on a looming demographic future in which it becomes increasingly difficult for young men to find partners. Through such interlacing of demographic projections, social-realism cinema, and media reporting, the "bare branches problem" (*guānggùn wèntí*; 光棍问题) has become a matter of concern in ways that highlight the frustrations of a growing group of especially socioeconomically disadvantaged young men living in rural areas who are unable to get married and have families (Jin et al. 2014).

When juxtaposed, *sheng nu* and *guanggun* as fertility figures highlight the particularities of China's contemporary mating gap. With increasing numbers of women gaining higher education degrees, thereby gaining access to higher paid jobs and possibilities for independent living until they find the right partners, *guanggun* are increasingly seen as, in a sense, "ineligible" for marriage in a highly competitive society. Films like Jie Hao's, alongside media reporting and governmental initiatives to address China's "marriage squeeze," condense concerns about the increasing difficulties men who would like to establish families are facing in the fertility figure of *guanggun*.

DINKs

Finally, in more recent years, we have seen how a third, perhaps more transnational fertility figure has emerged through popular media in China in the form of "DINKs" (*dīngkè yìzú*; 丁克一族)—double income, no kids. In 2019, Chinese Internet billionaire Jack Ma told staff at his online retail company, "To be able to work 996 is a huge bliss; if you want to join Alibaba, you need to be prepared to work twelve hours a day, otherwise why even bother joining?" ("Working 12 Hours a Day" 2019). A "996" working culture—working from 9:00 a.m. to 9:00 p.m. six days a week—has become in many ways synonymous with China's decades-long economic boom in its urban centers, as young professionals are expected to put in long hours to stay ahead in a highly competitive job market. Yet, the backlash to Ma's comments was swift, with many incredulous online posts on the social media platform Weibo, including, "Did you ever think about the elderly at home who need care, (or) the children who need company? If all enterprises enforce a 996 schedule, no one [would] have children" (Wang and Shane 2019; see also Pak 2021).

In one recent analysis of census data, an estimated 188 million DINK families were identified in China (Ning 2023), indicating that, for many couples, "childlessness" is a reality, whether by choice, because of the difficulties, pressures, and expenses of childrearing, or due to infertility (cf. Fong 2004; Xu 2013). When one user community on China's Sohu Internet platform asked young users whether they planned to have children, it received numerous responses highlighting rising living and childcare costs. Others referred to the intensities of parenting that they themselves had experienced as children during the one-child-policy era:

I'm twenty years old and I'm not married yet, but I've made up my mind that I don't want children after I get married. Why? Because I don't want to lose myself because of my child. I have an older sister, and my parents loved us very much since childhood. In my impression, parents put all their sustenance and hope in their entire life on their children. When they were young, they took care of me and my sister wholeheartedly, without

原创 **新的丁克一族正在兴起？几个95后新人的答案，很刷脑**

许多人都知道丁克这个词，指的是那种结婚了却不要生孩子的家庭。随着时代的变化，身边有不少95后的年轻人也兴起了类似的观点。为什么会这样呢？上次在知乎上面，有许多年轻人留言，主要有下面三个源因。

NO

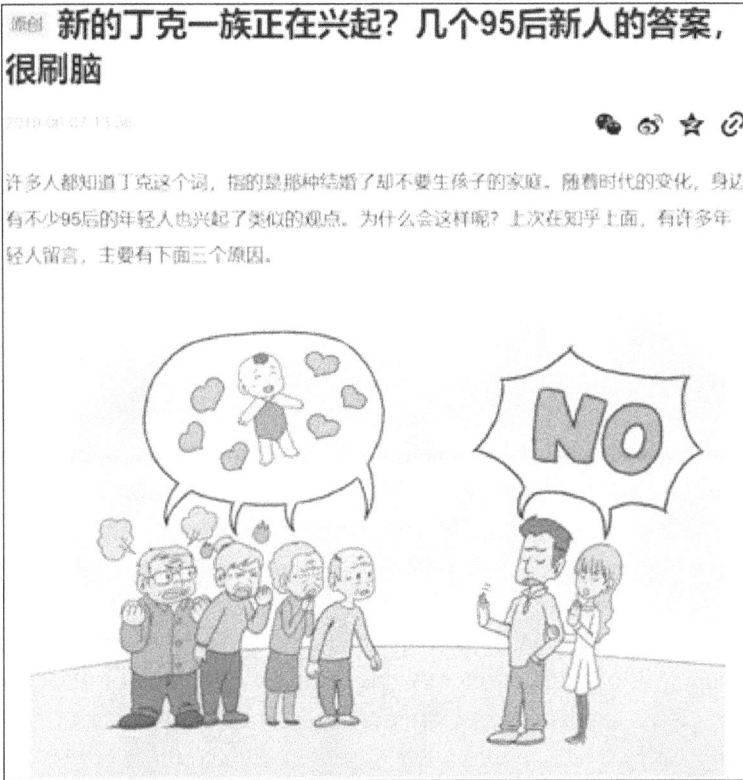

Figure 6.4. Screenshot of Blog Post "Is a New DINK Family Form Emerging? The Answers of Several Post-95 Newcomers Are Very Refreshing"

entertainment or career. I feel that they have no self in their lives, and they are all for their children. I don't want this kind of life. (Sohu 2019)

Couples who choose to live a *dīngkè yìzú* lifestyle have, perhaps predictably, been singled out as selfish and naïve, as commentators and experts question who will look after them as they age. In one response to the government's call to boost birth rates in China, Hu Jiye, a professor at China's University of Political Science and Law, went as far as suggesting that a social care tax be levied on this group, arguing that since "these DINK families have no offspring when they get old, and they want to take up societal resources, they should be taxed in the future" (Liang 2018).

Conclusion

Throughout East Asia, fertility rates have continued to fall, leading demographers to describe the region as one marked by "ultra-low fertility" (Jones 2019). In response, governments in countries like China, South Korea, Japan, and Singapore have initiated a slew of new pronatalist policies and programs in the hopes of boosting national birth rates. This chapter suggests that such reconfigurations of national reproductive biopolitics are unavoidably constitutive of fertility figures and vice versa, as sociodemographic figuration processes come to be culturally embedded. Stuart Gietel-Basten and colleagues recently pointed to the dangers of pronatalist policies, pointing out that "by promoting the childrearing role of mothers while ignoring men's contribution, top-down pronatalist policies and discourses tend to reimpose conservative family and gender roles and reverse progress on gender equity and rights for sexual and gender minorities" (Gietel-Basten, Rotkirch, and Sobotka 2022: 2).

Yet, pronatalist policies and the campaigns that promote them are but one, albeit important, element in the shaping of figuration processes. While such policies and governmental programs are often underpinned by the prognostic work of demographers and economists as published in scientific publications, we must also pay attention to the films, viral videos, social media posts, novels, and news reports that are equally important conduits in forming and circulating the narratives, stories, and accounts that generate fertility figures. As demographic subjects, fertility figures are both representative of a "demographic" and inherently demographic in the ways that they come to be socioculturally mobilized in efforts to account for fertility change. And, although China's demo-dystopic figures are often stigmatized, at a more quotidian and populist level, they circulate more ambiguously, representing an increasingly shared sense of popular frustration with state policies and the everyday challenges of making a living, getting by, and being respected. Their perpetuation through social media, film, media reporting, political speeches, and more highlights a kind of "fertility penalty" being paid by young people who no longer feel they can take for granted having even one child, a sentiment that is barometric of a series of experienced losses, from financial to environmental. And, while the figuration processes I highlight in this chapter are particular to China, with its unique history of family planning, fertility figures are found wherever we might look for them, always situated within national reproductive biopolitics.

REFERENCES

Blair, Sampson Lee, Timothy J. Madigan, and Fang Fang. 2022. "'Bare Branches': Involuntary Bachelorhood in China in the 21st Century." In *Mate Selection in China: Causes and Consequences in the Search for a Spouse*, 135–48. Leeds: Emerald Publishing.

Braidotti, Rosi. 2014. "Writing as a Nomadic Subject." *Comparative Critical Studies* 11(2–3): 163–84.

Chen, Feinian, and Guangya Liu. 2009. "Population Aging in China." In *International Handbook of Population Aging*, ed. Peter Uhlenberg, 157–72. Dordrecht: Springer Netherlands.

Deng, Xiaoping. 1984 [1979]. *Selected Works of Deng Xiaoping (1975–1982)*. Beijing: Foreign Languages Press.

De Zordo, Silvia, Diana Marre, and Marcin Smietana. 2022. "Demographic Anxieties in the Age of 'Fertility Decline.'" *Medical Anthropology* 41(6–7): 591–99.

Escobar, Arturo. 1995. *Encountering Development: The Making and Unmaking of the Third World*. Princeton, NJ: Princeton University Press.

Fong, Vanessa L. 2004. *Only Hope: Coming of Age under China's One-Child Policy*. Stanford, CA: Stanford University Press.

Franklin, Sarah, and Celia Roberts. 2006. *Born and Made: An Ethnography of Preimplantation Genetic Diagnosis*. Princeton, NJ: Princeton University Press.

Gan, Nectar. 2022. "'We Are the Last Generation': China's Harsh Lockdowns Could Exacerbate Population Crisis." *CNN*, May 16. https://edition.cnn.com.

Gietel-Basten, Stuart, Anna Rotkirch, and Tomáš Sobotka. 2022. "Changing the Perspective on Low Birth Rates: Why Simplistic Solutions Won't Work." *BMJ* 379: e072670.

Greenhalgh, Susan, ed. 1995. *Situating Fertility: Anthropology and Demographic Inquiry*. Cambridge: Cambridge University Press.

———. 2008. *Just One Child: Science and Policy in Deng's China*. Berkeley: University of California Press.

———. 2014. "'Bare Sticks' and Other Dangers to the Social Body: Assembling Fatherhood in China." In *Globalized Fatherhood*, ed. Marcia C. Inhorn, Wendy Chavkin, and José-Alberto Navarro, 359–81. New York: Berghahn.

Greenhalgh, Susan, and Edwin A. Winckler. 2005. "Governing China's Population: From Leninist to Neoliberal Biopolitics." In *Governing China's Population*. Stanford, CA: Stanford University Press.

Gui, Tianhan. 2020. "'Leftover Women' or Single by Choice: Gender Role Negotiation of Single Professional Women in Contemporary China." *Journal of Family Issues* 41(11): 1956–78.

Guilmoto, Christophe Z. 2012. "Skewed Sex Ratios at Birth and Future Marriage Squeeze in China and India, 2005–2100." *Demography* 49(1): 77–100.

Hao, Jie (director). 2010. *Single Man*. Independent Film.

Haraway, Donna J. 1996. *Modest_Witness@Second_Millennium. FemaleMan_Meets_OncoMouse: Feminism and Technoscience*. London: Routledge.

———. 2016. *Staying with the Trouble: Making Kin in the Chthulucene*. Durham, NC: Duke University Press.

Homanen, Riikka, and Mianna Meskus. 2023. "Population Anxieties in Constituting Nordic Welfare State Futures: Affective Biopolitics in the Age of Environmental Crises." *BioSocieties*, March 28.

Huang, Tianqi. 2022. "Road of No Return: Uncertainty, Ambivalence, and Change in IVF Journeys in China." *Medical Anthropology* 41(6–7): 602–15.

Inhorn, Marcia C. 2023. *Motherhood on Ice: The Mating Gap and Why Women Freeze Their Eggs*. New York: New York University Press.

Jiang, Quanbao, Zhen Guo, Shuzhuo Li, and Marcus W. Feldman. 2013. "The Life Cycle of Bare Branch Families in China: A Simulation Study." *Canadian Studies in Population* 40(3–4): 134–48.

Jin, Xiaoyi, Lige Liu, Yan Li, Marcus W. Feldman, and Shuzhuo Li. 2014. "'Bare Branches' and the Marriage Market in Rural China." *Chinese Sociological Review* 46(1): 83–104.

Jones, Gavin W. 2019. "Ultra-low Fertility in East Asia: Policy Responses and Challenges." *Asian Population Studies* 15(2): 131–49.

Keimig, Rose K. 2021. *Growing Old in a New China: Transitions in Elder Care*. New Brunswick, NJ: Rutgers University Press.

Kvernflaten, Birgit, Peter Fedorcsák, and Kari Nyheim Solbrække. 2023. "It's All about Kids, Kids, Kids! Negotiating Reproductive Citizenship and Patient-Centred Care in 'Factory IVF.'" *BioSocieties* 18(2): 261–81.

"Let People Dare to Give Birth to 'Two Children.'" 2018. *People's Daily*, August 6.

Liang B. 2018. 政法大学教授：不仅要设生育基金 还要对丁克征税 [Professor at University of Political Science and Law: Not Only Should We Set Up a Birth Fund, but Also Tax DINKs]. *Sina News*, August 17. http://finance.sina.com.cn.

Nie, Jing-Bao. 2011. "Non-Medical Sex-Selective Abortion in China: Ethical and Public Policy Issues in the Context of 40 Million Missing Females." *British Medical Bulletin* 98(1): 7–20.

Ning, Nicholas. 2023. "Why Many 'Double Income, No Kids' Couples in China Don't Want Children." *ABC News*, May 20. www.abc.net.au.

Pak, Jennifer. 2021. "Chinese Citizens Greet New 3-Child Policy with Humor." *Marketplace*, June 21. www.marketplace.org.

Sasser, Jade S. 2018. *On Infertile Ground: Population Control and Women's Rights in the Era of Climate Change*. New York: New York University Press.

SK-II (director). 2016. *SK-II: Marriage Market Takeover*. April 6. www.youtube.com.

Sohu. 2019. 新的丁克一族正在兴起？几个95后新人的答案，很刷脑_孩子 [Is a New DINK Family on the Rise? The Answers of a Few Post-95 Newcomers Are Very Refreshing]. June 7. www.sohu.com.

Song, Jing, and Yingchun Ji. 2020. "Complexity of Chinese Family Life: Individualism, Familism, and Gender." *China Review* 20(2): 1–17.

Stevenson, Alexandra, and Zixu Wang. 2023. "China's Population Falls, Heralding a Demographic Crisis." *New York Times*, January 17. www.nytimes.com.

Wahlberg, Ayo. 2016. "The Birth and Routinization of IVF in China." *Reproductive BioMedicine and Society Online* 2: 97–107.

———. 2018. *Good Quality: The Routinization of Sperm Banking in China*. Oakland: University of California Press.

Wahlberg, Ayo, and Tine M. Gammeltoft, eds. 2018. *Selective Reproduction in the 21st Century*. New York: Springer International.

Wang, Hao. 2023. "China's National Health Commission Bans Single Women from Freezing Eggs: With or Without Legal and Ethical Justifications?" *Journal of Medical Ethics Blog*, May 8. https://blogs.bmj.com.

Wang, Serenitie, and Daniel Shane. 2019. "Jack Ma Endorses China's Controversial 12 Hours a Day, 6 Days a Week Work Culture." *CNN*, April 15. www.cnn.com.

Whittaker, Andrea. 2022. "Demodystopias: Narratives of Ultra-Low Fertility in Asia." *Economy and Society* 51(1): 116–37.

Winddance Twine, France. 2017. "The Fertility Continuum: Racism, Bio-Capitalism, and Post-Colonialism in the Transnational Surrogacy Industry." In *Babies for Sale? Transnational Surrogacy, Human Rights, and the Politics of Reproduction*, ed. Miranda Davies, 105–22. New York: Bloomsbury Academic & Professional.

"Working 12 Hours a Day, 6 Days a Week Is a 'Huge Bliss': Jack Ma Draws Controversy with Call for '996' Work Culture." 2019. *Straits Times*, April 12. www.straitstimes.com.

Wu, Cangping. 1980. Hengliang renkou fazhan he jingji fazhan xiang shiying de keguan biaojun [An Objective Criterion for Measuring the Conformity of Population Growth to Economic Development]. *Renkou Yanjiu* [Population Research] 1: 32–38.

Xi, Jinping. 2022. *Report to the 20th National Congress of the Communist Party of China*. People's Republic of China. https://english.www.gov.cn.

Xu, Huijing (director). 2013. *Mothers*. Icarus Films. https://icarusfilms.com.

Xu, Jing 2017. *The Good Child: Moral Development in a Chinese Preschool*. Stanford, CA: Stanford University Press.

Yeung, Wei-Jun Jean, Sonalde Desai, and Gavin W. Jones. 2018. "Families in Southeast and South Asia." *Annual Review of Sociology* 44: 469–95.

Zhou, X. 2019. 40岁"剩女"：期待爱情 也做好独自过一生的准备 [40-Year-Old "Leftover Woman": Looking Forward to Love and Preparing to Live Alone]. February 11. *SINA News*, https://news.sina.cn.

Zhu, Jianfeng, and Dong Dong. 2018. "From Quality Control to Informed Choice: Understanding 'Good Births' and Prenatal Genetic Testing in Contemporary Urban China." In *Handbook of Genomics, Health, and Society*, 2nd ed., ed. Sahra Gibbon, Barbara Prainsack, Stephen Hilgartner, and Janelle Lamoreaux, 47–54. London: Routledge.

7

Resilient Pronatalism

Reproductive Politics among Jews in Israel

DAPHNA BIRENBAUM-CARMELI

The state of Israel was founded in 1948. Over the course of its seventy-five years of existence, the country's population grew twelvefold, from eight hundred thousand people to ten million. Israel's current population density is 421 people per square kilometer, similar to that of India (World Population Review 2023). The respective average figure in Organization for Economic Cooperation and Development (OECD) countries is seventy-five. Israel has also changed dramatically in many other aspects since its founding. The state's political economy shifted from socialism to high capitalism; financially, it progressed from an underdeveloped to a wealthy, high-tech economy; culturally, Israel's population transformed from predominantly secular to increasingly religious. Israeli men and women became better educated and increasingly engaged in the paid labor market.

Reproduction has also changed radically, with immense shifts in fertility, as depicted in this chapter. Assisted reproductive technologies (ARTs), which have been developing since the late twentieth century, were swiftly adopted in Israel and proliferated throughout the country. Soon, Israeli women became the world's most intensive users of in vitro fertilization (IVF) and of intracytoplasmic sperm injection (ICSI), the technological procedure through which a sperm is inserted into an egg in vitro, effectively forcing fertilization, thereby resolving many cases of male subfertility. This endorsement of ARTs has also resulted in substantial changes in local reproductive practices, now including gamete and embryo freezing, donation, and storage in combination with various technologies based on the IVF platform, as well as surrogacy. And yet, throughout, and despite, these transformations, the local reproductive vernacular remains intact, especially among Jewish Israelis, invariably favoring large families and encouraging natality. In this chapter, I trace Israel's evolving reproductive discourse and what I call its *resilient pro-natalism* through illustrative moments in its formation, maintenance, and consistency over the decades.

Reproduction in Israel's Early Years

Since the inception of Zionism, reproduction has been closely associated with the survival of the Jewish people. Early Zionist leaders, such as Dr. Arthur Ruppin (1876–1943), who helped shape the Jewish prestate settlement in Palestine, considered low fertility a sign of national decay and called for increased Jewish reproduction (Stoller-Liss 2003). In these prestate years of the 1920s and 1930s, however, Jewish families in the region significantly downsized from an average of 3.7 children to 2.1 (in 1938–1941), while Muslim women in Palestine had 9.42 children on average (1943–1954). With the British mandate's limits on Jewish migration and in the wake of the Holocaust, low Jewish fertility was construed as a "demographic threat" that called for prioritizing national demographic considerations over individuals' reproductive desires. Starting in 1943, national committees were formed with the explicit goal of encouraging natality among Jewish women. State campaigns emphasized the mental harm that single children sustain due to a lack of siblings and condemned women with few children as frivolous and egoistic, neglecting their crucial maternal contribution to the nation-building project.

Soon after the state of Israel was founded, it started awarding prizes to "heroine mothers" giving birth to their tenth child. Ironically, a local opponent to the prize emphasized that, rather than few families of ten, "We are interested in the third, fourth, and fifth child in every family in Israel." Another expert, in her mothers' guidebook, explained, "Every family should have at least three children: two, to account for the parents and the rest, for the fortification of the family and the race" (Miriam Aharonova, cited in Stoller-Liss 2003).

In 1954, the state formed its first social benefit: a twelve-week paid maternity leave. In the 1960s, it established the Natality Committee (1962) and the Demographic Center (1968) to encourage local Jewish reproduction, for "an increase in natality in Israel is crucial for the future

Figure 1. Total Fertility Rate (TFR) in Israel, by religion

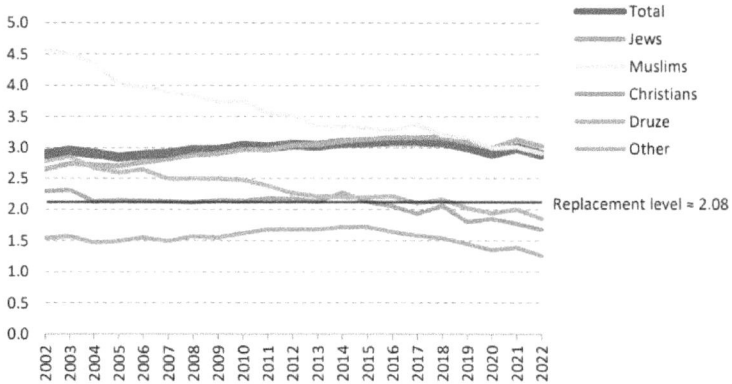

Source: Alex Weinreb, Taub Center | Data: CBS

Figure 7.1. Total Fertility Rate by Religious Group, 2002–2022. Credit: Alex Weinreb, Taub Center, Data: CBS, *Singer Annual Report Series State of the Nation Report: Society, Economy and Policy*, 2023.

of the whole Jewish people" (Doron and Kramer 1992; see also Barkai 1998; Portugese 1998).

At the same time, local Arab communities were experiencing major reproductive changes (see figure 7.1). As women's level of education and age at marriage rose and as more Arab women joined the paid labor force, women raised dramatically smaller families, moving from roughly 7.5 children per Druze woman and 4.8 among Christian women to two children per woman in the 2010s. Among Muslim women the shift was even starker, declining from an average of 9.4 children per woman in the 1960s to three today. Between 2002 and 2021, Arab women have decreased their families' sizes by about one-third, from 4.19 to 2.85 children per woman (Israel Central Bureau of Statistics 2022b). ARTs play a significant role in this downsizing. In the past few years, some Arab couples in Israel have resorted to ARTs in order to reconcile their plans for small families with their desires for sons (see Inhorn, chapter 1). Some Israeli Arab couples travel to the Palestinian Authority to pursue sex selection by means of IVF (which is illegal in Israel, with few, highly monitored exceptions). Using this advanced technology, despite having no reproductive impairment, these Arab couples technologically ensure the birth of sons without taking the "risk" of having large families. Says one Arab woman, "I don't want to end up like my mother, who had six daughters before she had a son" (Memmi 2012). Meanwhile this practice also contributes to the shrinking size of Israeli Arab families.

Assisted Reproduction and Resilient Pronatalism

The Jewish reproductive landscape is altogether different. Starting with a decline from 3.5 to 2.6 children per woman, between 1960 and the mid-1990s, Jewish women in Israel reversed course, with fertility levels rising by 19 percent, from 2.64 in 2002 to 3.13 in 2021 (Israel Central Bureau of Statistics 2022b). Today, despite a small decline of unclear significance, the fertility rate of Jewish Israelis is twice that of the OECD average—3.03 versus 1.65 children per woman.

Jewish pronatalism is commonly attributed to several factors: the Jewish commandment to "be fruitful and multiply," the Holocaust trauma that has conferred on Jewish reproduction heightened collective significance, and the view of childbearing as a way to alleviate fears of a minority population in a perennial regional war situation (Kahn 2000). Jewish population growth was thus constituted as a symbol of vitality for both the individual and the nation, a contribution to national revival, and a mode of self-realization.

The Israeli state has welcomed and actively supported ARTs since its early days, when the country's population included roughly two million people. In the late 1950s, Bruno Lunenfeld, an Israeli gynecologist and endocrinologist, played a key scientific and logistical role in the development of Pergonal, a potent fertility drug produced by Serono, the Swiss-Italian pharmaceutical company (Vertommen 2017). As part of Israel's involvement in the process, the Prime Minister's Office—notably, not the Ministry of Health—started to fund the drug for all Israeli women who needed it, as soon as it became available. Israel's population at that time included roughly two million people.

In the 1970s and 1980s, when IVF appeared on the reproductive scene, Israel was among its pioneer users. The first local "test tube baby," born in 1982, was the world's fifth (Birenbaum-Carmeli 2004). Soon, IVF proliferated throughout the country. Treatment was offered as part of the national health insurance and did not entail any payment or waiting. Women up to the age of forty-five, irrespective of their family status or sexual orientation, were eligible for treatment until they had two children with their current partner, if relevant, even if they had children from previous relationships. Preserved embryos could be transferred until the woman turned fifty-four. Treatment for the third child was funded by basic private health insurance. Israel's population in the early days of IVF was four million people, less than half its current size.

This generous funding underlies the exceptional use of the technology in Israel, which tops the list of world IVF consumption. Israeli women undergo roughly twice as many cycles as women in the second country on the list, usually one of the Scandinavian countries (Birenbaum-Carmeli 2016). IVF has also been normalized as a routine pathway to family founding. In a study of Israeli women undergoing IVF, 86 percent of the respondents replied to the open question, "How many treatment cycles would you be ready to undergo?" with, "As many as needed" (Birenbaum-Carmeli and Dirnfeld 2008). Newspaper articles praising women who have conceived after numerous IVF cycles enhanced their perseverance.

During the mid-1990s, Israel's ART sector underwent a major change, with the introduction of ICSI. As soon as ICSI became available, it received full funding and was added to standard IVF treatments in Israel. At this time, the number of IVF cycles nearly doubled (Birenbaum-Carmeli 2016), reflecting the expansion of IVF-ICSI as a treatment for male infertility.

With the rise of ARTs, reproduction has become even more prominent and presumably universal. In casual encounters, the question, "How many children do you have?" is posed directly, without first ensuring that the person has children at all. Women might be asked openly why they have only one child or "What are you waiting for?" even by strangers. Mothers of two, like myself, might also be asked, "Where is the third?"

Born and raised in Tel Aviv, I shared the pronatalist sentiment—and imperative—as did my friends, who graduated from universities and started working in the late 1990s, in demanding fields like medicine, computer science, law, psychology, and engineering. The desire to have children was universal and taken for granted. All but two of my friends had children in their late twenties. The remaining two underwent IVF and eventually gave birth to two and three children. The only exception was one friend who became a meditation guru in her twenties and disconnected from her previous social circles. None of my cohort of friends and further acquaintances has expressed doubts about becoming a parent, in any of our endless talks.

Childlessness was assumed to be not only involuntary but an utmost grief that justified every effort to overcome it. The idea of not wanting to have children—we have not known "such people" personally—was synonymous with egoism or mental disturbance. Adoption, of any kind, was present vaguely as an abstract option. All of my friends from high school, compulsory military service, and university have had children, most commonly, three. In several second-marriage families, the number rose to four. Two friends became single mothers, with one child each. I was among the very last to have children, following IVF, in the mid-1990s.

The history of the song "Children Are Joy, Children Are Blessing" encapsulates Israel's social climate. The song was first aired in 1976, when Israel's population was 3.3 million. Though its lyrics were intended to be an ironic commentary on the high local fertility, the song's significance was soon overlooked, and it became an anthem for large families, often sung at family celebrations and public events. The title has acquired a proverbial quality. Its representation of parenthood as life's paramount experience supersedes heteronormative families. Nearly fifty years after its release, in the 2014 Tel Aviv gay parade, "Children Are Joy, Children Are Blessing" was selected as the event's song, accompanying the parade's theme of "rainbow family life and equality." The special cover, produced for the event, was performed by famous Israeli transgender singer Dana International, thereby transgressing traditional boundaries of family, sexual orientation, and gender while at the same time performing from the familiar hymn book of compulsory procreative allegiance to the national fertility code.

Meanwhile, the 1990s also saw a large wave of Jewish emigration from the Former Soviet Union (FSU), heading primarily to the United States and Israel. The newcomers landed with just over one child per woman, on average. However, in the subsequent years, their fertility rates changed. About a decade after immigration, in 2000–2001, Jewish FSU immigrants in the United States had 1.21 children on average

TABLE 7.1. Fertility among FSU Immigrants and Jewish Women in Israel. Credit: Extrapolated from Konstantinov (2014: 16)

	FSU Immigrants			Jewish Women in Israel
	1991	2001	2013	2013
Birth rate per 1,000 women aged 15–49	35.6	45.4	60.3	89.4
TFR	1.31	1.56	1.95	3.11
		1.21 in the USA		

(Konstantinov 2014: 16). In Israel, the comparable figure was 1.56 (see table 7.1), suggesting that the environment might have influenced the immigrants' reproductive practices. By the year 2013, FSU immigrants in Israel had further enlarged their families to nearly two children each. Overall, the fertility rate of Jewish FSU immigrants in Israel, although still much lower than that of native Jewish Israeli women, increased by roughly 50 percent in the two decades following immigration.

This rise in fertility among immigrants to Israel was in line with the trend among the local native Jewish women, whose fertility rate rose by 19 percent between 1992 and 2015, from 2.64 to 3.13 (Israel Central Bureau of Statistics 2022b).

This pronatalist discourse remains vibrant in the new millennium. Several years ago, in the mid-2010s, seated in a car trapped in a traffic jam, with a highly educated family relative in his forties, I uttered, "Now imagine, in thirty years, next to every car lined up on the road, another car waiting." "Why would there be twice the cars?" he asked. "Because you have four children," I replied. My answer was met with dismissive silence. In Israel, it seems, one version of reproductive cause and effect—the role of fertility in nation building—is incompatible with another version of this same logic, that more children will mean more people. Several years later, in a professional meeting, a lawyer said off-record, "Ah, it's my dream to own a senior home; for the next fifty years, you'll have no worries, just more and more clients." I said, "Yes, but the same applies for kindergartens." Lumping the elderly together with children, my response was politely disregarded with what seemed like resentment. Shortly afterward, at an academic conference held in

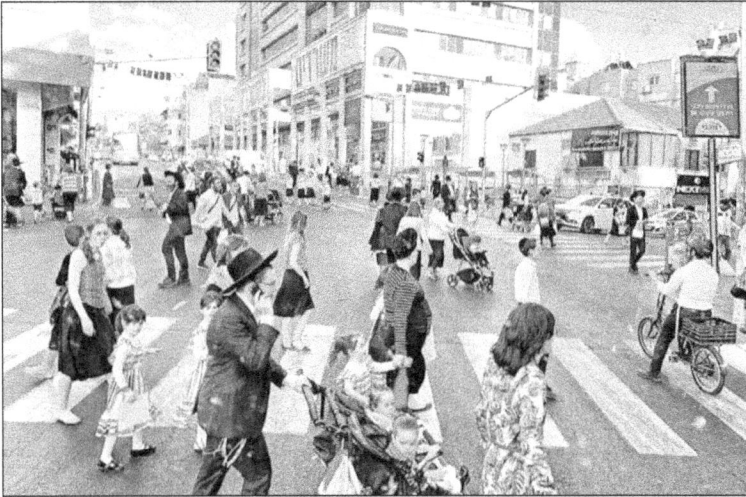

Figure 7.2. An Orthodox City Street in Israel

Israel, I mentioned that Israel's fertility rate was exceptional. The director of the hosting university started applauding, taking pride in the local fertility levels, and was soon joined by numerous members of the audience, students and professors alike. Lastly, a thirty-nine-year-old woman, who married at thirty-five and had three children, described her great hope to have a fourth child. When I gently raised the demographic concern, she smiled lightheartedly. "Look, it may not work [i.e., we may not succeed in having a fourth child], I don't know, but surely, demography won't be the reason."

In religious communities in Israel, the importance of parenthood is even greater. With roughly five children per woman in Israel's national-religious communities and nearly seven children per woman in Orthodox communities, these reproductive patterns are visible in towns and neighborhoods, where parents walk with baby strollers and groups of children in greater numbers than anywhere else (see figure 7.2). Personally, I face it in admission interviews with candidates for graduate programs in my own department of nursing. In these one-on-one encounters, every religious candidate, male or female, opens their self-presentations saying, "My name is ——, I am —— years old, and I have 2-3-4-5 lovely children," or else, ". . . and I don't yet have children." Recently, in my master's program class, there were two students in their

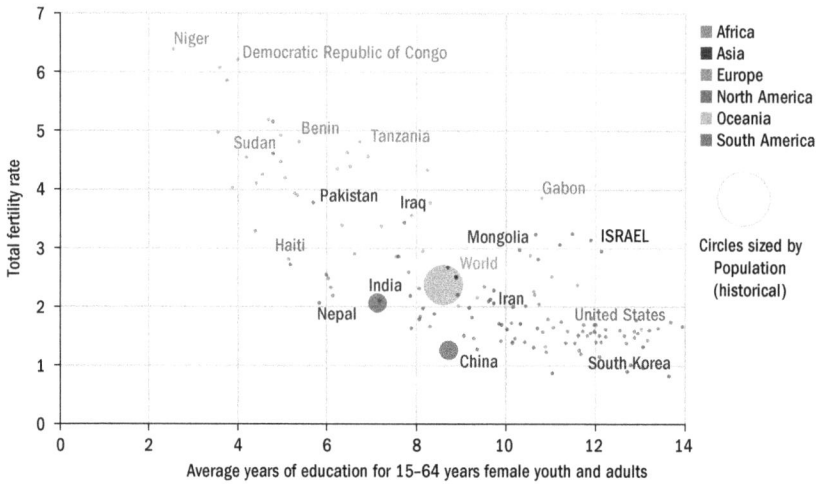

Figure 7.3. Women's Educational Attainment vs. Fertility, 2020. Credit: Our World in Data (n.d.).

midforties, one with eleven and one with thirteen children. Each had several grandchildren, and both were working full-time as midwives. For these religious Jewish nurses, parenthood is the supreme moral virtue. In the words of one graduate student, "This is our role, to bring as many souls as possible into the world."

Current reproductive practices of Israeli Jewish women are a world exception. They challenge circulating notions regarding direct links between women's employment and childbearing. Israeli women are highly educated. In 2018, Israeli women ranked third in the OECD in the local percentage of female population that has attained tertiary education (OECD 2019: Chart CO3.1.B). Also, in terms of labor market participation, Israeli women rank high, just below Norway (58.52 vs. 60.29) and above the United Kingdom (58.04), Germany (57.72), and Denmark (56.84). Among G7 countries, Israeli women's labor market participation is the third highest (Global Economy 2022). Even women's share in managerial positions in Israel is above the OECD (2022) average. Still, Israeli women have twice as many children as their European counterparts (see figure 7.3), standing out as a world reproductive outlier (Birenbaum-Carmeli 2021).

The accepted explanations of Israel's pronatalism, which focus on the religious commandment, Holocaust trauma, and regional security concerns, seem insufficient when fertility levels of Israel's Jewish women are juxtaposed with those of Jewish women in the United States, the world's second-largest Jewish community. The comparison reveals that at every level of religiosity, Jewish women have more children in Israel than in the United States (see table 7.2).

Israel's media has played an important role in maintaining this reproductive discourse, praising professionally accomplished mothers of numerous children. Dr. Naama Constantini, for instance, a female physician, head of sports medicine at the Tel Aviv University, and chair of the National Council for Women's Health at the Ministry of Health, has seven children with her husband, head of Pediatric Neurosurgery at Tel Aviv Medical Center, both secular Jewish doctors. In 2005, when Israel's population was approaching seven million with a population density of more than three hundred people per square kilometer—the OECD respective figure was thirty-five at the time—Dr. Constantini was cited in a newspaper interview: "We decided to have twelve children, but I was not quick enough. I wanted as many children as possible because I love children so much. If there is anything I am missing in my life, it's more children. We are all very close to each other. My mother has twenty-three grandchildren, and I grew up feeling that there is nothing like a close, supportive family. I, too, wanted this joy!" (Kroll 2005).

Moreover, Dr. Hanna Katan, an Orthodox female gynecologist specializing in fertility, is mother of thirteen. In a Passover interview in the country's most widely read daily, Dr. Katan stressed the precedence of family over career (Farkash 2009). She highlighted the advantages of large families over small families, saying that large families provide children with ample attention and support from siblings and allow them to

TABLE 7.2. Total Fertility Rates in Jewish Communities in the United States and Israel by Religiosity. Credit: *Pew Forum (2013: 35–46); ** Konstantinov 2015, p. 16

Difference (number of children)	Israel**	United States*	Total Fertility Rate
+1.0	3.17	2.1	Jewish average
+0.6	2.3 (secular)	1.7	Reform Jewish
+2.4	4.2 (religious)	1.8	Conservative
+3.0	7.1	4.1	Orthodox

develop social skills of cooperation and mutual consideration (Farkash 2009). She added, as a clinician, that being pregnant repeatedly "contributes immensely to the woman's body, as these women have lower rates of uterine, ovarian and breast cancers." The doctor described "Orthodox women with eight children, weeping in the clinic for not being able to conceive their ninth baby." She naturalized the desire for children, contending that the commandment to "be fruitful and multiply" is addressed to the man (not to the woman) because women have an innate desire for children. Dr. Katan ended the interview with (unspecified) studies' findings showing that older couples regret not having more children: "Only when we grow older, when the life race and career are behind us, do we realize the importance of the next generation. Not for the state, but for egoistic reasons, for children are truly a joy."

In 2011, Israel's population rose to 7.5 million. The advisor to the minister of the treasury published an article entitled "A Family with Eight Children Is a Sin" (Simhon 2011). The author, a professor of economics at Hebrew University, claimed that Israel's economy was still lagging behind those of similar, prosperous European economies because of its exceptional fertility and concluded, "The current government has performed important reforms. . . . But these changes are not enough to close the gap between us and the developed world, as long as we fail to convince, through open inter-sectorial dialog, that a woman who bears eight children sins against her own children and the entire society. . . . If only our leaders and opinion makers dare to raise the problem in its full force" (Simhon 2011). The article was attacked fiercely. In Israel's main Orthodox daily, a rabbi compared the author's proposition to Hitler's Final Solution and to

> hostile propaganda, familiar from dark regimes in history, that made a fascist demand to oppress the natural growth of the Jewish people, for the sake of the country. . . . It is well known that in all Haredi communities one meets thousands of families blessed with eight or more children . . . who will never appear in criminal records or in the vacuous world of secular youths, many of whom are gradually losing their human shape. . . . The reality is that Orthodox families with eight children enjoy much more gratification (*nahat*) from their offspring, for long years, much more than secular families of two or three children (and a dog) . . .

where children quickly turn their backs on their parents, contemptibly rejecting any value or ideal. (Globes Service 2011)

The centrality of parenthood persists in secular circles as well. As recently as 2016, the cover page of the holiday supplement of Israel's most widely read daily featured Geula Even, a forty-four-year-old esteemed television journalist, who had recently married a prominent Israeli politician. Even's interview was prompted by her front-page photograph, at the end of her fifth pregnancy, highlighting her beauty (see figure 7.4). Even was cited saying, "I've always envied large families. I admire women who have so many children. I literally worship any woman who manages to cope with such a hard and demanding work, especially those who have a career as well. . . . I hope so much we have more children, that we manage to make it" (Shir 2016).

Until the mid-2010s, I shared the pronatalist mindset of my fellow Israeli women and men and focused my research on the agony of individuals and couples who were struggling with infertility. In 2016, I was approached by Alon Tal, an Israeli professor of social policy, whom I had not known previously. Professor Tal invited me to join the Forum for Demography, Society, and Environment, which he was founding at that time. Embarrassing as it is for me to admit this, it was only at the forum's first meetings that I realized Israel's demographic outlook and the implications of its resilient pronatalism. For the first time, I was shocked to realize that the presumably small number of people added annually to the country's population was contributing to a colossal demographic problem.

Israel: Present and Future

Three times a year, on the festive occasions of the Jewish New Year, January 1, and Israel's Independence Day, all local media channels inform the public about the number of babies born, the number of incoming immigrants—all strictly Jewish—and the general growth of Israel's population that year. These figures are celebrated as evidence of national prosperity and success. Fertility treatments, including IVF and ICSI, are still being provided according to the rules of eligibility formed over four decades ago, leaving Israeli women in their place at the top of the world's

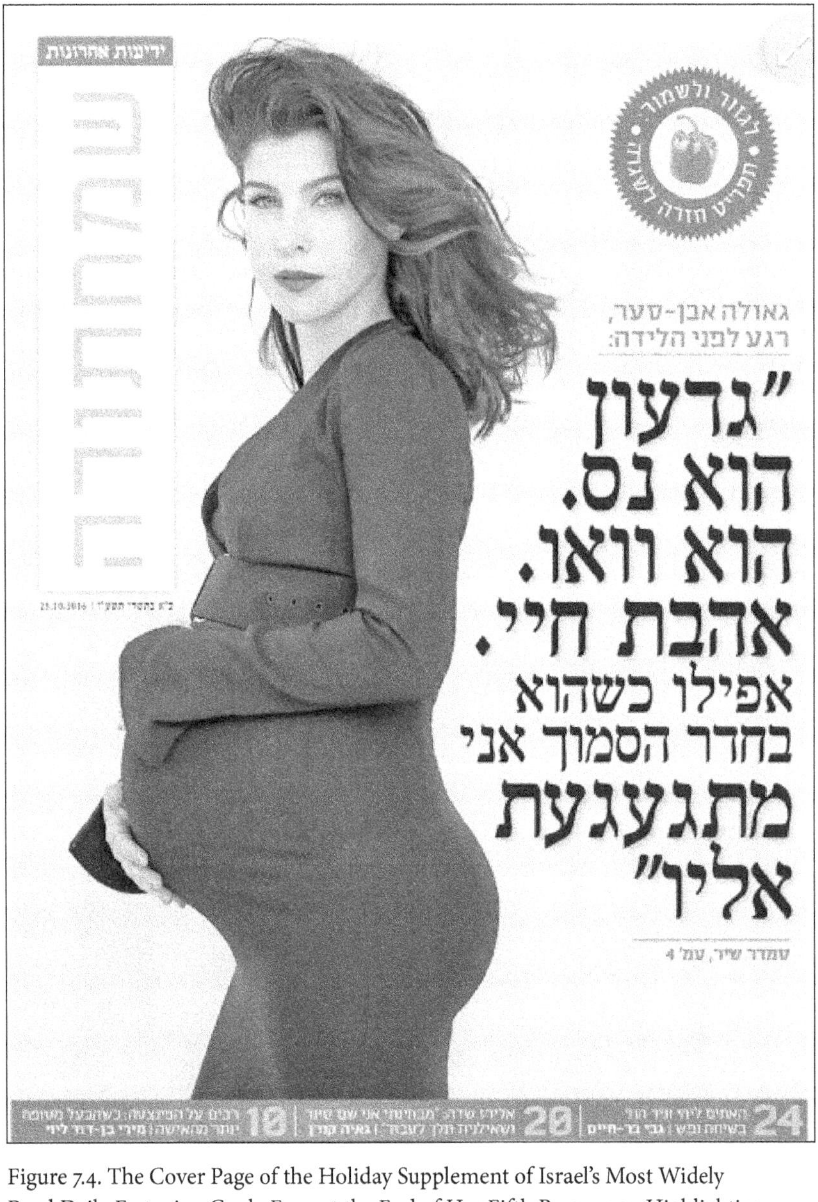

Figure 7.4. The Cover Page of the Holiday Supplement of Israel's Most Widely Read Daily Featuring Geula Even at the End of Her Fifth Pregnancy, Highlighting Her Beauty

users of the technologies. In many cases, women who marry relatively late use IVF in order to conceive their second or third child.

In the past few years, as the fertility reduction in developed nations has become more visible in the media, Israel's exceptional natality has gained even more public and media attention. In Israel's main nationalist-Orthodox daily, a rabbi (Navon 2021) asserted that "Europe is declining as a world force due to its shrinking population." He then cited the sorrowful pondering of a scholar asking "whether we are returning to a world wherein we'll have to consider euthanasia, encouragement of suicide, and terminating the lives of the elderly . . . [Israel, in contrast,] benefits from the Jewish birth miracle. . . . It is therefore painful to see that some people describe Israel's birth rate as a problem. . . . [A] people without children is a people that does not believe in its future, and vice versa regarding a people that loves children" (Navon 2021). Another article in the same nationalist-religious daily (Speiser 2022) investigated the link between fertility and the future of humanity. Juxtaposing Malthusian approaches with those that foresee the end of the world due to "frozen population growth," the authors ended with a citation of Elon Musk: "If people do not reproduce, society is going to crumble, remember my words."

Such perspectives hold firm ground also beyond religious circles. In an interview in Israel's most widely read newspaper (Zaga 2021), "Little Michal," a secular thirty-nine-year-old "entertainment empire with 3-4-5 shows a day, and mother of six," told her readers, "I want as many children as I can have, the more the better, whatever God gives me." A photo from the delivery room portrayed the good-looking career woman with her partner and their sixth child (see figure 7.5).

Having many children has remained a sign of moral virtue in Israel, across all social strata. In the liberal newspaper *Haaretz*, a recent headline declared, "Yaara is our sixth child. When she invites me to a trek with her, it's an honor" (Frank 2022). The speaker then explains that his wife, a physician, wanted six children, "probably because she is a daughter of Holocaust survivors." Both parents are secular, the daughter is highly ecologically aware, and the whole family is vegan.

Among my own relatives and friends, there are seven female physicians with three, four, or five children each. Each of these active and

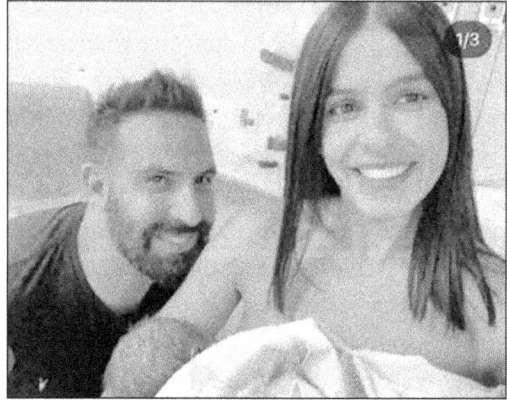

Figure 7.5. A Photo from the Delivery Room of "Little Michal," with Her Partner and Their Sixth Child

successful female physicians presents her large family as embodying her deep love of children. When I asked one mother of five how many children her two daughters, a doctor and a psychology student, were planning to have, she dismissed my question laughingly: "Birth control is not popular in our family." Although the environmentally conscious members of these upper-middle-class families recycle their waste, avoid disposable plasticware, and try to use clean energy, they, too, appear to share a carefully blinkered model of reproductive cause and effect. Having a large family continues to be perceived as achieving a singular moral virtue, while also fulfilling an existential duty, serving a public cause, and displaying the family's wealth. Such an ability to detach the nation's expansive reproductive orientation from its economic or environmental implications, and eventually, from its potentially debilitating influences on the lives of one's own offspring, prevails in Israel, also among couples living in the countryside as part of "returning to nature." Often, the incongruency is not consciously recognized, due to the limited capacity to acknowledge the environmental implications of natality.

In recent years, especially in the wake of COVID-19, local fertility has started to intrude more palpably into daily life. Israel's roads have become the most congested in the Western world, with an average driving speed of eleven kilometers per hour during rush hours (Dori 2016). Housing prices have more than doubled in the past decade. In 2022, Tel Aviv became the world's most expensive city, rendering it inaccessible to most of the country's population. One-third of Israel's children and more than half of Jerusalem's children live in poverty. Israel's education system is the most unequal in the OECD. Classes are crowded and students' achievements are deteriorating (Ben-Dor 2021). The land is literally full: visitors to national parks need to make early reservations. By the sea, every Israeli has an average of one centimeter of shoreline. Israel has become the third densest country in the OECD, after Korea and the Netherlands, but unlike these two low-fertility countries, Israel's population keeps growing. In 2065, Israel is predicted to reach 20 million people (Israel Central Bureau of Statistics 2017), roughly 922 people per square kilometer. The corresponding OECD figure is thirty-nine. Even if fertility rates declined to replacement level, much of this growth could not be halted because, as one demographer had explained, "The mothers have already been born."

The first signs of a change in perceptions of mandatory high fertility among Jewish Israelis may, however, be appearing. In the Israeli press, writers are beginning to associate infrastructure problems with unchecked reproduction. Challenges previously attributed to administrative causes, such as slow urban planning,[1] and construction or large classes and teachers' low salaries, are being increasingly contextualized within the country's steep population growth. Some well-educated secular Jewish Israelis are expressing doubt about having children.

Mainstream media sources are publishing articles with titles such as "Natality, Israel's Great and Silenced Problem" (Soreq 2021), "Such an Obvious National Suicide Is Something I Have Never Seen" (Perry 2022), or "Children Are Joy, but Have We Gone Too Far? The Giant Israeli Experiment of End Unknown" (Broitman 2022). The local fertility rate was called "unsustainable," "irreversible" (Broitman 2022), and "suicidal" (Perry 2022). Writers stress that "parents who care about their children's future should limit themselves to two children and rejoice in them," explaining that natality is "an acute problem that overshadows any other local problem" (Soreq 2021). Authors are protesting the silencing of the problem by scientists and politicians and politicizing the issue: "The more the Orthodox continue to give birth, while remaining segregated, withdrawn, and lacking general education, the greater the pool of right-wing voters" (Arlozorov 2022). A foreign correspondent commented, "Anyone who dares to raise the issue [of fertility] runs the risk of being accused of anti-Semitism" (Perry 2022).

Total Fertility Rate (TFR) of Jewish and Other Women, by Level of Religiosity, 1990–2021

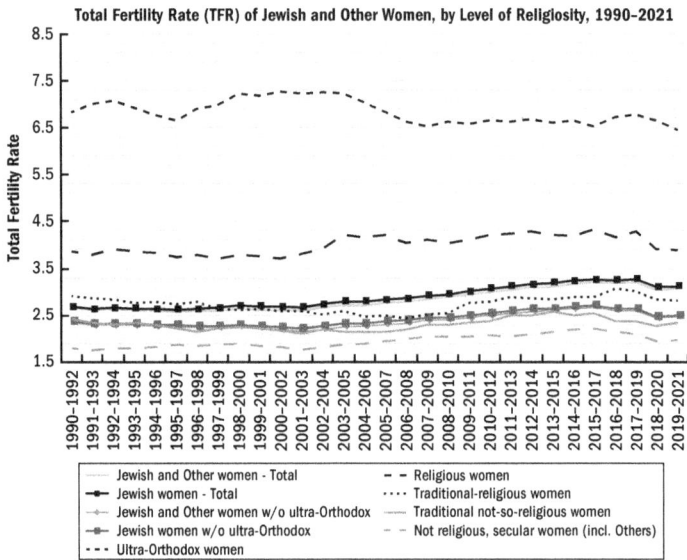

Figure 7.6. Total Fertility Rate of Jewish Women in Israel by Religiosity, 1990–2021.
Source: Israel Central Bureau of Statistics. 2022b. www.cbs.gov.il

Signs of debate surface at the practical level as well. In the 2021 discussions of Israel's Health Basket Committee, the proposal to fund egg
freezing due to nonmedical reasons was ranked as the lowest priority
and was therefore denied any public subsidy (Birenbaum-Carmeli 2023).
In the opposite direction, a year later, the same committee approved
IVF funding for male individuals or couples who undertake domestic
surrogacy (Efrati 2023). In February 2023, when the first baby was born
to a gay couple following domestic surrogacy, the main television news
edition stated, "One third of adult gay and lesbian couples in Israel have
children." Pronatalism is implied also more tacitly. For instance, on the
website of the association of the senior academic staff of Israeli universities, the standard travel insurance form lists, after the applicant's details
and their partner's, a list: Child 1, Child 2, Child 3, Child 4. On the other
hand, in a Zoom lecture to nine Israeli high-tech professional women
between the ages of thirty-four and thirty-six, only one participant had
children while the others were either hesitant about or resistant to motherhood. At the macro level, between 2018 and 2020, the total fertility
rate of Jewish Israeli women declined from 3.17 to 3.00. However, one

year later, in 2021, the figure rose again to 3.13 (Israel Central Bureau of Statistics 2022b). Possibly, the decline was linked to the COVID-19 pandemic. Regardless, among Orthodox women the figure has been relatively stable over the last decade with just under seven children per woman (Israel Central Bureau of Statistics 2022a).

From a different perspective, the right to parenthood—and even to grandparenthood—has been enshrined in pronatalist Israel, to a degree that at times counters children's best interests, highlighting the intergenerational factor as formative in Israel's resilient pronatalism.

Conclusion

Israel's resilient pronatalism acquires a particular manifestation in every local sector. Orthodox families willingly live in economic poverty for the sake of the esteemed virtue of raising families with seven children. Families with a nationalist religious conviction, who seek a somewhat higher standard of living, may choose to live as settlers in the Occupied West Bank, where housing is dramatically less expensive than elsewhere in Israel, so they can raise families of four to five children. Israeli women who start their families somewhat later often rely on state-funded ART in order to conceive. Women in their midthirties, without reproductive partners, increasingly undertake elective egg freezing, aiming to create an option for future parenthood. Israel's new reproductive order is thus rooted in its resilient pronatalism, but it expands even more broadly with the aid of ARTs, including both heterosexual and gay couples who can resort to domestic surrogacy, and unpartnered women and those who marry late, who make use of funded IVF or increasingly affordable egg freezing. In contrast, local Arab parents can opt for pre-implantation genetic diagnosis in order to ensure the birth of a son while keeping the family size small.

This resilient pronatalism fundamentally shapes Israeli reality. In the upcoming decades, working Israelis will have to provide for more children and simultaneously fund costly, intrusive IVF and ICSI, via the state. Furthermore, vast reproductive gaps among Israeli subpopulations mean that the more religious the sector, the more children they have and the faster it expands. The political map largely reflects these consistent differences. Following the November 1, 2022, elections, Israel's ruling coalition consisted, for the first time in the country's history, solely of religious and right-wing parties, all associated with the more observant-religious strata. Evidently, pronatalism is but one factor in the ongoing historical change. Still, it embodies the formative macrosocial impact that reproductive patterns may have under certain circumstances.

On a personal note, I must add that internalizing the demographic-reproductive concern is somewhat saddening for me. Becoming aware of Israel's demographic reality has modified my understanding. It has not changed, however, my memories or the environment I inhabit. Orthodox families of eight or twelve children are beyond my social circle and probably, therefore, beyond my emotional imagination. However, Israeli middle-class families of three or four children, whose homes are filled with children of various ages, are a reality I am used to appreciating, loving, and, yes, at times also envying. The vision of a two-child family, like my own, which is a perfect family in most of the developed world, feels, in Israel, small. At the macrosocial level, it is one more ecological toll that my wasteful generation has inflicted on its offspring.

In the year 2023, Israel faced two major crises: the internal political struggle over the country's democratic-Jewish character, followed by the October Hamas attack and subsequent war in Gaza. The ties between the political-military upheaval and the varying rates of fertility in different Jewish subpopulations in Israel can be read as a cause and probably also an effect of these stormy events. The social and political significance of these reproduction patterns will unfold in the coming years, as Israel paves its rocky road into the future.

NOTE

1 The majority of land in Israel is state owned and therefore depends on state funding to be released for construction.

REFERENCES

Arlozorov, Meirav. 2022. "The Future Is Here and It Does Not Look Promising: Haredi Demography Beats Israel." *The Marker*, November 3. www.themarker.com. [In Hebrew.]

Barkai, Haim. 1998. *The Evolution of Israel's Social Security System: Structure, Time Pattern, and Macroeconomic Impact.* Aldershot, UK: Ashgate.

Ben-Dor, Dan. 2021. "2021 Shoresh Guidebook." Shoresh Institution for Socioeconomic Research. https://shoresh.institute/. [In Hebrew.]

Birenbaum-Carmeli, Daphna. 2004. "'Cheaper Than a Newcomer': On the Political Economy of IVF in Israel." *Sociology of Health and Illness* 26(7): 897–924.

———. 2016. "Thirty-Five Years of Assisted Reproductive Technologies in Israel." *Reproductive BioMedicine and Society Online* 14(2): 16–23.

———. 2021. "Israeli Demography: A Composite Portrait of a Reproductive Outlier." *Israel Affairs* 27(6): 1053–81.

———. 2023. "Too Much Equity—Is There Such a Thing? The Public Discourse Surrounding Elective Egg Freezing Subsidy in Israel." *International Journal of Equity Health* 22(34). https://doi.org/10.1186/s12939-023-01831-8.

Birenbaum-Carmeli, Daphna, and Martha Dirnfeld. 2008. "In Vitro Fertilisation Policy in Israel and Women's Perspectives: The More the Better?" *Reproductive Health Matters* 16(31): 182–91.

Broitman, Doron. 2022. "'Children Are Joy, but Have We Possibly Gone Too Far?': The Giant Israeli Experiment Whose Consequences No One Can Foresee." *Calcalist*, January 14. www.calcalist.co.il. [In Hebrew.]

Dori, Oren. 2016. "11 Km/h and That's Just the Beginning: The Numbers behind the Transportation Catastrophe." *The Marker*, September 12. www.themarker.com. [In Hebrew.]

Doron, Avraham, and Ralph M. Kramer. 1992. *The Welfare State in Israel: The Evolution of Social Security Policy and Practice*. Boulder, CO: Westview Press.

Efrati, Ido. 2023. "The 2023 Health Basket: 350 Million Shekels Worth of Advanced Cancer Treatments and Children's Eyeglasses." *Haaretz*, January 18. www.haaretz.co.il. [In Hebrew.]

Farkash, Tali. 2009. "Easy for Her." *Ynet*, April 4. www.ynet.co.il. [In Hebrew.]

Frank, Dana. 2022. "Yaara Is Our Sixth Child: When She Invites Me on a Trip, It's a Great Honor." *Haaretz*, December 8. www.haaretz.co.il. [In Hebrew.]

The Global Economy. 2022. "Female Labor Force Participation: Country Rankings." www.theglobaleconomy.com.

Globes Service. 2011. "'*Yated Ne'eman*': Avi Simhon Proposes a 'Final Solution'—Eliminating Ultra-Orthodox Births." December 29. www.globes.co.il. [In Hebrew.]

Israel Central Bureau of Statistics. 2017. "Projections of Israel Population until 2065." May 21. www.cbs.gov.il.

———. 2022a. "Age-Specific Fertility Rates and Total Fertility Rate: Jewish Women—Ultra-Orthodox," Table 3. www.cbs.gov.il.

———. 2022b. "Live Births—Main Indicators, 2002–2021." www.cbs.gov.il.

Kahn, Susan Martha. 2000. *Reproducing Jews: A Cultural Account of Assisted Conception in Israel*. Durham, NC: Duke University Press.

Konstantinov, Vaclav. 2015. *Trends in FSU Immigrants' Integration in Israel over the Last Two Decades*. Jerusalem: Myers Brookdale JDC.

Kroll, Aviva. 2005. "A Phenomenon: The Top Decile No Longer Finds Two Children and a Dog Satisfactory, Not at All!" *Globes*, May 15. www.globes.co.il. [In Hebrew.]

Memmi, Sarah. 2012. "Sex Selection in Palestinian Society: A Pilot Study." *Lancet* 380, Supp. 1: S41.

Navon, Chaim. 2021. "'A Nation That Dwelleth Alone': The Nationalist Path Has Led Israel to Worldwide Success." *Makor Rishon*, April 14. www.makorrishon.co.il. [In Hebrew.]

OECD. 2019. "CO3.1: Educational Attainment by Gender." September. www.oecd.org.

———. 2022. "LMF1.6: Gender Differences in Employment." www.oecd.org.

Our World in Data. N.d. ""Women's Educational Attainment versus Ferility Rates, 1950–2020." www.ourworldindata.org, accessed September 7, 2024.

Perry, Dan. 2022. "I've Covered Tens of Countries: Such a National Suicide I've Never Seen." *Haaretz*, October 30. www.haaretz.co.il. [In Hebrew.]

Pew Forum. 2013. "A Portrait of Jewish Americans." www.pewforum.org.

Portugese, Jacqueline. 1998. *Fertility Policy in Israel: The Politics of Religion, Gender, and Nation*. Westport, CT: Praeger.

Shir, Smadar. 2016. "A Minute before the Fifth Birth: Geula Even-Saar Talks about Everything." *Ynet*, October 23. www.ynet.co.il. [In Hebrew.]

Simhon, Avi. 2011. "A Family with Eight Children Is a Sin." *The Marker*, December 28. www.themarker.com. [In Hebrew.]

Soreq, Naama. 2021. "Natality, the Great and Silenced Problem of the State of Israel." *Haaretz*, April 4. www.haaretz.co.il. [In Hebrew.]

Speiser, Elhanan. 2022. "Population Explosion or Population Depletion: Is the End of the World Approaching?" *Makore Rishon*, April 24. www.makorrishon.co.il. [In Hebrew.]

Stoller-Liss, S. 2003. "Here Is How I Raise a Zionist Baby: Constructing Israeli Mother and Baby by Parents' Guidebooks." *Iyunim Betkumat Israel* 13: 277–93. [In Hebrew.]

Vertommen, Sigrid. 2017. "From the Pergonal Project to Kadimastem: A Genealogy of Israel's Reproductive-Industrial Complex." *BioSocieties* 12: 282–306.

World Population Review. 2023. "Countries by Population Density: Countries by Density." https://worldpopulationreview.com.

Zaga, Bar. 2021. "Launching in the Delivery Room: Little Michal Is Mother of Six." *Ynet*, July 8. https://pplus.ynet.co.il. [In Hebrew.]

8

Fertility Paradoxes

Mexico's Shifting Reproductive Agendas

SANDRA P. GONZÁLEZ-SANTOS

"There are fertility clinics in Mexico! But, isn't Mexico a Catholic country? Isn't it overpopulated and poor? Don't they have more pressing health issues to address?" People have been asking me these questions since I began researching assisted reproductive technologies (ARTs) in Mexico in 2006. Many find the existence of ARTs in Mexico to be paradoxical, something absurd given the stereotypes that exist about the country. Explaining this paradox has been the center of my work, unpacking its elements and exploring how the ART industry has flourished in an overpopulated, culturally Catholic country, with 43.9 percent of its population living below the poverty line (CONEVAL 2023) and facing life-threatening conditions such as diabetes, hypertension, and malnutrition. Through a multisited ethnography, I have traced the political, economic, technological, cultural, and emotional entanglements that allowed the Mexican ART industry to develop and flourish (González-Santos 2020).

This chapter focuses on understanding Mexico's ART industry and the reproductive order it has created. I argue that the current reproductive order has been propelled by an aging population, below-replacement fertility rates, an increase in life expectancy, changes in family and gender dynamics, new abortion rights, a decrease in marriages and an increase in divorces, equal rights for same-sex marriages, and changes in women's place in society. These factors combine with stagnant high levels of poverty, a stratified healthcare system, and a neoliberal political economy. They have transformed reproductive medicine into a commodity, clinicians into service providers, and patients into consumers. The current reproductive order has created a number of fertility figures that sustain the invisibility of the vulnerable and the overvisibility of the elite.

This chapter explores the rise of this new reproductive order. Following a chronological narrative, it examines the *shifting reproductive agendas* key to the growth of the Mexican ART industry. In doing so, it identifies the combination of factors involved in the rapid growth of Mexico's infertility hypermarket and unpacks the dynamics of the current reproductive order. As I define it here, a reproductive agenda is the conjunction of public policies, infrastructures, knowledge sets, targeted populations, objectives, and methods developed and used to enact politics of reproduction by the state and the medical industry. I suggest that the current reproductive agenda includes elements of past agendas, while also being situated in the present. This combination is possible because past and present agendas align with and perpetuate the existing sociopolitical structure, which is extremely classist, racist, and gender unequal.

The Past

In what follows, I describe the agendas of the twentieth-century reproductive order, focusing on their objectives, whom they see as subjects of care and control, the infrastructure they built, and the purpose of their medical interventions. I highlight how they participated in placing infertility, reproduction, and family structure on the table for medical, social, and political discussion and management.

Puericultura and *Esterilología* (1930s–1970s)

After the Mexican Revolution (1910–1917), Mexico launched a national project to (re)build itself into a modern Western nation with a strong and healthy population. The state invested in developing public policies and building institutions designed to promote a pronatalist, eugenic, neo-Lamarkian reproductive agenda. The organizing paradigm was *puericultura*, the medical paradigm, rooted in eugenic ideas, that researched and studied the ways to conserve and improve the human species by focusing on the mother-child dyad from before pregnancy through the first years of a child's life. *Puericultura* became key in the solidification of gynecology and pediatrics in Mexico, in which managing reproduction was seen as the way to produce healthier individuals and a healthier population. *Puericultura* was central for the establishment of the *"gran familia Mexicana"* (great Mexican family): a family with a healthy mother-child dyad at its core, guided by medicine and overseen by a protective state. This family is captured in the logo of the Mexican Social Security Institute, established in 1943: an oversized eagle, representing the state, is swaddling a mother cradling and breastfeeding her child, representing the nation. There is no father in this fertility figure, only a safeguarding state overlooking a protective mother feeding a growing nation.

Physicians were given the power to evaluate who was "fit-to-marry," hence to reproduce. To get married, a couple had to present a medical certificate testifying that they had been evaluated by a physician, were found healthy enough to have offspring, and had received information about healthy reproductive practices. Physicians could withhold this certificate in cases of infertility, even though the condition was considered curable. *Esterilología* was the medical subspecialty focused on curing infertility.[1]

Puericultura's main subjects of control and care were women, particularly the "unfit-to-reproduce" women. This "unfitness" resulted from a classist and racist mindset, from viewing poor women with indigenous roots as having undesirable biological and social traits, and judging them ignorant because they consulted with midwives and traditional healers, whose ideas were considered remnants of an unhealthy and superstitious past. Eliminating such nonbiomedical ideas about reproduction remains a goal even today (Vega 2018).

Puericultura's task was to encourage women to follow a conscious maternity. This meant regularly visiting the hygiene centers where they could consult with healthcare providers trained in Western science and medicine. These centers exhorted women to follow their advice to ensure the health of their future babies. When puericulturists encountered extremely "unfit-to-reproduce" women, they encouraged them to refrain from reproducing or forcibly sterilized them (Castro 2021).

This pronatalist, but inherently racist, reproductive agenda was epitomized in Luis Echeverría's 1969 presidential campaign slogan: *"poblar es gobernar"* (to populate is to govern). *Puericultura* and *esterilología* were the official, professional pronatalist reproductive agendas of the time. Four years later, the national agenda on reproduction radically changed to endorse a strong family-planning campaign. How and why did this happen?

Family Planning (1960–1990)

By the 1960s, still in the middle of this pronatalist agenda, more than one hundred thousand Mexican peasants were gathering a wild yam called "*barbasco*," from which Mexican and North American scientists were synthesizing progesterone to make contraceptives, which more than two million women in the United States would eventually ingest in their daily contraceptive pill (Soto Laveaga 2009). At this stage, contraception in Mexico was used mostly by wealthy women who accessed it through the private sector.

On the other side of the border, demographers, politicians, and academics were fomenting a new reproductive concern. The Cold War heightened fears that the rapid population growth in less developed countries like Mexico would encourage illegal immigration to the United States, threaten the American way of life, and help socialist and communist ideals spread across Latin America (Stone 1953; Murphy 2017). These demographers, politicians, and academics argued in favor of investing in biomedical and sociological research on contraception and in family-planning campaigns in Mexico as a solution to this "population problem." These campaigns would educate people in reproductive matters, giving them tools to have fewer children. Particularly concerning were the "hyper-fertile-poor-urban" (and usually indigenous) women who were commonly described as "begging in the streets surrounded by little children." This trope is a reiteration of the "unfit-to-reproduce" woman of *puericultura* and continues today as a justification for limiting ART services in the public sector.

By 1974, the Mexican government had adopted the family-planning agenda and begun to establish its infrastructure, in some cases aided by organizations such as the Ford Foundation, the Rockefeller Foundation, and the Population Council. Article 4 of the Constitution and the Ley General of Población were written and amended, giving people the right to decide how many children they wanted to have and how and when to achieve this. These policies made the state responsible for offering free family-planning services in public institutions and allowed for the advertising and sale of contraceptive methods in public clinics. This constitutional article became central in the configuration of the ART industry in the next century.

Like *puericultura*, family planning involved problematic ways of providing contraception, particularly when it involved women (again) considered "unfit to reproduce." One strategy included systematically offering contraceptive methods at every single consultation with women, even when the visit was not gynecological. Another strategy was incentivizing healthcare providers to perform a minimum number of sterilizations, for which they received extra resources (Gutmann 2009). Sterilization procedures and intrauterine device (IUD) placements were usually performed after childbirth, miscarriage, or abortion, frequently without consent (Zavala de Cosío 1992). In rural areas, women were offered transportation to the nearest health center, where they were fitted with IUDs or sterilized, and then returned to their hometowns, all in the same day.

The government worked with renowned marketing firms and joined forces with the media to develop and broadcast family-planning campaigns designed to transform people's ideas about the ideal family size and the use of contraception. These campaigns appeared in the press, in public spaces, and on television. The advantages of having smaller families were commonly linked to affordability, using slogans such as "¿Pensando en el gasto? La familia pequeña vive mejor" (Thinking about costs? Small families live better lives) or "Pocos hijos para darles mucho" ([Have] fewer children to give them more). Campaigns also encouraged behavioral change. Playing on the idea of becoming fewer in number, they suggested becoming less macho, submissive, or corrupt: "Vámonos haciendo menos . . . machos . . . sumisas . . . corruptos" (Let's become less macho . . . submissive . . . corrupt). The fertility figure of the "small family" was depicted as mother, father, a son, and a daughter, as represented in the icon of the National Population Council.

Again, women were the main targets of these campaigns, which now situated them as active, responsible individuals, with opinions and ideas and capable of changing and improving their own and their families' lives. They were encouraged to plan their pregnancies, to wait until they were in stable emotional and economic relationships, and to have no more than two children, well spaced. Ironically, women were later told that they were infertile because they had waited until they had stable relationships and jobs and had prioritized their careers over motherhood. Placing women in charge of their reproduction was not always received positively by men; some felt they were being left out of the reproductive decisions. Hence, campaigns were redesigned to portray family planning as a couple's decision. Within the clinical context, physicians abandoned the interest in curing infertility, as suggested by *esterlilología*, and adopted the ideas of reproductive biology, which sought to control the hormones involved in reproduction. Reproductive biology, developed within the context of family planning, became the epistemological grounds for ARTs.

Present

The following reproductive agendas spanning the new millennium frame biomedical knowledge and technology as ways to manage, control, and, now, assist reproduction. They continue to include infertility, reproduction, and family structure in the medical, social, and political discussion. But they now occur in the context of globalization, rampant consumerism, free trade agreements, important political shifts, the Internet, and neoliberalism.

Globalization and Neoliberalism (1990s–2010s)

After twenty-five years of economic growth and infrastructure development, Mexico underwent repeated devaluations (in 1976, 1982, and 1994). This led the country to adopt a new import-export-based political economy, which required a profound adjustment of Mexicans' habits. A population of "weak consumers" had to be taught to buy, dispose, and consume (Morton 2003). A workforce accustomed to catering to its internal market now had to compete and satisfy the foreign consumer. A government that had spent years looking inward for stability and growth was now, for the first time, associating a better future with better relations with Washington (Fuentes 1993).

This radical shift was inscribed in the signing of the North American Free Trade Agreement (NAFTA) in 1993. Immediately, Mexico was overtaken by a tsunami of foreign influence through goods and television programs promoting ideas of individuality and consumerism. The neoliberalism that was being fashioned in Mexico defended individual liberty and protected the market, favoring private investments and industries while discouraging the welfare state, the protection of public goods, and the improvement of public services. For example, state investment in healthcare was reduced by 47 percent, and federal laws and regulations were adapted to facilitate foreign private insurance companies' and health services' participation in the national market; this boosted the growth of the private medical sector (Tamez González and Valle Arcos 2005).

Globalization and neoliberalism also influenced the reproductive agenda. In the past, the focus had been on the welfare of the nation, then on the well-being of the family. Now, the focus shifted toward the interests of the individual. Slogans emphasized new values—individualism, responsibility, empowerment, human rights, and gender equality—stressing the fact that family planning was an individual's decision and a good option to improve living standards (Nazar-Beutelspacher, Zapata-Martelo, and Vázquez-García 2004). Men became subjects of reproductive care and control in the late 1980s and early 1990s through campaigns promoting vasectomy as a contraceptive method and encouraging monogamy and the use of condoms to avoid HIV contagion. This was the first time the word "condom" was used in the media (Rico, Bronfman, and Chiriboga 1995; Gutmann 2009). Influenced by different social movements, the reproductive agenda began to expand beyond reproductive health, bringing in ideas and policies on reproductive rights in addition to concerns about maternal and child health, infertility, and sexually transmitted diseases. Although the reproductive agenda expanded beyond the notion of the "woman-of-reproductive-age-in-a-relationship" to include adolescents, young adults, and men, this fertility figure is still used within government documents in spite of its heteronormative, conservative implications and the bias this produces (Secretaría de Salud 2008).

The first ART services were established around 1985 in Mexico City (one private and one public) and Monterrey (one private), and they began reporting successful births in 1988. These clinics were central to the establishment and growth of the ART community. They published papers, organized conferences, invited foreign experts, and trained subsequent generations of ART specialists. NAFTA established favorable conditions for foreign clinics to consider Mexico as a potential market. Soon, a few clinics from the United States and Spain opened branches in Mexico or partnered with local ones. Although their organization and marketing strategies were unusual for Mexicans, local clinics ended up adopting these strategies, propelling the marketization and commodification of ART services in Mexico. These marketing strategies involved advertising on radio and television, in public spaces (billboards), and in the press, offering discounts, and working with banks for tailored loans. When the Internet arrived, clinics opened websites and, later, Facebook pages. The topic also inspired telenovelas as well as interviews with former users and stories of the rich and famous, all highlighting how the "ART-mother-to-be" endured everything to become a mother. Characterizing the ART woman as a "mother-at-all-costs" endorsed the Mexican mandate that women must be selfless and sacrificing mothers, wives, and daughters (Saldaña-Tejeda, Venegas Aguilera, and Davids 2017). These developments helped construct infertility as a common problem and ARTs as an acceptable solution (González-Santos 2020).

The first adopters of ARTs ventured into an unknown field with little information and support. This motivated them to create what they called a "fertility community," uniting patients, psychologists, and physicians. They set up websites and online support groups, and they organized events where practitioners and patients could meet. One of these early adopters took this idea one step further by organizing a trade show, Expofertilidad, held five times between 2007 and 2012 at the Mexican World Trade Center. These events offered a safe space where users and practitioners gave and received support and advice, experimented with resignifying what constitutes a family and what establishes kinship, and searched for the validation that their reproductive decisions were correct. This is where those using donated gametes would repeat, almost mantra-like, "S/he might not have your eyes, but s/he will have your gaze; s/he might not have your mouth, but s/he will have your smile."

Until this time, advertising healthcare, in the media or anywhere, was unprecedented in Mexico. Several physicians shared with me their discomfort with these marketing strategies. They were unsettled by the ways in which patients were transformed into clients, searching for the best deal, and physicians into salespeople, hawking their products. Nonetheless, this commercial edge engulfed the field of assisted reproduction, transforming it profoundly by the 2010s.

Current Reproductive Order

The year 2000 was significant for Mexicans, who participated in their first democratic election and had, for the first time in seven decades, a new governing party in office. Since then, three different parties have taken office, all favoring globalization, consumerism, and neoliberalism. The first two periods were won by the conservative party; this meant a cutback on the presence of family-planning campaigns in the media. Consequently, people were less informed about their contraceptive options and where to get contraceptives. Paradoxically, the struggle to legalize abortion also began in the year 2000, eventually succeeding in 2023. Abortion is now legal and free across Mexico in cases of pregnancy resulting from rape, and in ten of the thirty-two states it is legal without having to provide any justification, up to the twelfth week of pregnancy.

The struggle to legalize abortion occurred within a context in which teenage pregnancies were increasing. More than half of them involved sexual violence, and many included sexually transmitted diseases (Secretaría de Salud 2008, 2021). This rise in teenage pregnancy could also have been the result of a combination of a stigmatization of nonheterosexual forms of relationships (i.e., same-sex relationships) and sexual activity outside a formal union, with the availability of misleading information circulating in social media. This mixture erects barriers to acquiring and using contraception and having abortions, placing adolescents and queer individuals in vulnerable positions (Villalobos et al. 2020; Secretaría de Salud 2008, 2013, 2021).

For the past twenty years, each new administration has reported that the previous one reduced its investment in family-planning campaigns (Secretaría de Salud 2008, 2013, 2021).[2] These reports suggest that controlling fertility is no longer a matter of governmental interest. Mexico has arrived at the desired fertility rate—1.9 children per woman in 2020—so the perception is that there is no need for further action. While Mexicans have become fewer, they have also become older, with a median age of twenty-nine. Mexicans are living with chronic degenerative diseases like hypertension and diabetes; they marry less and divorce more; and more people work in jobs that do not offer social security. All this is transforming the way families can cope with caring for children, the elderly, and the sick (Myers and Vargas 2023). In the past, the extended family helped with these tasks, but this becomes more complicated as families shrink and age.

The ART industry has taken advantage of the government's loss of interest in fertility by controlling the conversation. For one, it has not made information accessible. It has been nearly forty years since the first clinics were established, and still unknown are the exact number of clinics that exist, the types of procedures they perform, and their outcomes. The Mexican Medical Association of Reproductive Medicine (AMMR), whose members are ART specialists, has never published this information. The National Sanitary Risk Commission (COFEPRIS), which inspects ART clinics in order to grant them licenses, has an unclear and difficult-to-access database, where clinics are not even listed by their commercial names. The Mexican Council of Gynecologists and Obstetricians should have a database of the ART specialists they certify, but having a certification is not the same as having a clinic. RedLara gathers information offered voluntarily by affiliated clinics,[3] but not all clinics are part of the network. Their latest report states that 188 clinics, located throughout fifteen countries, reported a total of 93,600 procedures; of these, thirty-eight were Mexican (sixty-three were in Brazil and twenty-eight in Argentina), and they performed 15,789 procedures (Brazil reported 39,142 and Argentina 20,054) (Zegers-Hochschild et al. 2020). This number contrasts with the 130 clinics COFEPRIS has listed and with the "80,000 procedures [that] are performed annually in Mexico," according to an ART specialist (Sánchez Cordero 2019).

The ART industry has helped to maintain the regulatory patchwork under which ART services operate. The first legislative bill was presented in 1999, and by 2020 there were more than thirty. Yet, not one has passed; thus there still is no federal law concerning ARTs. Currently, each clinic follows its own criteria concerning who is eligible for these services, what services are offered, and the content and structure of the consent forms and contracts (López et al. 2021). It is worth noting that not one bill has suggested prohibiting ART services. Most of them justify allowing ART services by appealing to Article 4 of the

Constitution, which stipulates that everyone has the right to form a family and to have access to health services. The objective of these bills has been to stipulate the criteria for who can access these services and for which reason (e.g., sex selection, avoiding genetic diseases, or social reasons). Presently, only some states have local regulations. Mexico City's regulation, for example, allows genetic manipulation to avoid the inheritance of undesirable genetic conditions, while Puebla's prohibits embryo selection, even if it is to avoid heritable diseases (González-Santos and Saldaña-Tejeda 2023).

After having many conversations with the policymakers and physicians involved in drafting some of these bills and after sitting in on the discussion over how to regulate ARTs, I see that regulating ARTs is not a priority. Currently, there is no clear advantage for the government nor the industry. Some of my interlocutors pointed out that one of the problems is the lack of resources to implement these laws (e.g., qualified staff); others told me that the religious lobby is against some parts of these bills, thus exerting pressure to hold back their approval; others say that it is not the right political time (Semmex 2022); and many simply agree that there is no interest or political gain. This uneven regulatory landscape contributes to the stratification of ART services and, with the advent of surrogacy, it is producing problematic scenarios for service providers and users (Saldaña-Tejeda et al. 2022). Surrogacy agencies, which proliferated in the past decade, are taking advantage of this regulatory patchwork and lack of oversight on fertility clinics. They act as translators between the Mexican legal and medical system (including the ART specialists, the gamete donors, and the surrogates) and their clients (Olavarría Patiño 2018).

The ART industry has also taken advantage of the difficulties of implementing laws concerning health-related advertisements, particularly when it comes to social media. In their first websites, clinics posted information about their staff's qualifications and basic information about infertility and the procedures they offered. With the emergence of social media, their online presence intensified, and their messages became more promotional, offering guarantee packages, assuring 100 percent success "or your money back," and narrating ARTs as almost risk free. They back up these claims with testimonies constructed through pictures and videos of former users. The pictures commonly have the (usually male) physician at the center, holding the baby or standing next to the mother with the baby. More recently, ART users have begun to chronicle their reproductive journeys through social media, turning into critics, evaluators, and promoters of these services. Although their stories tend to be more complex, showing the ups and downs, contrasting with the straightforward narrative told by clinics, they still commonly offer hope (that the procedure will eventually succeed) and rarely explore other ways of reproduction and kinship. They are now ART influencers, and some are now official spokespeople for the clinics where they achieved their goals.

The ART industry has also taken advantage of the marriage and reproductive rights granted to the LGTBQ+ community and the changes in family structure (more single parents), incorporating them into their client portfolios. For example, clinics now advertise egg freezing for young working women and sperm banks for single mothers-to-be; they offer lesbian couples a procedure called ROPA,[4] and they offer surrogacy to gay couples. Mexico is considered an attractive place to seek these services, particularly for North American customers, because it offers high-quality procedures at lower prices than those in the United States and because Mexico already has a history of being a destination for medical tourism. However, given the patchy laws and the particular way bureaucracy works in Mexico, (mainly foreign) intended parents commonly face unimagined (although documented) bureaucratic hurdles when trying to issue the newborn's identity papers. This has sparked negative press, legal battles, and bad experiences. It has also inspired media discussions concerning the autonomy of the women who are hired as surrogates and egg donors, contrasting their economic precarity with the affluence of those seeking their services, who are presented as wealthy, white, and foreign (GIRE 2015; Olavarría Patiño 2018).

The reproductive agenda sketched out by President López-Obrador's administration (2018–2024) was the latest example of how family planning has lost political priority. This agenda shifted from centering on family planning and contraception to dealing with sexual and reproductive health. Infertility became just one more line item in a list of concerns: sexual health, menstrual health, peri-/postmenopause, sexual dysfunctions, sexually transmitted diseases, cancers, and adolescent pregnancies (Secretaría de Salud 2021).

Reflections on Mexico's Reproductive Agendas

Physicians often told me that ARTs and contraception are two sides of the same coin. Exploring this perspective, I found that *esterilología* and reproductive biology (contraception) share an interest in understanding hormones and the processes involved in conception, in order to cure infertility and control fertility. However, as I see it, the ART industry promotes other intentions. Up until the 1980s, infertility had been constructed as a public health problem, with economic and social implications, that required public policy and state-financed research and institutions. The state first addressed underpopulation and then overpopulation, always framing its approach as beneficial for the nation. Then, influenced by globalization and neoliberalism, the idea of controlling fertility was reshaped by ideas of individual rights and desires, techno-fixes, and consumerism. Infertility became an individual, private, and personal matter. The ART sector abandoned the goal of curing infertility and now aims to give clients what they desire: children.

Three things unite these reproductive agendas. First, they use Western science to control fertility and exclude other forms of understanding reproduction held by many Mexicans (even when these are part of their culture) (Vega 2018). Second, they share a strong foreign influence, inspired by academics, politicians, and demographers from the United States, by alliances with foreign ART clinics and professionals, and by international surrogacy agencies. Third—and most important—they all invoke Article 4 of the Mexican Constitution: the right to have the desired family configuration. The shift from a health matter to a rights matter was accompanied by a shift in who controls reproduction. As described in the last section, in the twenty-first century the government lost interest in fertility matters, and the ART industry leaped into this vacuum by creating a market-favorable setting. This setting has allowed for the dissemination of false and exaggerated advertisement that cannot be critically read in the absence of trustworthy information regarding, for example, the number of ART cycles performed annually and the success rates of each clinic.

This market-favorable setting has intensified the stratification of ART services. Although ART services began simultaneously in the public and the private sectors, the former did not develop beyond a few services justified as training facilities, while the latter grew in size and scope. This made ARTs affordable for only a segment of the population, especially when the ART industry became part of the global and neoliberal cross-border healthcare market (particularly with the United States and Canada). The unequal access to ART services is displayed throughout private and public spaces, testimony to Mexico's class tensions. Two key examples illustrate this disparity. First, on the wall of a low-income house, located near a private hospital in a low-income neighborhood, hangs a billboard advertising a private ART clinic. People living in this house earn some extra money by renting their wall to an ART clinic whose services they could not afford. Second, wealthy ART users often turn to household employees for help with acquiring, managing, and administering fertility treatments, yet these employees could never afford these treatments for themselves. These homes are spaces where economic poverty and economic opulence clash, where those without access to certain goods and treatments are in direct contact with the healthcare they cannot afford. ARTs reveal the intermingling of economic disparities that sustains Mexico and that produces contained contempt, fear, resentment, and hatred but also wealth, opportunity, care practices, and an enigmatic and problematic stability.

Finally, the fertility figures produced over the years have transformed yet are still reproducing the invisibility of the vulnerable and the over-visibility of the elite. During the pronatalist period, the notion of the "*gran familia mexicana*," a heteronormative family that produced and raised several healthy children who would grow into hard-working citizens, predominated. This ideal family evolved into "*la familia pequeña vive mejor*," a heteronormative family with only two children. Then, during the twenty-first century, the notion of family became flexible enough to accept a variety of configurations, not only the heteronormative. All reproductive agendas have highlighted a set of contrasting figures: the poor-urban/rural-indigenous woman described as "hyperfertile" yet "unfit to reproduce," and the "fit-to-reproduce-young-urban-working-white woman," who needs to preserve her fertility by freezing her eggs. This categorization, still present today, is the epitome of the classist and racist disposition of Mexican political, economic, and social structures. A third set emerged within the neoliberal market when the patient-physician duo transformed into the "consumer-seller": the "ART influencer," the YouTuber, Instagrammer, and TikToker who documents and broadcasts their ART journey. These fertility figures co-inhabit the nascent global ART market, where skilled cheap laborers work alongside artificial intelligence technologies, all engrained in automated embryo assembly lines (González-Santos 2024).

Yet, the question remains: How could Mexico, being mostly Catholic, accept these reproductive agendas when they clearly go against the Catholic Church's mandates regarding reproduction? It is important to remember that in 1860, the Reform Laws (promulgated by Benito Juarez) took away many rights and duties held by the Catholic Church (such as marriage and birth certificates), denied Catholic clergy the right to vote, and expropriated their land and buildings. This was reiterated, first in the 1917 Constitution and then again during the Cristero Wars in the 1920s. Hence, throughout most of the twentieth century, Mexico's official relationship with the Catholic Church and the Vatican was practically nonexistent. This never meant that people could not practice religion; it simply meant that state and church were separate and the latter could not meddle in matters of the former. This started to change when, in 1992, President Carlos Salinas de Gortari reestablished official relations with the Vatican and changed the Constitution to allow clergy to vote. Since 2000, the presence and influence of the Catholic Church has slowly grown, but the laws that limit the church's official participation in the government are still in place. This does not mean that Catholic morality has no influence on policy, as the church sometimes adopts the path of pressuring conservative groups within the middle and upper economic segments of the population. In addition, it is important to note that assisted reproduction helps women become mothers, and it builds families. As I argue, this is central to Mexican life and belief systems; hence, it trumps the Vatican's prohibitions (González-Santos 2020).

Conclusion

The story I tell in this chapter leaves important things untouched.[5] It does not consider the number of families that are migrating so their teenage children will not grow up in the context of violence. It does not consider the number of maternal deaths that happen mostly in rural and indigenous communities. It does not consider the number of cases of obstetric violence instigated by discrimination, racism, and classism and that result in infertility. It does not consider the number of births overturned by femicides, the number of families broken by violence, or the number of children left orphans when their parents were forcibly removed. The part of the story I have told in this chapter addresses a reproductive agenda that presupposes life and that takes place in the context of biomedicine and biotechnology. But there is another side, one that lives in death and violence. Both sides make up Mexico's new reproductive order.

Mexico's new reproductive order is thus structured by a reproductive agenda based on life and a reproductive scenario based on death. It is a stratified order that brings together those who are unable to access even the basic elements of reproductive health (such as an IUD, a Pap smear, or an ultrasound) and those with access to the most innovative ARTs. It is an order that fits into the global ART market just as the Mexican industry fits into NAFTA, tailoring specific services for local consumers and others for foreign ones. It is an order guided by a market that works within a legal patchwork. It is an order that looks into the technological future, one with automated clinics with embryo assembly lines, mixing artificial intelligence and cheap labor. It is a neoliberal order that perpetuates racist, classist, and individualistic values and policies. It is an order that I still struggle to understand.

NOTES

1 This medical subspecialty was developed by a group of Mexican physicians concerned with infertility. They created the Mexican Association for the Study of Sterility, published a journal, and laid the groundwork for what would later be the Mexican Association of Reproductive Medicine, the association of ART experts.

2 At the beginning of every presidential term, the Ministry of Health publishes its specific plans of action to tackle health issues deemed a priority; this includes an evaluation of the situation left by the previous administration.

3 RedLara annually produces a report registering the number and type of procedures carried out by the subscribing clinics. These reports are published simultaneously in *Reproductive BioMedicine Online* and in the *Brazilian Journal of Reproductive Medicine*.

4 ROPA stands for Reception of Partner's Oocyte, where one becomes the genetic mother and the other the gestational mother.

5 I thank Abril Saldaña Tejeda for bringing this to my attention.

REFERENCES

Castro, Raúl. 2021. "Hacia una Sociología de la Anticoncepción Forzada en México" [A Sociology of Forced Contraception in Mexico]. In *Género y Sexualidad en Disputa: Desigualdades en el Derecho a Decidir Sobre el Propio Cuerpo Desde el Campo Médico*, 1st ed., ed. K. B. Bárcenas Barajas and R. Castro, 37–64. Mexico City: Universidad Nacional Autónoma de México.

CONEVAL. 2023. *Pobreza Multidimensional 2022*. August. www.coneval.org.

Fuentes, Carlos. 1993. "TLC, el Día Siguiente" [NAFTA: The Next Day]. *El País*. https://elpais.com.

GIRE. 2015. "Niñas y Mujeres Sin Justicia: Derechos Reproductivos en México" [Children and Women without Justice: Reproductive Rights in Mexico]. https://gire.org.mx.

González-Santos, Sandra P. 2011. "Space, Structure, and Social Dynamics within the Clinical Setting: Two Case Studies of Assisted Reproduction in Mexico City." *Health & Place* 17(1): 166–74.

———. 2016. "Peregrinar: El Ritual de la Reproducción Asistida" [Pilgrimage: The Ritual of Assisted Reproduction]. In *Reprodução Assistida e Relações de Gênero na América Latina*, ed. Cecilia Straw, Eliane Vargas, Mariana Viera Cherro, and Marlene Tamanini, 265–88. Curitiba, Brazil: Editor CVR.

———. 2020. *A Portrait of Assisted Reproduction in Mexico: Scientific, Political, and Cultural Interactions*. New York: Springer International Publishing.

———. 2024. "Creating Life: An Embryo Assembly Line." In *Beauty and Monstrosity in Art and Culture*, ed. Chara Kokkiou and Angeliki Malakasioti, 153–61. New York: Routledge.

González-Santos, Sandra P., and Abril Saldaña-Tejeda. 2023. "Contesting the 'No Rules' Label: ARTs in Mexico before and after the First MRT Baby." In *Reproduction Reborn: How Science, Ethics, and Law Shape Mitochondrial Replacement Therapies*, ed. Diana Bowman, Karinne Ludlow, and Walter G. Johnson, 143–70. Oxford: Oxford University Press.

Gutmann, Matthew C. 2009. "Planning Men out of Family Planning: A Case Study." *Sexualidad, Salud y Sociedad—Revista Latinoamericana* 1: 104–24.

López, Alma, Miguel Betancourt, Eduardo Casas, Socorro Retana-Márquez, Lizbeth Juárez-Rojas, and Fahiel Casillas. 2021. "The Need for Regulation in the Practice of Human Assisted Reproduction in Mexico: An Overview of the Regulations in the Rest of the World." *Reproductive Health* 18(1): 241.

Morton, Adam David. 2003. "Structural Change and Neoliberalism in Mexico: 'Passive Revolution' in the Global Political Economy." *Third World Quarterly* 24(4): 631–53.

Murphy, Michelle. 2017. *The Economization of Life*. Durham, NC: Duke University Press.

Myers, Robert G., and Daniela U. Vargas. 2023. "Atención a Niñas y Niños Menores de Cuatro Años en México Durante el Gobierno de AMLO: Análisis de un Cambio de Estrategia" [Care Given to Children under Four during AMLO's Administration:

An Analysis of a Change of Strategy]. *Revista Latinoamericana de Estudios Educativos* 53(1): article 1.

Nazar-Beutelspacher, Austreberta, Emma Zapata-Martelo, and Verónica Vázquez-García. 2004. "Population Policies and Women's Nutrition: A Study on Six Rural Communities in Chiapas." *Agricultura Sociedad y Desarrollo* 1(2): 147–62.

Olavarría Patiño, Maria Eugenia. 2018. "La Gestante Sustituta en México y La Noción de Trabajo Reproductivo" [The Gestating Substitute in Mexico and the Notion of Reproductive Work]. *Revista Interdisciplinaria de Estudios de Género de El Colegio de México* 4: 1–31.

Rico, Blanca, Mario Bronfman, Carlos del Rio Chiriboga. 1995. "Las Campañas Contra el Sida en México: ¿Los Sonidos del Silencio o Puente Sobre Aguas Turbulentas?" [The AIDS Campaigns in Mexico: "Sounds of Silence" or "A Bridge over Troubled Waters"?] *Salud Pública de México* 37(6): 643–53.

Saldaña-Tejeda, Abril, Alberto Aparicio, Sandra. P. González-Santos, Gabriela Arguedas-Ramírez, J. M. Cavalcanti, Melissa K. Shaw, and Laura Perler. 2022. "Policy Landscapes on Human Genome Editing: A Perspective from Latin America." *Trends in Biotechnology* 40(11): 1275–78.

Saldaña-Tejeda, Abril, Lilia Venegas Aguilera, Tine Davids, eds. 2017. *A Toda Madre. Una Mirada Multidisciplinaria a Las Maternidades en México* [A Toda Madre: A Multidisciplinary Perspective on the Maternities in Mexico]. Mexico City: Instituto Nacional de Antropología e Historia.

Sánchez Cordero, Olga. 2019. "La Legislación en Materia de Infertilidad y de Reproducción Asistida" [Legislation concerning Infertility and Assisted Reproduction]. August 5. Mexico City: Academia Nacional de Medicina de México.

Secretaría de Salud. 2008. "Programa de Acción Específico (PAE) Planificación Familiar y Anticoncepción 2007–2012" [Specific Plan of Action on Family Planning and Contraception 2007–2012]. Mexico: Ministry of Health.

———. 2013. "Programa de Acción Específica (PAE) Planificación Familiar y Anticoncepción 2013–2018" [Specific Plan of Action on Family Planning and Contraception 2013–2018]. Mexico: Ministry of Health.

———. 2021. "Programa de Acción Específico (PAE) Salud Sexual y Reproductiva 2020–2024" [Specific Plan of Action on Family Planning and Contraception 2020–2024]. Mexico: Ministry of Health.

Semmex. 2022. "Ley Aprobada Sobre Maternidad Subrogada en CDMX en 2010 no Fue Publicada" [The Approved Law on Surrogacy in Mexico City in 2010 Was Not Published]. *La Silla Rota. La Cadera de Eva*, February 23.

Soto Laveaga, Gabriela. 2009. *Jungle Laboratories: Mexican Peasants, National Projects, and the Making of the Pill.* Durham, NC: Duke University Press.

Stone, Abraham. 1953. "Problemas de Fertilidad, Esterilidad y Población" [Fertility Problems, Sterility, and Population]. *Estudios sobre Esterilidad* 4(2): 66.

Tamez González, Silvia, and Rosa Irene Valle Arcos. 2005. "Desigualdad Social y Reforma Neoliberal en Salud" [Social Inequality and the Neoliberal Health Reform]. *Revista Mexicana de Sociología* 67(2): 321–56.

Vega, Rosalynn A. 2018. *No Alternative: Childbirth, Citizenship, and Indigenous Culture in Mexico*. Austin: University of Texas Press.

Villalobos, Aremis, Leticia Ávila-Burgos, Celia Hubert, Leticia Suárez-López, Elvia de la Vara-Salazar, María I. Hernández-Serrato, Tonatiuh Barrientos-Gutiérrez. 2020. "Prevalencias y Factores Asociados con el Uso de Métodos Anticonceptivos Modernos en Adolescentes, 2012 y 2018" [The Prevalence and Associated Factors Related to the Use of Modern Contraceptive Methods by Adolescents, 2012–2018]. *Salud Pública de México* 62: 648–60.

Zavala de Cosío, María Eugenia. 1992. *Cambios de Fecundidad en México y Políticas de Población* [Changes in Mexico's Fecundity and Population Politics]. México: El Colegio de México/Fondo de Cultura Económica.

Zegers-Hochschild, Fernando, Javier A. Crosby, Carolina Musri, Maria do Carmo B. de Souza, A. Gustavo Martinez, Adelino Amaral Silva, José María Mojarra, Diego Masoli, and Natalia Posada. 2020. "Assisted Reproductive Techniques in Latin America: The Latin American Registry, 2017." *JBRA Assisted Reproduction* 24(3): 362–78.

9

Reproductive Rebellion

Challenging Authority and Seeking Autonomy in Iran's Fertility Regime

SORAYA TREMAYNE

In 2012, the supreme religious leader of the Islamic Republic of Iran, Ayatollah Khamenei, did something unusual. Addressing a conference on October 10, he admitted to an error: "One of the mistakes we made in the 1990s was population control. Government officials were wrong on this matter, and I, too, had a part. May God and history forgive us" (Karami 2012).

This chapter explores the historically shifting relationship among the Iranian state, religious leaders, and the country's younger generation of reproductive age in an effort to examine patterns of fertility choices, fertility change, and fertility control that have shaped the past 150 years of Iranian history. It first examines the uneven and often paradoxical impact of the Iranian state's long-term project of reshaping the nation's population through a series of shifting *fertility regimes*, the first of which was initiated in the late nineteenth century while the most recent continues today. To describe the new reproductive order in the Iranian context, this chapter tracks how Iranian state approaches to regulating the population have evolved through five distinct phases, each implementing policies and interventions that deliberately reverse the fertility regimes that preceded them. Currently, following a sharp decline in the birth rate, which has now fallen below replacement level, the state has adopted yet another new fertility regime based on pronatalist policies to reverse the current trend of two children per family, and thus to reverse population decline. However, more than a decade into this new regime, no significant success has been noted, with the population growth declining to current levels of 0.71 (Statista 2023).

This chapter asks what lessons can be learned from the long sequence of situated fertility transitions in Iran, particularly as they reveal the ongoing importance of women's empowerment in this process. Based on long-term research that I have carried out in Iran on various aspects of reproduction (Tremayne 2023), the chapter explores the underlying social and cultural factors responsible for the dramatic shift in child-bearing practices beyond the state's long-running rhetoric of pointing at economic hardship as the main cause of the fertility decline. The case studies, interviews, and reports in the media that are included here reveal the driving forces behind the reproductive decisions being made by the current generation of reproductive age. These examples are only a small portion, selected to convey the extent to which the current generation of reproductive age is resisting the state's coercive reproductive policies and thus contributing substantially to fertility decline. These examples also signal that *not* producing the number of children demanded by the state does not represent the disappearance of reproductive values per se; rather, it reveals a quest for reproductive autonomy.

To understand whether the fertility decline indicates a fundamental transformation, or disappearance, of traditional reproductive norms and values among young Iranians of reproductive age, this chapter takes a brief look at the seemingly polarized attitudes toward reproduction among Iranians. On one hand, most couples have limited the size of their families to one or at most two children, while a very small minority has also opted for voluntary childlessness altogether. Preference for a small-size family is shown to be widespread nationally and is not limited to certain layers of society, as the findings of several recent studies confirm. In one study, for example, researchers found that the steep fall in the Iranian birth rate across all sectors of society reflected a "similar attitude" of disinclination to have large families, or even any children at all: "Those couples who have just married show no inclination to have any children or perhaps just one. This tendency over the past decade illustrates that for women of urban and rural backgrounds, from different social classes, the poor and the rich, illiterate, and literate, all have a similar attitude to giving birth these days, leading to the downward trend in Iranian TFR (total fertility rate)" ("Iran's Population Crisis" 2013).On the other hand, over 20 percent of married couples (around four million) are known to be infertile and are desperately seeking treatment (Jannati 2021).

By adopting a comparative historical perspective, and through examining the social and cultural barriers to the success of the current state's policies, this chapter highlights the complexities and competing demands on people of reproductive age. It contemplates whether defying the state's plea for larger families may at some level comprise a form of resistance, or what I call *reproductive rebellion*, driven by social and political grievances. Is such rebellion by reproductive-age Iranians an act of dissent against the state's body politic? I suggest that the management of reproductive life in the context of the new reproductive order can no longer be accurately or meaningfully understood in terms of formal systems of authority, control, or (non)compliance with policymakers' directives. Instead, fertility has become a medium for a distinctive form of political expression and resistance. Furthermore, under the influence of feminism, women's agency has become increasingly central in determining the vicissitudes of a domain we might describe as "reproductive life," marking a definitive shift toward the feminization of reproductive politics.

This chapter draws upon four decades (1980 to date) of ethnographic fieldwork in Iran in different rural and urban areas, reflecting varying degrees of economic development, education, and political and religious conservatism. It also incorporates selected findings from fifteen years (2003–2018) of acting as an expert witness for Iranian asylum seekers in courts in the United Kingdom. My research over four decades with Iranians of different social backgrounds inside and outside the country has convinced me that social change rarely involves a complete departure from the fundamental cultural values and norms that have been built over centuries.

The Iranian State and Its Population Policies

In Iran, current attitudes toward childbearing are reactions to the long-term engagement of the state with population issues. According to Firoozeh Kashani-Sabet (2011), the interest of the state in achieving an ideal population size is not new and dates back more than a century to 1874. In total, between 1874 and 2023, the Iranian state introduced five different approaches, or fertility regimes, to regulate the population, each directing citizens to change their reproductive values and practices to meet population goals. Whether pronatalist or antinatalist, these campaigns share three common features. First, with the exception of Iran's current pronatalist policies, state campaigns did not rely on coercive measures to achieve their goals; instead, they relied on advocacy to promote reproduction as a core cultural value. To varying degrees, the government framed these efforts as empowering individuals to help build a strong nation. Second, these campaigns addressed women as key social actors responsible for the nation's reproductive life and thus positioned women of reproductive age as the main agents responsible for the success or failure of the policies (Tremayne 2023). Finally, these policies were projections of the state's nation-building ambitions. This chapter reviews these policies and traces the gradual shifts in Iranian fertility politics, through which the current reproductive order is emerging.

Five Demographic Ebbs without Flows

The Qajar Pronatalist Approach (1874)

Although no substantial information exists on the demographic characteristics of the population under the Qajar Dynasty (1785–1925), its overall health was seen as having depleted so alarmingly in the late nineteenth century that by 1874 the state actively attempted to improve the situation through promoting good hygiene. In lieu of explicitly encouraging pronatalism, the state focused on issues of maternal and child health, which became the core of a hygiene movement. In her account of Qajar interventions, Kashani-Sabet (2011: 5) argues that the state did not resort to formal laws regarding childbirth and that its arguments were not solely based on Western concepts. Instead, the state's discourse was based on the importance of mothers' health, which appealed to Iranians because such themes could be adapted to the more familiar Islamic injunctions regarding parenting and maternity. Moreover, the awareness of women's health and infant mortality, which significantly expanded during the nineteenth century, brought maternalism to the heart of contemporary Iranian thought, concepts of nationhood, and tasks of a modern government. Such prospects readily appealed to people, who accepted the state's vision willingly.

The Pahlavi Antinatalist Approach (1964–1968)

In the second major phase of Iranian fertility promotion, beginning almost a century later, the Pahlavi Dynasty (1925–1979) devised new policies linking population control to national prosperity and economic development. The first explicit policies were formulated in 1964 following census figures that confirmed rates of population increasing by 3.1 percent per annum (see table 9.1). After Iran's official participation in the Third International Population Conference in Bucharest in 1974, the state acknowledged the necessity of a family-planning program as a human right and emphasized its social and economic benefits for families and society (Roudi-Fahimi 2002, 2012). Women of reproductive age once again became the prime focus of a new set of policies that this time were antinatalist, with the improvement of maternal and child health reiterated as the vehicle for integrating their agency into the national interest. Despite these ambitious policies to slow population growth, however, the program did not prove as successful as anticipated, in part due to its top-down approach, which targeted the educated, urban middle classes (Hoodfar 1995, 2017; Ladier-Fouladi 1997, 2017; Abbasi-Shavazi, McDonald, and Hosseini-Chavoshi 2011).

The Theocratic Pronatalist Approach (1980s)

Yet another dramatic U-turn in Iranian fertility management took place within less than a decade. With the fall of the Pahlavi Dynasty brought about by the Islamic Revolution in 1979, the founder of the theocratic Islamic Republic, Ayatollah Khomeini, ordered all family planning programs to be closed during the 1980s. He explicitly encouraged larger families and reminded women that their role, above all, was to produce and raise as many children as possible (Hoodfar 1995, 2017). Again, although the new Islamic Republic refrained from introducing mandatory or coercive pronatalist policies, the religious authorities engaged in powerful rhetoric, alleging that family planning was a plot by Western powers designed to subjugate Islamic nations and limit the number of Muslims. The theocratic state lowered the age of marriage to nine for girls and fifteen for boys, increased maternity benefits, incentivized larger families, and outlawed sterilization and abortion. An additional justification for the new pronatalist fertility regime introduced in the 1980s was the outbreak of the Iran-Iraq War, which resulted in the heavy loss of approximately one million people between 1980 and 1988. Ayatollah Khomeini frequently encouraged the Iranian people in his public speeches to have larger families to replace "the army of 20 million" (Hoodfar 1995) lost in the decade-long conflict. This reversal of previous Iranian state fertility rhetoric appealed to conservative and religious groups, which disapproved of the antinatalist policies of the Pahlavi Dynasty, and the population growth surged.

The New Antinatalist Policies (1990–2011)

By 1986, the National Census confirmed that Iranian population growth had doubled in the space of two decades, rising to nearly 4 percent per annum and generating increasing state concern about the escalating economic costs of such rapid, unchecked growth. The heavy-handed pronatalist approach of the 1980s was once again reversed by the end of the decade and was replaced by a new state-sponsored antinatalist program, the Campaign for the Regulation of the Family. These new fertility policies, which began to be implemented in the late 1980s, eventually proved so successful over the ensuing decade that they halved the annual growth rate by 1996, and by 2011 the rate was nearly halved again, dropping from 2 percent in the late 1990s to 1.3 percent in 2011. This singular achievement won Iran the United Nation's Population Award and was described by leading Iranian demographers as "the largest and fastest" fertility decline ever recorded: "Confounding all conventional wisdom, the fertility rate in the Islamic Republic of Iran fell from around 7.0 per woman in the early 1980s to 1.9 births per woman in 2006. That this, the largest and fastest fall in fertility ever recorded, should have occurred in one of the world's few Islamic Republics demands explanation" (Abbasi-Shavazi, McDonald, and Hosseini-Chavoshi 2011: 7).

Key to Iran's singularly successful fertility-reduction regime between 1996 and 2011 was an exceptionally well-coordinated and all-encompassing state-sponsored family-planning program, which was culturally sensitive in its attempts to bring about fertility change in a society dominated by religious and political conservatism. The success of these policies also led Iran to become something of a "textbook case"

TABLE 9.1. Iran's Population according to Successive Censuses. Credit: Iran Statistical Yearbook (2016)

Census Year	Population	Average Annual Growth (%)	Populations Density/ square km²	Proportion Urban (%)	Household Size
1956	18,954,704	—	12	31.4	—
1966	25,785,210	3.1	16	~37.5	—
1976	33,708,744	2.7	20	47	5.02
1986	49,445,010	3.9	30	~54.0	5.11
1996	60,055,488	2	36	~61.0	4.84
2006	70,495,782	1.6	43	68.5	4.03
2011	75,149,669	1.3	46	71.4	3.55
2014	80,840,713	1.22	49	71.4	3

in fertility studies, and the subject of numerous detailed studies by academic scholars from a range of disciplines (Abbasi-Shavazi, McDonald, and Hosseini-Chavoshi 2011; Ladier-Fouladi 1997, 2017; Tremayne 2004). Importantly, many of these studies suggested that, in addition to their success in dramatically reducing fertility rates, these antinatalist policies left a lasting impact on the fertility perceptions, values, and practices of postmillennial generations, substantially redefining their outlook on childbearing in general.

Rather than resorting to coercive measures, the state chose a campaign of advocacy, carefully side-stepping any form of direct pressure on people to reduce the size of their family. Policymakers adopted this more subtle strategy to mitigate potential ire from conservative and religious leaders, who were more likely to reject antinatalist policies as thwarting God's will but whose support was key to the success of the program. Indeed, most senior clerics, including Ayatollah Khamenei, willingly cooperated and endorsed these antinatalist policies, which the Ayatollah, two decades later, referred to as his "mistake."

Two further factors played a crucial role in the success of these antinatalist policies. Rather than pointing fingers at women and holding them responsible for reducing the birth rate, the campaign enlisted their cooperation, positioning them as active players implementing much-needed changes. This strategic decision empowered women to make their own reproductive decisions and bolstered their ability to resist the often-coercive influences of conservative men, including their husbands (Hoodfar 1995, 2017; Tremayne 2006). In tandem with this strategy of female empowerment, an elaborate education program was launched, which imposed sex segregation and dramatically increased female school attendance and literacy. Parents from rural areas and religiously conservative sectors of society showed great willingness to send their daughters to single-sex schools. However, while one of the Islamic Republic's main objectives was to educate women to be good Muslim women and mothers, this policy yielded unexpected outcomes (Mehran 2003/4). For example, the significant increase in female literacy had several impacts on reproduction, including a rise in the average age of marriage, a marked increase in the divorce rate, and a dramatic decline in family size.

To illustrate the impact of the antinatalist policies on the younger generation, almost a decade into the start of the initiative, when I was on a mission working with the Iranian Bureau of Women's Affairs in 1997, several ultraconservative female employees of the bureau related that their children would come back from school and tell them, "Please don't have more than two children. We are ashamed to go to school and say that there are more than two children in our family." One pregnant woman said that her teenage daughter told her, "You are not a battery hen. Why are you having so many children?" It is this generation of offspring, who are now into their later stages of reproductive life, who refuse to bow to state demands to have children—which would reverse the very values that the state itself had anchored in them a few decades earlier. Effectively, the unalterable impact of these policies is erecting the greatest barrier to the success of the current pronatalist policies, even among conservative groups.

The Ultraconservative Pronatalist Policies (2011–Present)

The outstanding success of Iran's antinatalist policies, which were confirmed by the 2011 census to have yielded a total fertility rate below the replacement level, once again spurred the authorities into action. After the supreme religious leader's repentance, followed by then president Ahmadinejad blaming the antinatalist family-planning program as "a Western import" and "ungodly," the state fertility pendulum swung back once again, abruptly reversing its population policies for the third time in as many decades. The new pronatalist policies now emphasize procreation as a national imperative and encourage couples to have a minimum of three children. As part of its efforts, the state continues to release alarming figures on the aging population and the dangers of falling marriage rates, voluntary childlessness, and a dramatic rise in the divorce rate (Iran Project 2016).

The State's Population Repentance and the Citizens' Reproductive Rebellion

In November 2021, just three months into his presidency, Ebrahim Raisi submitted a bill to Parliament entitled "The Rejuvenation of the Population and the Protection of the Family," aimed at increasing population growth. The bill was approved in accordance with Article 53 of the Constitution by the joint commission without being debated in an open parliamentary session. Since the new law's enactment, the issue of population growth has taken top priority on the government's agenda. The state is dismantling all family-planning programs, banning all forms of contraception and prenatal ultrasound scans, and classifying abortion as a criminal offense—even in cases of severe fetal abnormality (*Saham News* 2023).

Instead, the state is incentivizing childbirth, by offering financial loans and extra leave to families who have more than two children, as well as exemption from compulsory military service for young men with more than two children. However, five years into the program, these efforts are proving unsuccessful. No significant national change in childbearing patterns has been recorded. This failure raises important questions about not only the role of the Iranian state and its history of contrasting fertility regimes and policies but also what the Iranian case can tell us about the deepening conflict between popular and theocratic, or grassroots and top-down, logics of reproductive cause and effect in the new reproductive order.

The consistent failure of the state's pronatalist policies has led the authorities to blame a conflicting variety of factors. Early in the current fertility crisis, the authorities regularly argued that economic hardship was the main cause of falling birth rates (Tremayne 2023: 117–40). However, this claim has been repeatedly contradicted by various studies, including from Iran Open Data (Iran Wire 2021), which confirmed that, while unemployment in Tehran was comparatively low in early 2020, the divorce ratio was still high. In contrast, rural areas with higher unemployment rates had some of the country's lowest divorce rates. Further into the crisis, the government changed tack and is now holding young couples responsible for failing to reproduce the number of children demanded by the state. In May 2023, vice president for women and family affairs Ensieh Khazali stated that "only 30 percent of cases refusing to have children are related to economic reasons, and the remaining 70 percent stems from the outlook to life and high expectations of young people for a luxurious lifestyle, and the fact that they are putting their individual interests above other priorities" (Mypersia 2023). Her statement provoked strong public reactions, ranging from anger and resentment to hopelessness, and even criticism of the government for depriving the next generation of a viable reproductive future. One Iranian lamented, "Even if we have the economic means of bringing children into this world and looking after them, what hope is there for their future in this country?" Another said, "A life without any hope is not worth living and our children will tell us you were wrong to bring us into this world" ("Iran Pushes" 2021). In the same interview, one young woman lambasted the state's draconian pronatalist policies by complaining that "the only thing [the state is] good at is intruding in people's beds. They have put their knee on people's necks and told them to have children." Another interviewee I spoke with went even further, claiming that "the state is using us as reproductive tools and slaves like the ones in *The Handmaid's Tale.*"[1] While the state's current pronatalist policies harm both men and women, women remain the ultimate target and casualty. The Office of the United Nations High Commission for Human Rights (OHCHR 2021) denounced them, noting that "it is shocking to see the extent to which the authorities have applied criminal law to restrict women's fundamental [reproductive] rights."

The authorities' perceptions notwithstanding, Iran's reduction in family size stems from a combination of accumulated factors and is not solely based on weakening reproductive norms. The findings of various studies show that, despite the ideational change toward a small family size norm of two children, the fertility behavior of Iranian women shows little to no preference for zero parity (Abbasi-Shavazi and Razeghi-Nasrabad 2010; Hosseini-Chavoshi, McDonald, and Abbasi-Shavazi 2007).

The Plight of the Involuntarily Childless

The reproductive behavior of young Iranians reducing the size of their families to a maximum of two children is only half of the story, however. Alongside these couples are many who suffer from involuntary childlessness and desperately seek infertility treatment. The rate of involuntary childlessness in Iran, which has a population of around 89 million (Worldometers 2023), is estimated at around 20 percent of all married couples, or about four million (Jannati 2021). As a result, the state saw another opportunity to boost population growth by helping infertile couples conceive via assisted reproductive technologies (ARTs). Policymakers moved to make infertility treatment, previously mainly in the hands of the private sector, one of their new pronatalist priorities. State-sponsored infertility treatment clinics have opened in deprived areas of the country, with health insurance providers instructed to cover the costs of the infertility treatment, including in vitro fertilization (IVF), in an effort to boost the birth rate through improved fertility care (Tremayne and Mehdi Akhondi 2016). Although the insurance providers are supposed to cover the costs of up to five cycles of IVF, depending on the age of the couple seeking treatment, there is no evidence showing that this coverage has been implemented. And despite this seemingly helpful initiative, the state's heavy investment in promoting ARTs does not seem to be contributing significantly to population growth. While infertile couples welcome the provision of free fertility treatments, policymakers fundamentally misunderstand the scope of their effects. According to infertility clinic practitioners, the maximum success rate of children born through the use of ARTs is 20 percent, or twenty thousand children per month. This number is a negligible contribution to the numbers required to replenish the declining population. Even if successful couples returned to have a second child, which few do, this figure will remain below the numbers required. The likelihood of a third round of ARTs is remote. Therefore, the state's calculation to have infertile couples produce families with more than two children is more optimistic than practical (Morshed-Behbahani et al. 2020). Interestingly, recent personal communication from practitioners at the infertility treatment clinics in Iran shows that many fertile couples, who already have children and who are facing severe economic hardship, are being lured by the state's promises of financial help and other incentives and are approaching infertility treatment clinics asking the clinics to help them have twins or even triplets. However, personal communications with several infertility clinics and reports in the media confirm that many of these families, who heeded the state's demands and had more than three children, naturally or through ARTs, have never received any acknowledgment or help from the state.

The study of infertility provides an invaluable lens through which to view the broader context of reproduction by shedding light on whether and to what extent reproductive values and practices have been altered, and whether these changes are responsible for the continuing decline in population growth. The persistence of the centrality of reproduction as the embodiment of family, kinship, marriage, and fertility, underpinning society and ensuring its stability, remains paramount in Iranian society, a fact that is also shown by Marcia C. Inhorn's extensive work in the Arab Middle East on infertility and ARTs (Inhorn 2006; Inhorn et al. 2017). These observations illustrate the persistence and extent to which an infertile couple's kin group influences—and even shapes—its reproductive decisions. Such involvement was evident among the infertile women in my study, especially within conservative layers of society, some of whom would not have minded remaining childless but were forced to submit to relentless pressure or even threats from their in-laws to seek treatment or face divorce, as well as violence by their husbands and often from their own kin group too. Furthermore, these pressures are not limited to infertile women but also exist, albeit to varying degrees, in cases of fertile women. For example, one young woman casually and matter-of-factly mentioned to me, "I had one child so that I could cross it off my 'to-do list.'" This woman sounded apologetic about becoming a mother, and her statement revealed that she had done so to rid herself of the relentless pressures she faced from her family, kin, and society in general to reproduce. The "to-do list" is an illustration of the complexities and competing demands people of reproductive age face. It is noteworthy that the demands of the state for its citizens to have more chidren are not included in the "to-do list" of the current generation of reproductive-age Iranians. It is these persisting cultural norms and values, and not the state's carrot-and-stick-policies, that motivate or even pressure both fertile and infertile couples to reproduce.

Population Complexities

While declining population growth is not unique to Iran, and indeed now characterizes most countries around the globe, Iran's experience is unique and thus instructive. For 150 years, through the rule of two dynasties and a theocratic republic, Iranian fertility regimes have sought to shape population trends. During these years, three governments adopted five policies, each contradicting the previous one and expecting citizens to adjust their reproductive values and practices to suit the state's body politic. Three of these reversals took place under the Islamic Republic's rule and within a span of forty years, with the antinatalist policies of the 1980s to 1990s standing out for their exemplary accomplishments and current pronatalist attempts floundering. Even the positive components of the current program, such as the provision of infertility treatment, do not seem to have made any meaningful contribution to increasing population growth.

However, a far graver miscalculation responsible for the failure of the current policies is in its relationship with women. Rather than seeking their cooperation, the state has adopted brutal measures to force them to have children, by blocking their access to any form of contraception and to the technologies that ensure the health and the safety of the fetus, such as prenatal genetic screening tests. In doing so, the state is deliberately trying to disempower women and prevent them from controlling their reproductive lives. However, the presumption that coercion will turn back the clock and make women reverse their childbearing practices has backfired dramatically. In response, instead of losing power over their reproductive lives, women have adopted various strategies, from ignoring and bypassing the authorities to actively defying them, which have eroded the power of the state. For the generations of reproductive age, especially for women, the ground has shifted beyond the fight for their reproductive rights and has become a reproductive rebellion, involving a battle for autonomy and human rights. The refusal to reproduce has become one of the most effective weapons in the hands of the generations of reproductive age to confront the power of the state. This defiance reached its peak following the death of a young woman, Mahsa Amini, in 2022, while in police custody for not wearing her headscarf (*hejab*) properly, which triggered the "Women, Life, Freedom" movement in Iran.

In considering whether the dramatic decline in childbearing practices means an irreversible transformation of reproductive norms and values, several points emerge. First, what may seem to be a contradiction in values and behavior between those who choose childlessness and those who are infertile and want to have children, is not about reproduction per se and whether or not to have children. As contemporary Iranian demography indicates, each couple continues to have an average of two children (Behjati-Ardakani, Navabakhsh, and Hassan Hosseini 2016). Those who choose not to have any children form a small minority. The demand of the state to have more than two children—which, as we have seen, is powerfully promoted and legally reinforced—is evidently being subverted. Meanwhile, the (often unrelenting) pressures of family, kin, and social norms likewise enjoin higher fertility, but not sufficiently to meet the level demanded by the state. In other words, it is not that childbearing values have disappeared among the younger generations but that having children is more a matter of choice in terms of timing and the number of children desired.

Conclusion

Two distinct themes emerge from this chapter. First, as the history of state involvement with the country's population makes clear, no lessons have been learned by the current autocratic Iranian state, which believes that the exercise of force is the only mechanism sufficient to achieve its goals. Analysis of the ebbs and flows of the population in Iran shows that, while four out of the five policies had a moderate to high degree of success, none adopted a coercive strategy. It also shows that it was the antinatalist policies that achieved exemplary success, an achievement that would have been unthinkable given the prevailing traditional norms and values attached to having large families at that time.

In contrast, by imposing its draconian pronatalist policies, the current Iranian regime acts under the misapprehension that it can bring citizens to their knees using force. Moreover, there is a stark contrast between the Qajar Dynasty's approach from 150 years ago, which encouraged population growth by improving the health of the population and thus succeeded in gaining popular support, and that of the current state, which is flagrantly sacrificing the health of the population in order to increase population growth at all costs, yet failing to do so.

Second, the findings of this chapter show that the question of reproduction has superseded that of mere childbearing and embodies the social, cultural, and political aspirations and grievances of the younger generations of Iranians, in particular of women. It is clear that most women's rejection of the state's demands for more children does not indicate the disappearance of reproductive values but rather is a show of reproductive rebellion, a sense of defiance and determination to assert their autonomy and retain control over their own lives. From this new perspective, not only does reproduction become a means of continuity, but women's bodies become a means of protest, strategy, and power, while also conforming to persistent cultural, but not political, forces. While the future of Iran's population decline remains unclear, it seems certain that forcing citizens to reproduce is not a game that the state is likely to win.

NOTE

1 Published in 1985, *The Handmaid's Tale* by Margaret Atwood is a futuristic dystopian novel that details a near-future theonomic totalitarian state.

REFERENCES

Abbasi-Shavazi, Mohammad Jalal, Peter McDonald, and Meimanat Hosseini-Chavoshi. 2011. *The Fertility Transition in Iran: Revolution and Reproduction*. New York: Springer.

Abbasi-Shavazi, Mohammad Jalal, and Hajieh Bibi Razeghi-Nasrabad. 2010. "Patterns and Factors Affecting Marriage Interval and First Birth in Iran." *Journal of Population Association of Iran* 5(9): 75–107.

Behjati-Ardakani, Zohreh, Mehrdad Navabakhsh, and Seyed Hassan Hosseini. 2016. "Sociological Study on the Transformation of Fertility and Childbearing Concept in Iran." *Journal of Reproduction and Infertility* 18(1): 153–61.

Hoodfar, Homa. 1995. "Population Policy and Gender Equity in Post-Revolutionary Iran." In *Family, Gender, and Population in the Middle East: Policies in Context*, ed. Carla Makhlouf, 105–35. Cairo: American University of Cairo.

————. 2017. "Turning Back the Clock: Population Policy and Human Rights in Iran." *Routledge Handbook on Human Rights and the Middle East and North Africa*, ed. Anthony Tirado Chase, 230–42. London: Routledge.

Hosseini-Chavoshi, Meimanat, Peter McDonald, and Mohammad Jalal Abbasi-Shavazi. 2007. "Fertility and Contraceptive Use Dynamics in Iran and Its Low Fertility Regions." Australian National University, DSRI Working Paper No.1.

Inhorn, Marcia C. 2006. "'He Won't Be My Son': Middle Eastern Muslim Men's Discourses of Adoption and Gamete Donation." In *Medical Anthropology Quarterly* 20(1): 94–120.

Inhorn, Marcia C., Daphna Birenbaum-Carmeli, Soraya Tremayne, and Zeynep B. Gurtin. 2017. "Assisted Reproduction and Kinship in the Middle East: A Regional and Religious Comparison." *Reproductive BioMedicine and Society Online* 4: 41–51.

Iran Project. 2016. "Single Child Families Challenge Iran's Population Growth." *The Iran Project* (blog). http://theiranproject.com.

"Iran Pushes for Baby Boom by Curtailing Access to Contraceptives and Abortions." 2021. *Middle East Eye*, December 5. www.middleeasteye.net.

"Iran's Population Crisis Awaits Iranian People." 2013. Tabnak, September 24. www .tabnak.ir. [In Persian.]

Iran Statistical Yearbook. 2016. Ministry of the Interior, Statistical Centre of Iran. www. amar.org.ir.

Iran Wire. 2021. "Figures Show a Province-Level 'Great Divide' in Divorce Rates in Iran." September 2. https://iranwire.com.

Jannati, Amir Naser. 2021. "About 20% of Iranian Couples Have Infertility Problems: Expert." *Tehran Times*, November 5. www.tehrantimes.com.

Karami, Arash. 2012. "Khamenei on Population Control: 'May God and History Forgive Us.'" *Al Monitor*, October 17. www.al-monitor.com.

Kashani-Sabet, Firoozeh. 2011. *Conceiving Citizens: Women and the Politics of Motherhood in Iran*. Oxford: Oxford University Press.

Ladier-Fouladi, Marie. 1997. "The Fertility Transition in Iran." *Population: An English Selection* 9: 191–214.

————. 2017. "La Nouvelle Politique de Population de la Republique Islamique: Enjeux et Defies" [The New Population Policy of the Islamic Republic: Issues and Challenges]. *Bulletin de l'Association de Géographies Français* 94(4): 587–99.

Mehran, Golnar. 2003/4. "Gender and Education in Iran." Paper commissioned for the EFA Global Monitoring Report, *Gender and Education for All: The Leap to Equality*.

Morshed-Behbahani, Bahar, Minoor Lamyian, Hassan Joulaei, and Ali Montazeri. 2020. "Analysis and Exploration of Infertility Policies in Iran: A Study Protocol." *Health Research Policy and Systems* 18(5). https://doi.org/10.1186/s12961 -019-0505-3.

Mypersia. 2023. Report on Interview with Prime Minister's Deputy for Women and Family Affairs. Instagram, May 12. https://t.me/mypersia24/25911. [In Persian.]

OHCHR (United Nations Office of the High Commission on Human Rights). 2021. "Iran: Repeal 'Crippling' New Anti-Abortion Law—UN Experts." November 16.

Roudi-Fahimi, Farzaneh. 2002. "Iran's Family Planning Program: Responding to a Nation's Needs." *Population Reference Bureau* 31: 1–8.

———. 2012. "Iran Is Reversing Its Population Policies." *Viewpoints* 7, August 28, Woodrow Wilson International Center for Scholars.

Saham News. 2023. June 2. https://t.me/sahamnewsorg/88266. [In Persian.]

Statista. 2023. "Iran: Population Growth from 2012 to 2022." www.statista.com.

Tremayne, Soraya. 2004. "And Never the Twain Shall Meet: Reproductive Health Policies of the Islamic Republic of Iran." In *Reproductive Agency, Medicine, and the State: Cultural Transformations in Childbearing*, ed. Maya Unnithan-Kumar, 181–202. Oxford: Berghahn.

———. 2006. "Modernity and Early Marriage: A View from Within." *Journal of the Middle East Women's Studies* 2(1): 65–94.

———. 2023. *Inconceivable Iran: To Reproduce or Not to Reproduce.* Oxford: Berghahn.

Tremayne, Soraya, and Mohammad Mehdi Akhondi. 2016. "Conceiving IVF in Iran." *Reproductive BioMedicine and Society Online* 2: 62–70.

Worldometers. 2023. "Iran Population (Live)." July 16. www.worldometers.info.

10

Rethinking Demography

Assisted Reproduction and the "Proximate Determinants of Fertility" Reexamined

NITZAN PERI-ROTEM

Translating reproductive cause and effect into demographic formulas that can be used to predict fertility change across different societies and historical periods has been crucial to demography since its inception. Accurately identifying "intermediate determinants of fertility"—a set of social, biological, and behavioral variables better known today as the "proximate determinants of fertility"—plays a key role in not only measuring but also defining the key causal elements of fertility change. This chapter revisits the work of Kingsley Davis and Judith Blake, who first introduced a framework to measure causal determinants of fertility change in the 1950s, and examines the way such demographic models have evolved over time. In addition, it offers suggestions as to how such models might be redefined in the context of the new reproductive order.

Rarely can one point to a single article that has truly redefined an entire field of research. Kingsley Davis and Judith Blake's (1956) publication, "Social Structure and Fertility: An Analytic Framework," which robustly argued the scientific case for a comparative sociology of fertility, is, however, one example of just such a paradigm-shifting study. Their groundbreaking article laid the foundations for the new field of social demography by proposing a specific mechanism for understanding how societal factors influence fertility patterns. Highlighting the importance of the unique social and historical contexts—and in particular the "social structures" that shape variations in fertility (Davis and Blake 1956: 211)—Davis and Blake introduced the term "comparative sociology of reproduction" to describe a systematic approach to the analysis of fertility change that took into account what they called "intermediate variables," through which not only social, institutional, and economic but also cultural factors could "influence" or "condition" fertility.

Since its initial publication, Davis and Blake's model of "intermediate variables" has radically transformed demography and led to the growth of new demographic subfields, including anthropological demography, and the study of what Susan Greenhalgh (1995) described as "situated fertility." Indeed, Greenhalgh's call, mentioned in the introduction to this volume, for greater attention to the specific historical and cultural influences on fertility is in many ways a direct extension of Davis and Blake's model. As we shall see in this chapter, the study of "intermediate variables" quickly became an established methodology that transformed the ways core fertility and population data sets are compiled by leading organizations, such as the United Nations, and how they are interpreted in national and international research exercises, such as the World Fertility Survey.

In this chapter, I review the origins and influence of the theory of the "intermediate variables," which later became known as the "proximate determinants of fertility," arguing for a need to revisit this concept more vigorously in the context of the new reproductive order. In what follows, I highlight the existing limitations of the proximate-determinants model in its definitions of who is likely to conceive and who is considered infertile. In addition, I argue that assisted reproductive technologies (ARTs) should be incorporated into the model, given their increasingly global spread and their impact, not only on fertility outcomes but also on other reproductive and social perceptions and behaviors. Other ways in which the proximate-determinants model could be improved are by situating it within the broader cultural, economic, and political context of given societies, as well as bridging across the disciplinary boundaries of the sociology and biology of fertility. Finally, the interrelationships between sociocultural factors and fertility should be seen as recursive, or cyclical, rather than unidirectional, since fertility trends are not only influenced by, but also shape, existing social perceptions, which in turn alter reproductive behaviors.

The Intermediate Variables

Davis and Blake defined "intermediate variables" as those mechanisms "through which any sociocultural factors influencing the level of fertility must operate" (Davis and Blake 1956: 211). All three elements of this definition are crucial: the intermediate variables are shaped by (1) factors of social organization, such as cultural or institutional structures; and (2) influential beliefs, or normative social practices; but (3) they must be those, and only those, that can directly affect biological fertility and thus fertility levels. This means that the intermediate variables must directly affect the "three necessary steps" of successful biological reproduction, namely, intercourse, conception, and gestation followed by birth. Davis and Blake consequently categorized "intermediate variables" into three main types: (1) "intercourse variables" include determinants of coital exposure (such as age at entry into union, celibacy, union dissolution, and sex frequency); (2) "conception variables" (including contraception use, fecundity, and infecundity); and (3) "gestation variables" (miscarriage or induced abortion).

The basic idea of this three-part typology of the intermediate variables is to identify and characterize a *limited* set of variables that can be isolated as channels, or mechanisms, through which any other influences at the societal level, be they cultural, socioeconomic, or environmental, can affect fertility. The aim is thus to open up the study of fertility to more systematic analysis of the determining impact of variations in social organization: "In order to study the effects of institutional factors," the authors note, "one needs to break down the reproductive process itself so as to distinguish clearly the various mechanisms through which, and only through which, any social factor *can* influence fertility" (Davis and Blake 1956: 234, original emphasis). Therefore, any attempt to make causal explanations about the ways in which sociocultural conditions affect fertility should involve these intermediate variables.

In total, Davis and Blake identify eleven subcategories of "intermediate variables" within their three main categories, each of which can be assigned a positive or negative value in the effort to determine its influence on fertility. It is also assumed that all eleven variables exist in all societies, so there cannot be a question of whether any one of them is present or not, leaving instead only the question of how—or in particular, how much—it is influencing fertility levels. Thus, they explain, "One cannot say, as is frequently implied in the literature, that some of these variables are affecting fertility in one society but not in another. *All* of the variables are present in *every* society. This is because, as mentioned before, each one *is* a variable—it can operate either to reduce or to enhance fertility. If abortion is *not* practiced, the fertility-value of variable number 11 is 'plus.' In other words, the absence of a specific practice does not imply 'no influence' on fertility, because this very absence is a form of influence" (Davis and Blake 1956: 212, original emphasis).

Over time, Davis and Blake's model has both evolved and been adapted by many demographers seeking to achieve a similar goal by using the concept of intermediate variables. In 1978, for example, demographer John Bongaarts created a simplified quantifiable model based on Davis and Blake's intermediate determinants of fertility, for which he coined the term "proximate determinants of fertility." In contrast to Davis and Blake (whose "intermediate variables" he considered too numerous and complex to reliably quantify), Bongaarts's model included "only a small number of conceptually distinct and quantitatively important intermediate fertility variables" (Bongaarts 1978: 106) that could more reliably be measured. His revised typology of eight variables relates strictly to women of reproductive age and in a formal union and falls under three main categories of "fertility factors": (1) "exposure factors" (the proportion of women who are in a marital [or other] union); (2) "deliberate factors" (the proportion of married couples using contraception or abortion); and (3) "natural marital factors" (including lactation,[1] intercourse, infertility, and miscarriage). Bongaarts offered a mathematical equation by which overall fertility, or TFR (total fertility rate), can be calculated by simply multiplying "total fecundity" by all the proximate variables,[2] arguing that this "should explain 100 percent of variation in fertility" (Bongaarts 2015: 536).

Criticism of the Proximate Determinants of Fertility

Despite being one of the most widely used demographic instruments for both measuring and projecting fertility rates worldwide, the proximate-determinants-of-fertility model has also attracted criticism regarding its underlying assumptions, operationalization, and reliability. As this volume argues, these shortcomings also point to much wider and more macrolevel shifts in reproductive cause and effect, including the influence of new reproductive technologies and increasing fertility precarity, among other factors shaping what we are calling "the new reproductive order."

A Misleading Formula?

Bongaarts's model of the proximate determinants of fertility initially gained popularity among demographers due to its simplicity and relatively modest data requirements. Rather than eleven, or even eight, there were only four main vector variables required to estimate the fertility rate of a given population: the proportion of women in consensual unions, the proportion using contraception, the number of abortions women have had by the end of their reproductive years, and the average length of breastfeeding. For example, in a 1992 review article evaluating several different methodologies for measuring the impact of proximate determinants on fertility, demographer Kia Reinis concluded that the Bongaarts model performs well when used to run random computational simulations but much less effectively when it is applied to real populations. Reinis argued not only that the assumptions underlying the model and its formula were "too heroic and simplistic" but that the "very poor estimates" of fertility that resulted from these failures "should serve as a sober warning to those who compute indices and believe that they adequately measure the fertility-reducing impact of the proximate determinants of fertility" (Reinis 1992: 325).

Due to the overreliance on what have been criticized as the false premises of this predictive formula, both Bongaarts's and other models of the intermediate determinants of fertility may lead to a narrow or simplistic view of fertility behavior and to neglecting the societal context that shapes and interacts with them. This criticism of an overly formulaic approach has similarly been voiced by Davis and Blake themselves, as Judith Blake noted in an interview from 1989, more than thirty years after the publication of their work: "The whole point of the [1956] article was to say, 'if you want to look at sociocultural influences on fertility, then you have to be aware of what they operate through and that these are the variables they operate through.' I think nobody would ever have accused us of thinking that what we wanted to do was to just look at those variables. So it ends up that something like that provides people with a very mechanical way of looking at things. It's unfortunate that that's happened" (PAA Oral History Project 2005: 106). However, Blake has also acknowledged the paradoxical nature of the proximate-determinants model, which aims to account for the entire variation in fertility rates across societies, while disregarding the complex relation-ships between fertility behavior and social and cultural factors: "And yet a non-mechanical way, for all those countries with all that's going on, would not have been possible" (PAA Oral History Project 2005: 106).

In sum, the quantified model of the proximate determinants of fer-tility, which builds upon but also condenses Davis and Blake's already foreshortened framework, is now accused of having shifted attention away from the very same intricate relationships between sociocultural aspects and fertility behavior that the concept of "intermediate vari-ables" was designed to illuminate. The more formulaic the model has become, the more deceptive the focus on measuring the effect of a lim-ited number of variables on fertility outcomes. In exchange for ease of calculation and a "heroic" formula, it appears the baby has possibly been thrown out with the bathwater.

Whose Sexual Activity Counts?

Much of the criticism of Bongaarts's model of the proximate deter-minants of fertility involves issues of empirical definition and measurement. One area of concern raised by critics is the measure of what is known as "sexual exposure"—meaning, more precisely, the occurrence and frequency of unprotected heterosexual intercourse. In a major review article evaluating twenty years of proximate-determinant models, published in 1998, demographer John Stover (1998) argued that Bongaarts's measure is biased as it excludes sexually active women who are not in unions, while also overestimating sexual activity among those who are married.

More than fifteen years later, Bongaarts has partly accepted Stover's proposal to revise the sexual-exposure measure to include sexually ac-tive women outside formal unions, in addition to all married women of reproductive age (Bongaarts 2015). Nevertheless, this measure may still be subject to bias, given that not all married women are sexually active, and the frequency of sexual intercourse clearly varies across and within populations as well as over time (Peri-Rotem and Skirbekk 2023; Stover 1998; Twenge, Sherman, and Wells 2017).

An additional challenge to this measure is the difficulty of account-ing for various sexual practices that have different consequences for the risk of pregnancy, including the use of withdrawal or non-penile-vaginal intercourse. These factors, justifiably or not, are classified as "conception variables" in Davis and Blake's intermediate-variables framework. However, in most cases, there are insufficient data to estimate their contribution to fertility trends. In sum, there is no consensus on who should be considered as sexually active, nor on the effect of sex frequency on the likelihood of conception.

Measuring Infertility

Defining and measuring infertility has been another subject of considerable controversy in the debate over proximate-determinants-of-fertility models and beyond. When assessing levels of "pathological infertility" or "sterility," Bongaarts has used a measure based on the proportion of women who are childless at the end of their reproductive years, i.e., between the ages of forty-five and forty-nine (Bongaarts, Frank, and Lesthaeghe 1984). However, he has also and more recently argued that, since the 1990s, sterility variations between populations (at least those that are included in the Demographic Health Survey) "have become small enough to be ignored" (Bongaarts 2015: 543). Therefore, according to Bongaarts, there is no longer any sufficient justification—or necessity—to include an index of sterility in the proximate determinants of fertility.

In contrast to Bongaarts, who used a measure of lifetime childlessness, Stover's (1998) measure refers to both lifetime and current infertility, by including women who have not given birth in the last five years, while being in union without using contraception. Using this more nuanced measure, Stover found evidence of substantial differences across regions in levels of infertility. For example, the proportion of infertile women was found to be higher in Asia and Africa than in Latin America (Stover 1998).

A more recent study led by the health psychologist Jacky Boivin, which assessed the prevalence of both current and lifetime infertility, was also able to identify divergent levels of infertility across populations with varying levels of development, showing a range of 4 percent to 17 percent in the prevalence of current infertility (measured as a delay in twelve months or more in conception) among women between the ages of twenty and forty-four (Boivin et al. 2007). Furthermore, the contributing factors to infertility vary significantly between more and less developed countries. In the latter, infection from sexually transmitted diseases and poor reproductive care form the main drivers of infertility, while in more developed countries, there are (increasingly) higher rates of age-related infertility (Boivin et al. 2007; Datta et al. 2016; Inhorn and Patrizio 2015; Larsen 2003).

It should be noted that both the prevalence of infertility and its contributing factors are not stable and tend to change over time. For example, the postponement of first birth, which increases the risk of age-related infertility, has also been found to rise in less developed countries, including in Africa and Latin America, partly as a result of increasing labor market opportunities for women (Gyimah 2003; Rosero-Bixby, Castro-Martín, and Martín-García 2009). Furthermore, what is known as the female "reproductive window," or in other words, the life course period when women are considered at risk of becoming pregnant, has changed over time. In the past 150 years, in many populations there has been a decrease in the average age of menarche, while the age of menopause has either remained stable or increased (Skirbekk 2022). In addition, developments in ARTs have further stretched the limits of the biological reproductive lifespan, by enabling, in some cases, postmenopausal women to become pregnant and give birth (Billari et al. 2007; Banh, Havemann, and Phelps 2010). As the use of ARTs is constantly growing, the limits of the reproductive lifespan may further expand.

The Role of Assisted Reproductive Technologies

While the proximate-determinants model has been adjusted to address the increasing disconnection between sexual activity and marriage, the recent revisions have yet to consider the role of ARTs in shaping fertility trends. The use of ARTs, which facilitated new pathways of family formation, has rapidly risen in virtually all parts of the world over the past four decades; in some countries, babies born following ART use comprise nearly 8 percent of all children born in a given year (Chambers et al. 2021).

ARTs are unique in the context of the intermediate determinants of fertility, as they provide a way to reproduce independently from heterosexual intercourse, although they can influence and be influenced by other intermediate variables. For example, having the option to become a parent without a partner from the opposite sex may influence norms, perceptions, and strategies of family building (Inhorn et al. 2018; Pralat 2018), which could potentially alter patterns of union formation and dissolution. Also, the increased availability of ARTs as a form of treatment for age-related infertility can lead to extended use of contraception in order to postpone childbearing, and vice versa (Szewczuk 2012). Finally, while in some regions the access to ARTs is highly limited, this does not mean that it bears no consequences on the reproductive aspirations, intentions, and behaviors of these populations (Inhorn and Patrizio 2015).

Beyond Statistical Modeling

What can we therefore learn by revisiting the proximate determinants of fertility in light of recent technological, social, demographic, and environmental developments? And, how can we address caveats in the existing framework?

Considering the Broader Picture

The criticism of the quantified models of the proximate determinants of fertility highlights the importance of considering the broader picture of the relationships between structural and cultural conditions and fertility behavior. This approach is not new and has already been put forward by the American social demographer Calvin Goldscheider (1971, 2006), who argued that in order to understand the fertility behavior of different groups, one should take into account the broader social organization of that group, including norms and values that guide daily life and the way these norms are reconstructed and reinforced alongside social and political changes.

The need for a more comprehensive approach for understanding fertility change is further stressed by Susan Greenhalgh (1990, 1995), who offered an analytic framework—a political economy of fertility—that can be seen as an extension to the intermediate-variables thesis. One of the underlying assumptions of this framework is that factors affecting fertility operate at both micro (community, regional) and macro (national, international, global) levels, and that these elements are interconnected.

According to this framework, fertility change is not only a product of long-term social, economic, political, and cultural processes, but it is also shaped by the interactions between structure and agency, and between environment and behavior (Greenhalgh 1990).

A similar approach can be applied when one examines the influence of top-down policies aimed at influencing fertility levels of a given society. In a recently published article in the medical journal *The BMJ*, demographers Stuart Gietel-Basten, Anna Rotkirch, and Tomáš Sobotka (2022) argue against "simplistic" target-driven population policies, which often use narrowly oriented and harmful interventions, including restricted access to abortion, contraception, and sexual education, as seen in chapter 9 of this volume on Iran. These policies, they argue, not only have a limited effect on fertility but also have potentially detrimental consequences for gender equality, human rights, and sexual and reproductive health (Gietel-Basten, Rotkirch, and Sobotka 2022). Recent examples include the tightening of abortion restrictions in Poland in 2021, followed a year later by the overturning of the constitutional right to abortion by the United States Supreme Court. A recent study from Poland found evidence that the added restrictions to abortion have led to a decline, rather than an increase in fertility levels (Matysiak and Van der Velde 2023). In order to understand this counterintuitive outcome, one needs to acknowledge the interconnections between the different intermediate determinants of fertility and the wider political, economic, and social context. While changes to abortion policy are likely to influence decisions about pregnancy termination, they may also affect individuals' actions that would lead to (or prevent) a pregnancy, including sexual activity and/or contraceptive behavior, depending on the circumstances (Levine 2004). Therefore, fertility cannot be simply manipulated by means of altering one or more of the proximate determinants, and their effect on fertility must be understood in relation to the wider social setting.

Reframing Sociobiological Interactions

The classification of societal-level factors as indirect determinants of fertility and biological-physiological factors as direct determinants creates a divide between social and biological factors that may influence fertility, while also preserving the idea of "natural" fertility as a kind of neutral bottom line. In recent years, an increasing number of studies have addressed the interaction between socioeconomic and biomedical characteristics in relation to fertility, and these have indicated the complex nature of these interactions (see, for example, Hobcraft 2006; Kulathinal and Säävälä 2015; and Mills et al. 2021). Some of these studies have found that socioeconomic factors are equally as important to the realization of fertility intentions as epidemiological factors, and sometimes more so. For example, a study from Australia found that highly educated women were most likely to realize their intention to have a child within four years, while other biomedical measures, including self-rated health, body mass index, and smoking status did not have a significant effect on the realization of fertility intentions (Beaujouan et al. 2019). Similarly, a study from Britain shows that (women's) education remains an important predictor of couples' fertility outcomes after controlling for health indicators and other demographic factors (Peri-Rotem 2023).

These studies demonstrate the complex relationships between socioeconomic, biomedical factors and fertility and the difficulty in disentangling biological, social, and cultural explanations of fertility outcomes. Health factors may act as both indirect and direct determinants of fertility and are closely intertwined with socioeconomic factors. For example, lower-educated women are more likely to smoke than higher-educated ones (Cutler and Lleras-Muney 2010; Pampel, Krueger, and Denney 2010), and smoking is associated with earlier age of menopause and reduced fecundity (Gold et al. 2013; Sharma et al. 2013). In addition, higher-educated women are more likely to use preventive medicine, which is linked with improved reproductive health (Cutler and Lleras-Muney 2010; Murto et al. 2017) and are also more likely to seek medical help when experiencing infertility and to use ARTs (Bunting and Boivin 2007; Datta et al. 2016). The positive association between education and reproductive health holds across a wide range of high- and low-income countries (World Health Organization 2009).

Thus, the interaction between socioeconomic status and health factors, which is shaped by macrolevel social, economic, and political forces, may lead to different fertility outcomes. However, current demographic research has only begun to explore these intersections.

Directions of Influence

One of the most important insights to be gained from recent studies that demonstrate the complex relationships between multiple factors that influence fertility is that these factors also interact with each other. More than any other recent insight from demography, this "interactivity" factor significantly complicates the "intermediate" or "proximate-variable" approach, while also showing why it may have extensive unrealized potential.

As we have seen, in the proximate-determinants-of-fertility model, the mechanism of influence is understood as unidirectional and the analytic, or causal, focus on the effects of societal factors on fertility outcomes via the behavioral and biological intermediate variables is linear. While both Bongaarts and Davis and Blake recognize the codependencies between the different intermediate variables, neither framework considers other directions of influence between the different components of the model. For example, existing fertility patterns, resulting from specific social, economic, or political developments, can shape individuals' lifestyles, norms, and attitudes about the ideal or intended family size, which in turn lead to behaviors that support these fertility intentions. This kind of recursive relationship between fertility and social norms, including kinship, gender, and parenting norms, is crucial to the low-fertility-trap hypothesis initially proposed by a team of European demographers (Lutz, Skirbekk, and Testa 2006) and recently popularized by the British reproductive biologist Robert John Aitken (2022) in his book, *The Infertility Trap*. According to the low-fertility-trap hypothesis, once fertility falls to "lowest-low" levels (i.e., below 1.5 children per woman), it is less likely to rise back up again, due to both demographic and social mechanisms, which reinforce each other (Lutz, Skirbekk, and Testa 2006). In this model—as in the Changing In-Fertilities Project (CIFP) that led to this volume—it is perceptions of fertility change that themselves are understood to have a transformative, causal effect on fertility beliefs, intentions, and behaviors, and in turn feed back into the same fertility dynamics they are responding to. Thus, as new generations grow up in a low-fertility environment and become used to its particular lifestyles and economic expectations, family-size norms and preferences adjust accordingly. Similar processes may occur at the individual level, as people may change their fertility preferences following childbirth (Sennott and Yeatman 2012). Among demographers, and in particular advocates of the fertility-trap hypothesis, various "tipping points" can be reached, driven by feedback loops that not only drive but accelerate certain directions of change. This has been exemplified in the afterlife of China's one-child policy.

Taking such considerations into account can contribute to developing new and elaborate applications to the proximate determinants of fertility. For example, we might envisage potential mechanisms of influence in the interrelationships between education and fertility, while incorporating the contribution of health indicators and ARTs alongside key intermediate determinants of fertility.

Figure 10.1 shows the path diagram of such a hypothesized "circular" relationship between education and fertility. One of the most intensively studied areas of fertility "cause and effect," the relationship between increased women's education and fertility decline, is also one of the main preoccupations that led John Bongaarts to develop his intervention-oriented simplified models of "key" fertility factors to begin with. As figure 10.1 shows, the relationship between education and fertility is assumed to be mediated by the proximate determinants of sexual activity (linked to patterns of union formation, including delayed marriage) and contraceptive use, as well as by differential use of assisted reproduction and health factors. However, it is worth noting that many of these factors, including occurrence and timing of marriage, contraceptive use, and health, are also likely to affect educational achievements. In addition, if all of the intermediate factors are assumed to be correlated (e.g., ART use is associated with health, sexual exposure, etc.), then the resulting picture is more of an interactive fertility matrix, or set of recursive loops, than a set of arrows mapping the influence of one-way fertility "drivers" or "determinants." For example, and as argued by Reinis (1992) in her critiques of Bongaarts's model already mentioned above, contraception use is likely to be influenced by fertility behavior, i.e., the number of children a woman already has, yet such an action—arguably among the "simplest" of family-planning measures to detect—cannot be factored into the classic unidirectional formula of the intermediate variables.

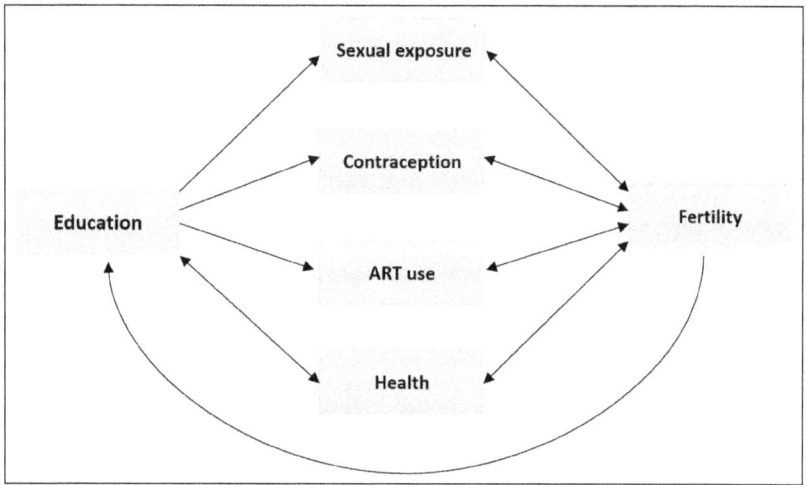

Figure 10.1. Path Diagram Modeling Hypothesized Relationships between Education and Fertility

Long description: A path diagram showing unidirectional arrows from education on the left to sexual exposure, contraception, and ART use and a bidirectional arrow between education and health. Bidirectional arrows link sexual exposure, contraception, ART use, and health in the middle to fertility on the right-hand side. A unidirectional arrow links fertility to education.

Conclusion

Both the proximate- and intermediate-determinants-of-fertility frameworks and their corresponding models have significantly shaped the way demographers study, theorize, and analyze fertility patterns. These influential frameworks have been continuously adjusted and modified over the past seven decades, and the debate about their uses, shortcomings, intentions, and strengths is in many ways a map of the history of demography itself. This chapter has highlighted some of the key points of controversy, including the argument that the oversimplified model of the proximate determinants of fertility may become so formulaic as to obscure exactly the added social complexities such models were originally designed to help illuminate. Nonetheless, the ways in which these variables are defined and measured, as well as the inclusion and exclusion of variables within the proximate-determinants framework, have had far-reaching implications for how we interpret different fertility behaviors and understand fertility change over time and space. For example, definitions of who is infertile and who is at risk of becoming pregnant are still shaping and being shaped by social norms and expectations regarding who *should* become pregnant. Furthermore, the uneven global spread of reproductive technologies poses new challenges to understanding the biological limits to reproduction and the role of ARTs in shaping fertility behavior in different societies.

Thus, in this chapter, I have proposed some adjustments to the proximate-determinants framework, including the need to consider the wider social settings in which the fertility determinants operate. This approach builds on ideas presented in Davis and Blake's original framework but can be used to understand the implications of current policies on fertility behavior. Other adjustments include the incorporation of ARTs as an additional intermediate variable and a health indicator that may be defined as either a direct or indirect determinant of fertility, due to its potential to influence both fertility and societal-level factors. Finally, defining the model as recursive, or as a fertility matrix, involving different and coproductive directions of influence, may lead to more authentic representations of the complex interrelationships between the different variables that determine fertility change.

These adjustments, however, are not without limitations and may pose new empirical and theoretical challenges; both ART use and health may be measured in multiple ways, and their effects on fertility are undoubtedly less straightforward compared to the "classic" intermediate determinants. For example, some of the births that followed the use of assisted reproduction may also have happened without it. In addition, the mechanisms linking health factors with fertility are not well understood. It should also be noted that, while these adjustments call for more elaborated modeling of the determinants of fertility, which would take into account the wider social context, it is not possible to include all potentially relevant factors. Nonetheless, rethinking the proximate determinants of fertility can promote the exploration of new research avenues and contribute to a better understanding of the causes and consequences of fertility in a rapidly changing world.

NOTES

1 Exclusive breastfeeding has been found to delay the return of ovulation following childbirth. However, the effectiveness of breastfeeding as a method of contraception varies significantly across societies and is found to be weaker in countries with higher economic development (Lethbridge 1989; Todd and Lerch 2021).

2 Total fecundity is the hypothetical total fertility rate that would be observed if the inhibiting effects of the proximate variables are removed, i.e., in the absence of contraception, abortion, and lactation, and assuming that all women are married or in unions. Total fecundity is typically estimated at around fifteen births per woman (Bongaarts 1978, 2015).

REFERENCES

Aitken, R. John. 2022. *The Infertility Trap: Why Life Choices Impact Your Fertility and Why We Must Act Now*. Cambridge: Cambridge University Press.

Banh, David, Dara L. Havemann, and John Y. Phelps. 2010. "Reproduction beyond Menopause: How Old Is Too Old for Assisted Reproductive Technology?" *Journal of Assisted Reproduction and Genetics* 27(7): 365–70.

Beaujouan, Éva, Anna Reimondos, Edith Gray, Ann Evans, and Tomás Sobotka. 2019. "Declining Realisation of Reproductive Intentions with Age." *Human Reproduction* 34(10): 1906–14.

Billari, Francesco C., Hans-Peter Kohler, Gunnar Andersson, and Hans Lundström. 2007. "Approaching the Limit: Long-Term Trends in Late and Very Late Fertility." *Population and Development Review* 33(1): 149–70.

Boivin, Jacky, Laura Bunting, John A. Collins, and Karl G. Nygren. 2007. "International Estimates of Infertility Prevalence and Treatment-Seeking: Potential Need and Demand for Infertility Medical Care." *Human Reproduction* 22(6): 1506–12.

Bongaarts, John. 1978. "A Framework for Analyzing the Proximate Determinants of Fertility." *Population and Development Review* 4(1): 105–32.

———. 2015. "Modeling the Fertility Impact of the Proximate Determinants: Time for a Tune-Up." *Demographic Research* 33(19): 535–60.

Bongaarts, John, Odile Frank, and Ron Lesthaeghe. 1984. "The Proximate Determinants of Fertility in Sub-Saharan Africa." *Population and Development Review* 10(3): 511–37.

Bunting, Laura, and Jacky Boivin. 2007. "Decision-Making about Seeking Medical Advice in an Internet Sample of Women Trying to Get Pregnant." *Human Reproduction* 22(6): 1662–68.

Chambers, Georgina M., Silke Dyer, Fernando Zegers-Hochschild, Jacques de Mouzon, Osamu Ishihara, Manish Banker, Ragaa Mansour, Markus S. Kupka, and G. David Adamson. 2021. "International Committee for Monitoring Assisted Reproductive Technologies World Report: Assisted Reproductive Technology, 2014." *Human Reproduction* 36(11): 2921–34.

Cutler, David M., and Adriana Lleras-Muney. 2010. "Understanding Differences in Health Behaviors by Education." *Journal of Health Economics* 29(1): 1–28.

Datta, J., M. J. Palmer, C. Tanton, L. J. Gibson, K. G. Jones, W. Macdowall, A. Glasier, P. Sonnenberg, N. Field, C. H. Mercer, A. M. Johnson, and K. Wellings. 2016. "Prevalence of Infertility and Help Seeking among 15000 Women and Men." *Human Reproduction* 31(9): 2108–18.

Davis, Kingsley, and Judith Blake. 1956. "Social Structure and Fertility: An Analytic Framework." *Economic Development and Cultural Change* 4(3): 211–35.

Gietel-Basten, Stuart, Anna Rotkirch, and Tomáš Sobotka. 2022. "Changing the Perspective on Low Birth Rates: Why Simplistic Solutions Won't Work." *BMJ* 379: 1–5.

Gold, Ellen B., Sybil L. Crawford, Nancy E. Avis, Carolyn J. Crandall, Karen A. Matthews, L. Elaine Waetjen, Jennifer S. Lee, Rebecca Thurston, Marike Vuga, and Siobán D. Harlow. 2013. "Factors Related to Age at Natural Menopause: Longitudinal Analyses from SWAN." *American Journal of Epidemiology* 178(1): 70–83.

Goldscheider, Calvin. 1971. *Population, Modernization, and Social Structure.* Boston: Little, Brown.

———. 2006. "Religion, Family, and Fertility: What Do We Know Historically and Comparatively?" In *Religion and the Decline of Fertility in the Western World*, ed. Renzo Derosas and Frans van Poppel, 41–57. Dordrecht: Springer.

Greenhalgh, Susan. 1990. "Toward a Political Economy of Fertility: Anthropological Contributions." *Population and Development Review* 16(1): 85–106.

———. 1995. *Situating Fertility.* Cambridge: Cambridge University Press.

Gyimah, Stephen O. 2003. "Women's Educational Attainment and the Timing of Parenthood in Ghana: A Cohort Perspective." *PSC Discussion Papers* 17(4): 1–28.

Hobcraft, John. 2006. "The ABC of Demographic Behaviour: How the Interplays of Alleles, Brains, and Contexts over the Life Course Should Shape Research Aimed at Understanding Population Processes." *Population Studies* 60(2): 153–87.

Inhorn, Marcia C., Daphna Birenbaum-Carmeli, Lynn M. Westphal, Joseph Doyle, Norbert Gleicher, Dror Meirow, Martha Dirnfeld, Daniel Seidman, Arik Kahane, and Pasquale Patrizio. 2018. "Ten Pathways to Elective Egg Freezing: A Binational Analysis." *Journal of Assisted Reproduction and Genetics* 35(1): 2003–11.

Inhorn, Marcia C., and Pasquale Patrizio. 2015. "Infertility around the Globe: New Thinking on Gender, Reproductive Technologies, and Global Movements in the 21st Century." *Human Reproduction Update* 21(4): 411–26.

Kulathinal, Sangita, and Minna Säävälä. 2015. "Fertility Intentions and Early Life Health Stress among Women in Eight Indian Cities: Testing the Reproductive Acceleration Hypothesis." *Journal of Biosocial Science* 47(5): 632–49.

Larsen, Ulla. 2003. "Infertility in Central Africa." *Tropical Medicine and International Health* 8(4): 354–67.

Lethbridge, Dona J. 1989. "The Use of Breastfeeding as a Contraceptive." *Journal of Obstetric, Gynecological, and Neonatal Nursing* 18(1): 31–37.

Levine, Philip B. 2004. *Sex and Consequences: Abortion, Public Policy, and the Economics of Fertility*. Princeton, NJ: Princeton University Press.

Lutz, Wolfgang, Vegard Skirbekk, and Maria Rita Testa. 2006. "The Low-Fertility Trap Hypothesis: Forces That May Lead to Further Postponement and Fewer Births in Europe." *Vienna Yearbook of Population Research* 4: 167–92.

Matysiak, Anna, and Lucas van der Velde. 2023. "Tightening of Abortion Laws and Fertility." Paper presented at the annual meeting of Population Association of America, New Orleans, Louisiana, April 13.

Mills, Melinda C., Felix C. Tropf, David M. Brazel, Natalie van Zuydam, Ahmad Vaez, eQTLGen Consortium, BIOS Consortium, Human Reproductive Behaviour Consortium, Tune H. Pers, Harold Snieder, John R. B. Perry, Ken K. Ong, Marcel den Hoed, Nicola Barban, and Felix R. Day. 2021. "Identification of 371 Genetic Variants for Age at First Sex and Birth Linked to Externalising Behaviour." *Nature Human Behaviour* 5: 1717–30.

Murto, Tiina, Yngve Agneta, Skoog Svanberg Agneta, Altmäe Signe, Salumets Andres, Wånggren Kjell, and Stavreus-Evers Anneli. 2017. "Compliance to the Recommended Use of Folic Acid Supplements for Women in Sweden Is Higher among Those under Treatment for Infertility Than among Fertile Controls and Is Also Related to Socioeconomic Status and Lifestyle." *Food & Nutrition Research* 61(1): 1–7.

PAA Oral History Project. 2005. *Demographic Destinies: Interviews with Presidents and Secretary-Treasurers of the Population Association of America, by Jean van der Tak* 1(3). Washington, DC: Population Association of America.

Pampel, Fred C., Patrick M. Krueger, and Justin T. Denney. 2010. "Socioeconomic Disparities in Health Behaviors." *Annual Review of Sociology* 36: 349–70.

Peri-Rotem, Nitzan. 2023. "Education, Health Indicators, and Fertility Outcomes: A Longitudinal Analysis of Couples in Britain." *Longitudinal and Life Course Studies* 15(1): 109–32.

Peri-Rotem, Nitzan, and Vegard Skirbekk. 2023. "Religiosity, Sex Frequency, and Sexual Satisfaction in Britain: Evidence from the Third National Survey of Sexual Attitudes and Lifestyles (Natsal)." *Journal of Sex Research* 60(1): 13–35.

Pralat, Robert. 2018. "More Natural Does Not Equal More Normal: Lesbian, Gay, and Bisexual People's Views about Different Pathways to Parenthood." *Journal of Family Issues* 39(18): 4179–4203.

Reinis, Kia I. 1992. "The Impact of the Proximate Determinants of Fertility: Evaluating Bongaarts's and Hobcraft and Little's Methods of Estimation." *Population Studies* 46(1): 309–26.

Rosero-Bixby, Luis, Teresa Castro-Martín, and Teresa Martín-García. 2009. "Is Latin America Starting to Retreat from Early and Universal Childbearing?" *Demographic Research* 20(9): 169–94.

Sennott, Christie, and Sara Yeatman. 2012. "Stability and Change in Fertility Preferences among Young Women in Malawi." *International Perspectives on Sexual and Reproductive Health* 38(1): 34–42.

Sharma, Rakesh, Kelly R. Biedenharn, Jennifer M. Fedor, and Ashok Agarwal. 2013. "Lifestyle Factors and Reproductive Health: Taking Control of Your Fertility." *Reproductive Biology and Endocrinology* 11(66): 1–15.

Skirbekk, Vegard. 2022. *Decline and Prosper! Changing Global Birth Rates and the Advantage of Fewer Children.* Cham, UK: Palgrave Macmillan.

Stover, John. 1998. "Revising the Proximate Determinants of Fertility Framework: What Have We Learned in the Past 20 Years?" *Studies in Family Planning* 29(3): 255–67.

Szewczuk, Elizabeth. 2012. "Age-Related Infertility: A Tale of Two Technologies." *Sociology of Health & Illness* 34(3): 429–43.

Todd, Nicolas, and Mathias Lerch. 2021. "Socioeconomic Development Predicts a Weaker Contraceptive Effect of Breastfeeding." *PNAS* 118(29): 1–6.

Twenge, Jean M., Ryne A. Sherman, and Brooke E. Wells. 2017. "Declines in Sexual Frequency among American Adults, 1989–2014." *Archives of Sexual Behavior* 46: 2389–2401.

World Health Organization. 2009. *Promoting Adolescent Sexual and Reproductive Health through Schools in Low Income Countries: An Information Brief.* Department of Child and Adolescent Health and Development. Geneva, Switzerland.

PART III

In-Fertile Economies

The chapters in this section focus on the political economy of in-fertility in a world in which markets for fertility services and products, as well as new and old forms of reproductive labor, continue to expand rapidly. The ART industry in today's new reproductive order is characterized by three important features. First, the delivery of IVF services has become increasingly commercial and transactional in nature, as well as increasingly profit driven. The IVF industry is not only growing but consolidating under the influence of investment capital. Second, the ART industry is highly international and mobile. IVF delivery exists transnationally within a *global reproscape*, in which people, technologies, money, human body parts (e.g., eggs and sperm), and human biodata (e.g., based on fertility measures) move across national borders. Third, the ART sector requires the recruitment and scaling up of increasing amounts of reproductive labor. Millions of workers, performing highly diverse forms of reproductive service work, now participate in the complex global ART industry, including IVF physicians, embryologists, clinic managers, couriers, donors, surrogates, and fertility brokers. These frontline fertility providers are in turn backed up by a vast new industry of in-fertility enterprise, ranging from financing and insurance services to online support and information portals.

To begin to understand the *fertinomics* of this new reproductive order, it is critical to identify the key values shaping the new industry. "Fertility efficiency" is one of the leading discourses now found in an increasingly financialized and commercial ART sector, which promotes increased automation, reduced labor costs, and various treatment "add-ons" to extend fertility and enhance clinic profitability (chapter 11). The mobility of the ART sector at the heart of the new reproductive order can be clearly seen in the rapidly changing logistics of reproductive workflows, supply chains, and managerial strategies involved in the "mobile reproductive labor" of "fly-in fly-out" (FIFO) clinicians in sub-Saharan Africa—a region once devoid of IVF clinics, but now becoming one of the fastest-growing ART markets in the world (chapter 12). Resource-poor post-Soviet nations are also encouraging new forms of reproductive labor, as seen in Georgia's new class of "motherworkers," or surrogates who participate in "housewifization" in order to support their own families through remunerated domestic confinement (chapter 13). Finally, it is important to recognize the new reproductive economy of human biodata in the world today. In the nation of Finland, a profitable human biodata "goldmine" is being developed, although it reflects long-standing "repropolitical anxieties" about population control and a haunting history of eugenic sterilizations (chapter 14). Taken together, these thought-provoking chapters on in-fertile economies speak to multiple forms of exploitation and extraction—of data, labor, human bodies, and body parts made profitable. Ultimately, we see the ways in which stratified reproduction and reproductive injustices live on within the new reproductive order's political economy.

11

Fertility Efficiency

Rationalizing Reproductive Extensions in Financialized IVF

LUCY VAN DE WIEL

In the last decade, one of the key changes in the assisted reproduction field is the extension of fertility along a number of axes: extending the fertile years with frozen eggs, extending the in vitro fertilization (IVF) cycle with so-called add-on technologies, and expanding the fertility sector with new financial investments. Each of these extensions illustrates how fertility perceptions and practices are changing within an IVF sector that is itself transforming in line with new business imperatives.

The introduction of egg freezing has enabled the extension of the reproductive lifespan to later ages—as well as the precaritization of fertility at earlier ages—and broadened the indication for fertility treatment to women without an infertility diagnosis. Meanwhile, new reproductive technologies for testing, screening, and predicting future fertility and viability, such as time-lapse embryo imaging and preimplantation genetic testing, have extended the IVF cycle with additional treatment steps. These technologies, moreover, represent a key shift toward the automation of IVF, as they incorporate new data-driven, artificial intelligence, and cloud-based approaches to predicting embryo viability and future fertility.

These developments are situated within a broader expansion of the IVF sector. Since its emergence during the neoliberal and privatizing reigns of Thatcher and Reagan, the fertility sector has been a relatively privatized industry (Franklin 2022; Harris 2006). Yet particularly in the last decade, private equity investors have become interested in the fertility field. As a result, the fertility sector is increasingly financialized, pointing not only to the marketization of reproduction in private fertility clinics but also to the fertility clinic itself becoming an object of investment that can be bought and sold for a return. The effects thereof on the commercial-clinical infrastructures of IVF provide an important backdrop for contemporary reimaginings of fertility.

Drawing on these three interrelated trends, this chapter introduces the concept of *fertility efficiency* to explore how the sector is reshaping perceptions of fertility and, conversely, how changing perceptions of fertility are reshaping the sector. This concept emerged from a series of twenty-one semistructured interviews with fertility professionals—including medical directors, embryologists, and consultants—that took place in 2019–2022. They were conducted in person and online (Zoom) and drawn primarily from the United States, the United Kingdom, and the Netherlands. When discussing key changes in the fertility sector in the last decade, participants expressed strong views on these shifts toward financialization and automation. Some welcomed the investment in and scaling up of the fertility sector, while others raised concerns about exploitation, overtreatment, and commercialization. Yet what was recognized across these fault lines was the significance of the concept of "efficiency" in rationalizing the key changes in the fertility sector today.

Directly addressing the question of how "IVF technologies are not only responding to but also changing the ways in which fertility and infertility are perceived and practiced" (Franklin and Inhorn, Introduction), the references to improving efficiency reflect a renegotiation among IVF professionals of what constitutes fertility and how it is changing in the face of new market and technological developments. This notion of fertility efficiency emerged in my conversations with fertility professionals as a locus of contestation, in which several fault lines in contemporary IVF—public/private, independent/consolidated, old/new generations, status quo/innovative distinctions—were amplified. In this chapter, I focus on three dimensions of efficiency—scalar, automated, and treatment efficiency—which not only represent material shifts in the organization of contemporary IVF but also reflect a change in the logic that both underlies the very understanding of fertility itself and drives the emergence of a more financialized and automated new reproductive order.

Scalar Efficiency

The last decade has seen a significant shift from the prevalence of smaller independent IVF clinics to the creation of larger fertility groups. This move toward consolidation is often driven by private equity investments, which use mergers and acquisitions as a method for increasing the value of IVF clinics. These investors typically aim to "exit" and sell the fertility company for more money after about five to seven years. The emergence of these larger fertility groups reflects the expectation that the return on investment (ROI) can be increased by "scaling up" IVF.

Scalar efficiency references the promise of creating value through economies of scale, centralizing services, and standardizing practices between clinics. The fertility professionals I spoke with had strongly divergent opinions on this development, with some seeing it as a desirable business practice that improves fertility treatment and others raising concerns about the effects of consolidation on patient care and medical autonomy. Still others became disillusioned by working in these large fertility groups and set up their own independent clinics as alternatives. Yet all fertility professionals with whom I spoke agreed that consolidation was prevalent in IVF. One US-based medical director illustrated this by telling me, "Look, I'm running a pretty successful IVF center here in New York City, and I'm getting probably I would say, especially in the last year or two, at least one or two emails a week from people who want to talk to us about buying us." Given that consolidation has changed the organizational structure of the IVF sector across the globe, it warrants critical reflection.

Many people in the field, especially those working in independent clinics or public hospitals, have raised concerns about consolidation. Pasquale Patrizio and colleagues, for example, argue that it poses a threat to smaller and not-for-profit clinics and can lead to a monopoly situation (Patrizio et al. 2022). They cite the example of Australia, arguing that a monopoly of three large networks has led to rising costs, decreasing live birth rates, and decreasing patient satisfaction. Due to the investors' need for ROI, affordable treatment options are less promoted and less available, while add-on treatments are disproportionately popular. Preimplantation genetic testing, for example, occurs in 30 percent of private IVF cycles, but only 0.5 percent in academic IVF cycles—a trend that is mirrored in the US context (Borsa and Bruch 2022). Larger fertility groups also tend to invest more in marketing—particularly to increase patient and cycle numbers. This is particularly relevant for egg freezing, in which presumably fertile women become candidates for infertility treatment (Patrizio et al. 2022).

Conversely, proponents of private equity investments emphasize the benefits of the increased efficiency of their consolidated clinics. One North American medical director, for example, explains, "I think I see industry money as actually positive where I think most fertility doctors see it as negative. The reason I see it as positive is because I see inefficiencies in the system that anybody from a business, logistics mind will fix right away." He argues that private equity brings him "not just more money, also the logic and insights, to watch through the flows, to actually see it as processes and get feedback." This statement expresses that what is at stake here is not only a matter of money but also a shift in interpretation: a different way of seeing. This director understands the private equity investments as introducing a logic through which the fertility clinic and the assisted reproductive process can be seen as "flows" and "processes" that can be "fixed" by making them more efficient.

Although the claim is often made that private equity does not affect (clinical) practice, most fertility professionals I spoke with highlight the significant changes that are made in the name of efficiency. One North American IVF consultant and investor explained that the influx of private equity investments is both motivated by, and intensifies, the promise of ROI through increased efficiency and the optimization of IVF:

> Private equity, God bless them, are the most predictable people. They are absolutely agnostic to what they invest in. They look for high-margin businesses where the profit is very high relative to the price of the production of what they're doing. . . . They can find businesses, combine them, in some cases find efficiencies that they can use to drive the cost of running the business down, and then, just the way the private equity industry is structured, which is usually ten-year closed-end funds, find someone to sell it to. . . .
>
> So, something like IVF, which is a high-margin business, very decentralized, lots of inefficiency built in, because it was never looked at from an efficiency standpoint. Because, frankly, the pricing was pretty. . . . You could just pass out anything you wanted to your patients because you were focusing mainly on wealthy patients. There's enormous potential for other markets there. So, private equity sees this.

The "enormous potential for other markets" he is referring to is the large group of people who could be fertility patients but cannot afford IVF. He suggests that making the IVF cycle more efficient could make the treatment more affordable and thereby more accessible to a larger group of people:

> The biggest opportunity is not in what you [the private equity investor] do, which is consolidating the existing marketplace. It's addressing the ten times bigger marketplace that's not being addressed at all right now.
>
> So, let's try to make the procedure more available. . . . We do that by using technology. All the IVF centers, certainly in the [United States] but in a way everywhere around the world, they're all artisanal kitchens. Everyone's doing it their own way with their own vocabulary and their own protocols. We've never really had an effort to optimize the process in a way that defines a best practice and [that] is able to produce it and provide it at an affordable way to a much, much larger group of patients. So, actually, it's kind of a free market democratization.

The notion of democratization is widespread in the new private equity–backed fertility groups. The idea that ROI-driven increased efficiency will also translate into lower prices and more accessibility for patients is built on a vision of an optimized assisted reproductive process that requires less labor, lower costs, and less time.

This idea of IVF optimization—in which IVF optimizes reproduction and technological innovations optimize the IVF cycle—is driving large investments into the fertility industry. This consultant describes a mutually reinforcing process, in which the promise of the future growth of the fertility market attracts investors, who in turn require "efficiencies" to "drive the cost of running a business down" to enable further growth: "It makes a lot of sense . . . to have maybe a very good, high-functioning clinic merge with the smaller clinics that are in other geographic areas that may not be offering the same quality of service. They merge. They export the best practices to the lower-functioning clinics. And suddenly you're raising the quality of care for everybody." Consolidation is here described as a means of improving quality of care by exporting and harmonizing best practices between clinics. Collaboration or sharing best practices does not necessarily require an organizational merge. Yet this statement reflects the prevalent euphemistic framing of business decisions in the fertility field, in which the changes driven by new pressures on achieving ROI are presented as improvements for patients or staff.

Notwithstanding this optimistic presentation, the shift toward larger fertility groups divides opinion among fertility professionals. One medical director in the United Kingdom who previously worked in larger private equity–funded fertility groups speaks directly to the pressures and priorities associated with private equity (PE) investments in IVF:

> I'm sure each PE firm is different, but you have a different set of priorities. So the priority, ultimately, if you're owned by private equity, becomes showing growth and returning value. And the main purpose of PE, usually, is to generate growth. PE firms don't want to buy a clinic that makes a million pounds every year profit, they want a clinic that makes a million-pound profit the first year and twenty-million-a-year profit by year five. . . . So what then happens, is you have your business nipped and tucked to show great growth. Especially just before the sale.

He explains that private equity investment positions profit growth as the key priority for clinics. The sale of a clinic, as the moment when the ROI gets determined, becomes central to the timeline of a fertility company. At this point, the growth in profit can be increased by having a fertility business "nipped and tucked." Rather than democratizing treatment with reduced costs for patients, efficiency here functions to improve returning value for the investors.

A North American medical director, who speaks favorably of private equity investments, suggests what such nipping and tucking might mean: "So I live this [private equity investment] every day. It is a good thing. I think competition is great, it makes us all better. I think medicine is highly inefficient, and it is labor-intensive, and it is physically intense, and I think that big business is good for removing waste. For trimming the fat. For improving efficiency." While the UK-based medical director raised concerns about the focus on growth and the presale cuts in the clinic to increase ROI, this medical director presents these as means for improving fertility care. Continuing the cosmetic surgery metaphors, the earlier "nip and tuck" is here "trimming the fat." Focusing on profit growth does not conflict with providing good patient care, but rather "makes us all better" because it "improves efficiency."

This strategic use of the word "efficiency" is quite interesting. Whereas the explicit mention of a profit motive is incongruent with the "priceless" value of reproduction and the active "de-commodifying" of reproductive transactions (Thompson 2005: 255; Smietana 2017), the framing of business imperatives as a means of improving efficiency is much less controversial. What is the rhetorical and structural work that the framing of private equity–backed fertility companies as more "efficient" does?

The nipping and tucking that medical directors described included reducing the time patients spend with doctors by increasing their time with other, lower-paid staff such as nurses and administrators; decreasing administrative labor through digitalization and automation; and harmonizing practices across different branches within the fertility group. Concerning this last point, one UK-based medical director describes, "When you acquire, as an investor, new clinics . . . there's always that sort of thought: can you harmonize them so that the less efficient ones learn from the more efficient ones? And believe you me, the latest ones to accept harmonization are the medics. Embryologists are very, very, compliant; they are happy to follow protocols, and as long as there are protocols in place, they don't have this fixation about their practice—medics do." Here the notion of efficiency motivates a harmonization of practice between clinics. This approach often means that medical professionals, whether doctors or embryologists, have less autonomy over their practices, which become more protocol driven. Although this medical director says the embryologists are compliant, those embryologists interviewed were already aware of, and concerned about, these developments. One embryologist reflected, "Of course I know private clinics that have been bought by such large fertility companies. Yes, if I speak with my colleague who works there, they just get all the things and they have to work with them. These are no longer the choices of the embryologists themselves."

When no longer the choice of the embryologists themselves, the decision making that was previously determined in the lab is now controlled by boards of management and so-called business-doctors, as one Dutch fertility specialist calls them: "The most important problem is that it is no longer doctors who run a practice, but 'business-doctors.'

Not people with a medical degree, but people with an MBA are the ones who make decisions." Likewise, a UK-based medical director reflected, "It got to the point where I wasn't comfortable with some of the decisions made. There were some decisions made that impacted significantly, clinically, that were made by nonclinicians, just made by people up in the managerial office."

In this sense, the move toward scalar efficiency can also entail a transfer of power. With the shift from independent clinics to large fertility groups, decision-making powers typically move from medical professionals to health managers. In order to understand what is at stake and what conceptual shifts are implicated in this transfer of power and move toward efficiency, it is important to consider its effects on automation, labor, and the treatment cycle itself.

Automated Efficiency

Automation is at the heart of the appeals to increase efficiency in the fertility clinic. The promise of new technologies designed to improve the clinic's efficiency by digitizing, datafying, and automating IVF is ubiquitous. As a result, patients increasingly encounter the clinic through digital platforms as bookings, patient support, and medical records move online. Likewise, embryologists are increasingly handling screens alongside Petri dishes, as labs are automated with AI-driven time-lapse incubators, cloud-based preimplantation genetic testing, and robotic cryopreservation systems—with the specter of the "IVF-in-a-box" a key point on the imagined horizon of next-gen ARTs. New fertility companies appeal to investors by sketching a cloud-based and platformized future for assisted reproduction that uses digital technologies to increase scale, meet the needs of a new generation of patients, and cut costs compared to the analogue, in-real-life clinics and the highly skilled practices of "embryology and its still-artisanal sense of craft" (Franklin 2013: 286).

These moves toward automation and datafication are often presented as a means of increasing efficiency in a way that benefits both patients and personnel. New digital fertility companies such as Apricity, billed as an online clinic, Kindbody, which seeks to decrease costs by digitizing its services, and Progyny, the fertility insurer that harnesses data to increase its influence, tout automation as a means of changing the face of assisted reproduction. The new business models for these fertility companies seek to cut costs by automating the clinic, collecting data, or adopting an online intermediary role in a platformized fertility economy (Van de Wiel 2019, 2022).

Recognizing this drive toward automated efficiency in IVF, a US-based medical director explained that he "believe[s] in the utilization of technology to improve both clinical efficiency and efficacy." Likewise, a UK-based medical director highlighted the automation of the embryology lab as an important means of making fertility clinics more efficient: "Making the process more efficient is probably automating what you can automate. . . . There is some equipment, like time-lapse incubators, which to a lot of people they are very inefficient because the utility of time-lapse technology is still debatable. . . . Artificial intelligence is somehow bringing new utilities to this specific field, but at the end of the day, for example in my clinic, we use it a lot, because it reduces the workload in the embryology lab a lot."

The technology referenced here, time-lapse embryo imaging, is an add-on technology for embryo selection that patients typically pay extra for (Van de Wiel et al. 2020). It is one of the most popular embryo-selection technologies introduced in the last decade, riding the wave of the booming "business of manufacturing and sorting maybe-babies" (Wahlberg and Gammeltoft 2018: vii). The time-lapse system takes regular images of developing embryos and uses this visual data to predict which one is most likely to develop into a healthy baby. Patients may encounter the time-lapse embryo videos, thereby engaging with "a new form of reproductive bioinformation that provide[s] important insights into the making of new reproductive knowledge and experience" (Hamper and Perrotta 2023). While time-lapse embryo imaging is widely discussed, studied, promoted, and sold for this predictive function to improve IVF success rates, this quotation highlights that this goal may in fact be secondary. Rather, from the clinic's point of view, the reduction in workload and increased efficiency of the lab is reason enough to implement this technology. This point was echoed by a US-based medical director, who explained, "Time-lapse embryology likely doesn't help the top 10 percent of IVF clinics in the world because they have such skilled embryologists that they can glean from standard approaches. But for many it allows for remote embryo monitoring and makes the experience much faster." By moving embryo monitoring online and automating embryo observation in this way, clinics can thus adopt new embryological technologies in the name of efficiency—even if they may be presented to patients as a means of improving live birth rates.

Besides embryo selection, automation innovation also occurs in relation to cryopreservation. One example that was introduced in Europe for the first time in 2022 is TMRW's automated cryopreservation technology. This company uses robotics to store frozen eggs, sperm, and embryos. As the number of eggs and embryos that clinics store rises, TMRW aims to use robotics to tackle the increasingly complicated logistics of cryopreservation. Particularly referencing the rising popularity of egg freezing, they received a £153.5 million investment to automate egg storage (Crunchbase 2023). A UK-based medical director described,

> [There is the] mommy robot and the baby robot. The baby robot sits in your IVF clinic. It looks like a big Costa coffee machine—it's very cool. Your embryologist looks into it, it reads their retina, in terms of ID checking . . . then the drawer pops out, you put the embryos in, it's like an ATM. . . . The robot . . . puts them in a very specific spot in the storage vat, and the robot always knows where they are and how many are in there, so your auditing is much easier.
>
> And then there's a mother robot . . . which will be in an off-site warehouse on the M25, a big cryobank, and then there's a courier company that will take the embryos or eggs from the baby robots in each of the clinics—it will be derisking for the clinic potentially, saving a lot of floor space—and they'll go off to the mother robot and be stored there.

The automation is described as a means of improving efficiency, not only by saving floor space in the clinic but as a means of avoiding legal risk associated with sample mix-ups and auditing standards.

In addition, as a US-based investor explains, it is also understood to limit labor costs: "The robot does inventory automatically. Instead of having a PhD-level embryologist . . . walk into the room with the thirty tanks with the clipboard and a pencil." As TMRW is implementing robotics systems for cryopreservation logistics, time-lapse embryo imaging seeks to automate embryo incubation, and Merck and Genea distribute automated vitrification machines—all these innovations represent elements of a vision in which the embryological process becomes increasingly automated.

Prelude, one of the largest US-based fertility groups, which was founded with a $200 million private equity investment, is behind a new project to integrate the abovementioned automation technologies and create a machine called Overture. Backed by major tech investors, such as Susan Wojcicki (CEO of YouTube) and Anne Wojcicki (CEO of 23andme), it aims to create a so-called IVF-in-a-box in the name of efficiency and under the slogan "fertility automated." One UK-based medical director describes the technology: "Floor space is expensive. Getting that Overture and putting it on a desk here would be much cheaper, much more efficient. Also, I won't need four highly paid embryologists. I'll only need one tech [to] put the eggs in one side, the sperm in the other, take the embryo out five days later. Or if I want to set up IVF in Indonesia, or in Tanzania, again I won't need to build a super-expensive IVF lab. I just plug in in my garage to my IVF lab-in-a-box, and I'll be able to do IVF. It's amazing." While Overture is not a technical reality, the story of its promise of a more efficient IVF lab in the future is generating large amounts of capital. As these investments play a key role in determining what is researched and developed, this drive toward a vision of automated efficiency is shaping the future of IVF.

The move toward automation dovetails with the related preoccupation with labor efficiency in contemporary IVF. Not only are new technologies introduced to reduce labor costs, but the focus on efficiency also shifts the division of labor within the clinic. One North American medical director said the following about private equity's impetus to fix "inefficiencies in the system": "So . . . let's say it takes me one hour to see a new patient. . . . Now, fifteen, let's say twenty minutes of that is actually pretty repetitive. I think the last twenty minutes could be like, 'Lucy it was really nice meeting you. You're now going to meet with my head nurse who will walk you through how we do everything we talked about.' So now I have forty minutes, and now I can see sixteen patients." This director describes the efficiency-focused reorganization of the clinic staff with an example of reducing a doctor's time spent with a patient, thereby allowing the doctor to see more patients a day. In this example, a "business, logistics mind" entails a set of translations and numericizations that become the basis for decision making within the clinic. The prioritization of certain measures of success—whether annual patients per doctor or live-birth rates—organizes the logic of efficiency by which a clinic is run.

While scalar efficiency pointed to the transfer of power from doctor to (finance) manager, automated and labor efficiency hints at a broader speculative narrative about future IVF, with a vision of IVF as "demedicalized," technologized, and untethered from the previously central position of the fertility doctor. According to one UK-based medical director,

> When you see an introduction to AI for clinical decision making, automation, miniaturization, it's all being changed, and in my view becomes demedicalized. I think there will be very few REIs (reproductive endocrinologists) running clinics. I think that a lot of them will be owned by big businesses. The nurses will do embryo transfers and egg collection; nurses are much cheaper and just as good, so I think the old-fashioned medical model long-term in the future will change and I think you see entrepreneurs . . . who come into this who understand scale, who understand growth, and [who] don't particularly have a high opinion of doctors. They see a different future. They might be right.

Treatment Efficiency

The logic of efficiency also directly structures what fertility and infertility mean in the clinical context. Rather than treatments to circumvent infertility, reproductive technologies may also be used to make embodied fertility, i.e., the process of getting pregnant itself, more efficient. One North American medical director, for example, describes how some of his patients "need [his] services" because they could not otherwise conceive, but recognizes that "a bigger part of the field is about efficiency," which deals with "improve[ment]" rather than "need." He elaborates:

> There is certainly a sector of the field where humans are not that efficient as creatures in terms of reproduction. And so, if you say to someone, listen, you've got a 5 percent chance . . . per month and I think in the next year and a half it may work for you, which means the majority of patients will probably conceive without help. So, do they need treatment? No. But

will people accept waiting a year and a half? No. So there's a lot of . . . intervention for efficiency's sake. You see this as a massive trend.

This explanation frames both human bodies as "not that efficient" and IVF as an intervention that can improve on that inefficiency. The medical director suggests that business incentives contribute to this "massive trend": "What they don't tell you is the business side of the field. . . . To say, yes, you can do [intrauterine insemination (IUI)] but it's a 12 percent chance. You sure you don't want to do IVF, just jump right into it, it's 50 percent chance? So, this tool is used a lot of times to show people the most efficient thing." As a variation of what I have elsewhere called a "calculus of fertility" (Van de Wiel 2020a: 101), the per-cycle chances of various treatment options function as the organizing logic for understanding fertility in this context. Approached in this way, a higher per-cycle chance—sometimes translated into a reduced estimated "time to live birth"—favors a more intense approach to treatment (IVF rather than IUI; IUI rather than waiting) and thereby aligns with the "business side of the field." Conversely, referencing the per-cycle live-birth chances as the key metric for reproductive success renders other considerations, such as the risks of overtreatment or overpayment, invisible. In the context of stronger drives to increase revenue, it is important to scrutinize whether particular presentations of infertility may rationalize faster and more costly engagements with reproductive technologies.

Fertility professionals have to navigate claims to patient autonomy in the face of these changing perceptions of fertility. The metricization of fertility treatment as chances per cycle and potentially reduced "time to live birth" can motivate patients to undergo more treatments sooner. One North American medical director described a recent shift toward a broader indication for fertility treatment: "First of all, there's patient autonomy. My body, I don't want to wait, you know, another five months. Versus what's, you know, appropriate. [S]everal years ago . . . our dictum was we would only treat patients with infertility. And what that did, effectively though, was rule out a lot of individuals, including LGBTQ community, including single women, including use of donor sperm, so that's really evolved. Especially when we get into, 'cause you want to be consistent, into egg freezing for fertility preservation." Initially, only infertility was an indication for treatment to avoid the overtreatment of people early in their fertility journeys. But this practice proved to be exclusionary toward the LGBTQ community and single women and no longer held after the introduction of egg freezing, which is aimed at fertile people. Now, as the indication for treatment has "evolved," the use of IVF to decrease time to live birth continues to pose dilemmas for fertility professionals. According to one, "Whether that woman who wants to get pregnant a little faster . . . is allowed to take advantage of that, if you will, gets into issues of autonomy, choice, risk. Now, [if] people come in and say, 'We haven't been trying yet, but we want to do IVF,' we would try to dissuade them. . . . But, is it six months or five months or seven months or nine months, you know? . . . That point is moving." The moving point of fertility treatment for "efficiency's sake" represents an ongoing shift in the way fertility is perceived as something that can be "sped up" with the aid of reproductive technologies. Reproductive technologies thus represent a more efficient alternative to technologically unassisted conception—which may be relevant to a much larger group of people who are trying to conceive and want to optimize their chances.

While IVF and IUI thus become tools for increasing fertility efficiency by reducing the time to conception, egg freezing is framed as a means of making fertility more efficient by extending this time. Particularly, US-based fertility companies that specialize in egg freezing promote the procedure to presumably fertile women and encourage early freezing as the most efficient option (Van de Wiel 2020b). While early egg freezing is presented as a way of improving frozen egg quality and quantity, it nevertheless runs the risk of overtreatment, overmedicalization, and the accumulation of high storage costs over the years. The associated marketing of egg freezing may reframe fertility as itself precarious and as at risk of losing its efficiency without timely interventions (Van de Wiel 2020a). This precariousness of fertility may be articulated in tandem with an understanding of egg freezing itself as a "hope technology" to counteract future fertility loss or "a technology of despair" and "repair" to counteract relationship dissolution (Inhorn et al. 2022).

Both the cases of early IVF and early egg freezing reflect how the shift from treating infertility to treating fertility inefficiency opens up a much bigger potential patient population that aligns with growth-based business incentives. When efficiency logic becomes a driving force in large-scale reforms in the fertility sector, it also affects the rationale for treatment and, by extension, the framing of fertility itself.

Conclusion

This chapter has highlighted how a logic of efficiency has become widespread in the fertility field. Various modes of scalar, automated, and treatment efficiency, often driven by the need to increase ROI, underlie structural and consequential shifts in the organization of contemporary assisted reproduction.

The underlying logic of efficiency is expressed as a drive to lower costs by reducing (high-paid) labor per cycle, standardize practices across clinics, and decrease the costs associated with clinical space— whether through technological innovations or by outsourcing parts of the treatment. Complementing these reductions, there is a drive to increase automation in embryology, logistics, and administration and to move both in-person practices and data online. These shifts may be seen as chafing against the decidedly unbusinesslike rhetoric within which reproduction has traditionally been couched, or they may be seen as commonsense approaches to running contemporary healthcare. Yet what is at stake here are subtle shifts that entail profound changes to the way in which assisted reproduction is organized.

The drive toward a scalar efficiency, which promotes growth in order to benefit from economies of scale, is visible in the significant consolidation in the field. Yet at a more profound level, the drive to increase growth and scale can also become expressed as a new interpretative framework for understanding fertility in line with the logic of efficiency. The treatment efficiency expressed in people's motivations for undergoing treatment may align with the logic of efficiency, while the quantification of fertility practices in line with the investors' priorities position certain metrics (e.g., cycle numbers) as markers of success and incentivization—which take on a new power to steer the future direction of a clinic.

In this way, efficiency logic can also entail a transfer of power. Whether mobilized as "common sense" or as a means of establishing a "win-win" situation, efficiency logic can rationalize a shift of power from a traditional GP-type model of physician-led independent fertility clinics toward one in which those who adjust and drive the levers of efficiency—management and investors—assume a more central and powerful role in running the clinic. This power can be expressed through quantified metrics of efficiency, which direct both the profession and the patient toward a model that aligns fertility care with a speculative return on investment. In all of these ways, the influx of capital drives the emergence of a new reproductive order in which ART businesses reframe in-fertility as in-efficiency precisely because of the logics of efficiency and ROI through which they themselves are built.

REFERENCES

Borsa, Alexander, and Joseph Dov Bruch. 2022. "Prevalence and Performance of Private Equity–Affiliated Fertility Practices in the United States." *Fertility and Sterility* 117(1): 124–30.

Crunchbase. 2023. "TMRW Life Sciences." www.crunchbase.com.

Franklin, Sarah. 2013. *Biological Relatives: IVF, Stem Cells, and the Future of Kinship.* Durham, NC: Duke University Press.

———. 2022. *Embodied Progress: A Cultural Account of Assisted Conception.* 2nd edition London: Taylor & Francis.

Hamper, Josie, and Manuela Perrotta. 2023. "Watching Embryos: Exploring the Geographies of Assisted Reproduction through Encounters with Embryo Imaging Technologies." *Social & Cultural Geography* 24(9): 1557–75.

Harris, Lisa. 2006. "Challenging Conception: A Clinical and Cultural History of In Vitro Fertilization in the United States." PhD dissertation, Ann Arbor: University of Michigan. https://deepblue.lib.umich.edu.

Inhorn, Marcia C., Daphna Birenbaum-Carmeli, Ruoxi Yu, and Pasquale Patrizio. 2022. "Egg Freezing at the End of Romance: A Technology of Hope, Despair, and Repair." *Science, Technology & Human Values* 47(1): 53–84.

Patrizio, Pasquale, David Albertini, Norbert Gleicher, and Arthur Caplan. 2022. "The Changing World of IVF: The Pros and Cons of New Business Models Offering Assisted Reproductive Technologies." *Journal of Assisted Reproduction and Genetics* 39(2): 305–13.

Smietana, Marcin. 2017. "Affective De-Commodifying, Economic De-Kinning: Surrogates' and Gay Fathers' Narratives in U.S. Surrogacy." *Sociological Research Online* 22(2): 163–75.

Thompson, Charis. 2005. *Making Parents: The Ontological Choreography of Reproductive Technologies.* Cambridge, MA: MIT Press.

Van de Wiel, Lucy. 2019. "The Datafication of Reproduction: Time-Lapse Embryo Imaging and the Commercialisation of IVF." *Sociology of Health & Illness* 41(S1): 193–209.

———. 2020a. *Freezing Fertility: Oocyte Cryopreservation and the Gender Politics of Aging.* New York: New York University Press.

———. 2020b. "The Speculative Turn in IVF: Egg Freezing and the Financialization of Fertility." *New Genetics and Society* 39(3): 306–26.

———. 2022. "Disrupting the Biological Clock: Fertility Benefits, Egg Freezing, and Proactive Fertility Management." *Reproductive BioMedicine and Society Online* 14(March): 239–50.

Van de Wiel, Lucy, Jack Wilkinson, Pantelitsa Athanasiou, and Joyce Harper. 2020. "The Prevalence, Promotion, and Pricing of Three IVF Add-Ons on Fertility Clinic Websites." *Reproductive BioMedicine Online* 41(5): 801–6.

Wahlberg, Ayo, and Tine M. Gammeltoft, eds. 2018. *Selective Reproduction in the 21st Century*. Cham, UK: Springer.

12

Mobile Reproductive Labor

Fly-in Fly-out Clinicians, Batched Patients, and
Extraction in African Assisted Reproduction

ANDREA WHITTAKER AND TRUDIE GERRITS

In the first ten days, Kampala is our biggest center . . . We
were doing between forty-five and sixty [cases] on a monthly
basis within ten days. We were doing [egg] extractions, then
[embryo] transfers [on] Day Three, but again that's because
we needed to be somewhere else, and then the next place
was Tanzania. [In Tanzania,] we were doing between ten and
fifteen, sometimes twenty [cases], so we could do those all
within a five- to six-day period. Then Zambia was midway,
sometimes twenty-five to thirty [cases]. So basically, it was
back-to-back in a thirty-day period; we would spend about
twenty-three days on doing the work in different countries,
and then seven days preparing for the next. . . . So we guys
just come in a day before the [oocyte] retrievals. So we
would fly in with direct flights. . . . So some of those clinics
we made sure that we did retrievals just in two days. . . . That
allows us to fit within the window.
—Billy, an embryologist from Eastern Africa describing his
working regime traveling across several countries

In this chapter we examine the movements of clinical specialists, such as
in vitro fertilization (IVF) physicians and embryologists, their motivations and experiences, and the forms of labor that assist in developing,
maintaining, and profiting from transnational markets in sub-Saharan
Africa. We concentrate on two forms of what we call *mobile reproduc-*
tive labor that characterize the socio-technical organization of these

clinics: the work of "fly-in fly-out" (FIFO) clinical staff involved in assisted reproduction and the use of "batching" as a means to efficiently organize IVF cycles in situations where time and services are limited.

"Fly-in fly-out," or "FIFO," is a term derived from the labor practices of the extractive industry of the Australian mining sector, where miners undertake FIFO work (although not necessarily flying per se), spending short periods of intense work at geographically isolated locations and then returning to their homes for breaks in between. This allows for constantly rotating shifts of staff to work in the mines in areas without elaborate physical and social infrastructures. It allows for mining to take place in locations that otherwise lack the skilled workforce for this purpose.

In applying this term to our informants, we deliberately draw upon suggestions of the work of traveling clinicians and scientists involved in IVF as another form of extractive industry involved in the transformation of raw material (Nahman 2013)—in this case, bodies and oocytes—to create economic values (profit), while at the same time creating affective values (care, pregnancy, children, parenthood). Such FIFO travel by medical staff takes place both to expand clinics' reach and market share into places where there is a shortage of local medical expertise and to allow increased access to these services. The dual logics of economic profit and improving access organize the nature of this work. Hence assistance for reproduction carries a tension between improving access and improving profits, seen as starkly inherent in the organization of work in clinics in limited-resource settings in sub-Saharan Africa. FIFO clinicians express an altruistic desire to assist patients in underresourced countries to expand assisted reproductive services—trying to create a new reproductive order of viable IVF clinics on the continent. But they also extract value from their work, as they invest in new clinics and make money from batched patient cohorts, or patients who are scheduled to arrive in the clinic at the same time and whose eggs are being extracted simultaneously to allow efficient and profitable time and staff management. But this extraction may not lead to successful pregnancy, and it does not always benefit patients.

By focusing on these movements and the infrastructures they involve, our chapter draws attention to the critical role of mobilities in the current provision of services to infertile patients in sub-Saharan

Africa. We propose that assisted reproduction can be seen as involving flows of people, materials, and capital continuously in motion. The movements inherent in assisted reproduction have been characterized by Marcia C. Inhorn as constituting a global "reproscape," referring to "a new world order characterized not only by circulating reproductive technologies (technoscapes), but also by circulating reproductive actors (ethnoscapes), and their gametes (bioscapes), leading to a large-scale global industry (financescapes)" (Inhorn 2015: 23). The movement of patients allows access to care, while the movement of medical staff allows access to patients and profit. Because of the unequal distribution of clinics across sub-Saharan Africa, many patients depend upon the movements of medical staff for their care, and patient care is structured in particular ways as a result.

In this chapter we also draw attention to the new forms of labor that have arisen within this global reproscape, crucial to maintaining access and profit. The nature of assisted reproductive technology (ART) work involves the coordinated and parallel efforts of a number of people, including patients, gamete donors, medical specialists, embryologists, facilitators, and couriers. It also requires transport, clinical, and laboratory infrastructure, and material objects such as culture media, pharmaceuticals, and laboratory equipment. The work is oriented toward hoped-for, but highly speculative, future outcomes of pregnancies and live births. Much of this specialized work occurs inside consultation rooms and laboratories and is invisible to patients. Here we examine forms of mobile reproductive labor—work that maintains and creates value in cross-border reproductive markets across sub-Saharan Africa. The organization of work within these clinics is influenced by the scarcity/availability of certain expertise—in particular embryologists—and the need for time, material, and cost efficiencies.

Access to ARTs in Sub-Saharan Africa

Access to ARTs is deficient across many countries in sub-Saharan Africa (Inhorn and Patrizio 2015). Multiple structural barriers limit access to quality fertility services, and where services are available, treatment is usually only affordable for the wealthiest people (Gerrits 2016). The International Federation of Fertility Societies noted at least 210 clinics in the region, with the largest number of clinics in South Africa, Nigeria, and Ghana (Allan et al. 2019; Dyer et al. 2020).

Multiple structural barriers limit access to ART in sub-Saharan Africa. No government provides financial support for ARTs, specialized fertility doctors and embryologists are scarce, and only a few academic centers provide publicly funded treatments, hence access is stratified by economic status (Botha, Shamley, and Dyer 2018). Previous studies show how travel is a means through which patients access ART services, including particular procedures, because they mistrust the quality of ART clinics in their home country (Hörbst 2016; Inhorn 2015; Gerrits 2018), or to avoid the stigma of infertility (Bochow 2015; Moll et al. 2022).

Yet little has been written about the movements of clinicians and other specialists in ARTs. One of the first mentions was by Bob Simpson (2016), who described "IVF troubadours" in Sri Lanka. These are international experts, in particular embryologists, flying into the country and "performing at great expense and with little regulatory oversight" (Simpson 2016: 10). Inhorn (2015: 40) describes the clinic she studied in Dubai as an example of "medical cosmopolitanism," headed by a physician originally from India and staffed with clinicians from the Middle East, Africa, South and Southeast Asia, and Western Europe. In Uganda and Ghana, Hörbst and Gerrits (2016a, 2016b) describe how the clinic founders trained and/or worked as IVF doctors in the United Kingdom or Germany, and staff in their clinics come from various countries and continents, reflecting both colonial bonds (with the United Kingdom and Germany) and postcolonial connections (Ghana was involved in study exchange programs with socialist countries like Cuba and Poland). The scarcity of embryologists in Ghana and Uganda affected the functioning of the clinics, the daily organization of the lab work, and the conduct of lab procedures. This phenomenon was most visible in the Ugandan clinic, which featured a rotation of experts from five different countries.

Ethnographic Methods

This chapter is based upon interviews undertaken as part of a larger project on emerging markets of assisted reproduction in sub-Saharan Africa and builds upon our earlier work. The project included 117 interviews undertaken between January 2022 and September 2023, with a variety of key informants from across sub-Saharan Africa (South Africa, Uganda, Mozambique, Namibia, Tanzania, Ethiopia, Cameroon, Zambia, and Ghana), including interviews and observations and involving site visits to three public and six private clinics in South Africa (in Pretoria, Johannesburg, Nelspruit, and Cape Town) between September and October 2022. A subset of these interviews included eight clinic staff members who regularly undertook FIFO travel as part of their work. This subset included one IVF physician, five embryologists, one clinic manager, and one patient coordinator who traveled with patients from one country to another. With permission, semistructured interviews were undertaken, either face-to-face (during fieldwork in South Africa) or via Zoom or WhatsApp. All names are pseudonyms. Ethical clearance was granted by Monash University and the University of the Witwatersrand, as well as by the participating clinics.

South Africa is an important "reprohub" (Inhorn 2017) for sub-Saharan Africa, with twenty-two clinics that are considered Centres of Excellence by the South African Society for Reproductive Medicine and Gynaecological Endoscopy (SASREG) and at least an additional eight clinics where other fertility specialists consult. Three public clinics offer training for a limited number of laboratory scientists and IVF specialists from across the region.

Clinicians and Mobile Knowledges

Many clinicians and embryologists in Africa gain qualifications and experience in assisted reproduction through mobilities. Except for a few trained in South Africa, most of the clinicians and embryologists we interviewed had traveled to centers in Europe and the United States at some point in their careers. Mobile clinicians cross not only geographical boundaries but different health systems, regulatory systems, practices, and economic resources, bringing these diverse experiences back to clinics in Sub-Saharan Africa. These professionals cultivate wide professional and social networks, later reinforced through travel to international conferences, clinic visits, and consultations.

Many staff members embody the global reproscape, along with the financial benefits and career opportunities it affords. For example, Eric is an embryologist from Ethiopia who moved to Australia and undertook a master's in clinical embryology in 2018. He then moved to Bangkok and worked in a private clinic for six months, before returning to Ethiopia to establish a clinic. To do so, he collaborated with his Australian trainers, who helped plan the clinic, which was funded by a US university through US contacts from the hospital, was built by an Indian company, and now employs infertility specialists trained in Egypt and other embryologists trained in India.

Specialists from the Global North also travel to sub-Saharan Africa as consultants to provide expertise, help set up clinics with colleagues, or volunteer as medi-tourists. Such movements occur between sub-Saharan African countries as well. Our South African interlocuters had trained other clinicians in Zimbabwe, Namibia, Gabon, and Kenya, and the embryologists had equipped and trained staff in laboratories in Namibia, Zimbabwe, Kenya, and Uganda. In many cases these specialists own or have shares in the new clinics they helped establish, suggesting that the decision to start clinics and train staff is motivated both by genuine professional commitment to increase access to ARTs in countries with no services and by financial incentives. Local clinics in Ethiopia, Tanzania, or Namibia are thus microcosms of the global reproscape, with clinics linked intimately to global trends, practices, and aspirations.

Regular FIFO Work

Apart from sporadic inputs in sub-Saharan Africa, IVF clinicians and embryologists may also be involved in regular FIFO work. Such clinical staff travel regularly to provide services in affiliated "satellite" or "sister" clinics: branches of major clinics in South Africa that supply regular services for a limited range of IVF procedures. The movement of IVF specialists and embryologists between clinics on a regular schedule is a business model designed to overcome a shortage of medical specialists and hence expand access to a limited range of services to patients in a particular country. Local staff handle the recruitment and administration of local patients and, depending on whether a gynecologist is available, may oversee the initial assessments, with test materials returned to the main clinic for processing. FIFO specialist staff from the main clinic travel regularly to serve these satellite clinics. One specialist from South Africa was described as "flying all over Cameroon and Nigeria" on a regular schedule of visits as he oversaw cycles. Other clinics in South Africa had satellite clinics in Namibia, and staff members drive six and a half hours there regularly every two months for ten to twelve days of ART work. Another embryologist we interviewed, Peter, travels from Cape Town to Windhoek in Namibia every three months for a week at a time, reflecting, "We fit in a whole bunch of people into one week and we only go up every now and then."

Nelly, a clinical director we interviewed, runs clinics in Uganda, with sister clinics in Zambia, Tanzania, and Rwanda (although that clinic has since closed). She described her FIFO work: "We had two teams, so we had our clinical team and the embryologists—the embryologists actually traveled quite often because they went to the different facilities doing the transfers and so on. I traveled—it depends, so for instance, when we were just opening a facility like in Lusaka in Zambia, I would probably travel every two weeks just to stay on top of all the operational requirements that would be needed. But after a hospital is established I'd go quarterly." Clinic staff we interviewed were generally positive about the experience of FIFO work. South African fertility specialist Dr. Teo enjoyed his regular trips to Namibia as a respite from his usual work regime. In his normal practice in South Africa, he usually does gynecological surgery three days a week in addition to teaching and managing ART treatment cycles. Dr. Teo enjoys the regular interludes in Namibia, reflecting, "All I do in Namibia is consultations—if I'm there for the cycles then I would do retrievals in the morning, and then there [are] . . . one or two consultant scans, and then a few days later the transfers happen. So, it's a much more laid-back day for me, so I'd probably be done, most days, if it's a busy day I'll probably be done by about 4:00 p.m." The absence of gynecological surgery facilities means that these cases are referred to South Africa.

Staff members viewed their travel as providing a valuable service. Helene, the coordinator in a Cameroonian clinic, declared, "I love [my work] dearly, I am passionate about it, I am always next to the patient, that comes naturally." However, the staff are also aware that it can only reach a limited part of the population that is able to access these treatments at a higher cost. For example, Dr. Teo saw his work as meaningful in that he was treating people who otherwise might not be able to access such technologies. He reflected, "In . . . Africa, most people that actually need ART services cannot actually afford it, you know, that's the reality . . . they just can never get to. So, yeah, so trying to reach out . . . there's a lot of work going on, trying to get the sort of facilities and those things available to people who otherwise would not reach [them]."

While clinics are motivated by their ability to provide care to local populations, they are also motivated by profit. Clinics would often decide to expand services into other countries, through satellite clinics, based on financial considerations. For example, Nelly explained the decision to expand her clinic's services to Tanzania, Rwanda, and Zambia:

> It came down to how many patients from those countries we were seeing at the local branch. So the more patients we saw from Tanzania, that gave us an indication okay, there's demand there. Oftentimes when we would start a new branch—because in the initial start-up capital wasn't too much, you'd just start as a clinic and so you were able to test the market so to speak, so it wasn't a huge barrier to be able to do that. . . . But also population size, we considered the population size, we considered the paying power—at the end of the day IVF is costly and also because we are a foreign entity for all these other countries. What are the economic benefits to us as coming in as investors? How can the money move around?

Similarly, as Peter mentioned, the decision by their South African clinic to set up a satellite service in Namibia was made in order to counter the same move by a competing clinic so as to ensure they would still maintain their market share of Namibian patients. According to Peter, "What pushed us to open it was that our competitors in Cape Town opened a clinic up there. . . . As soon as they opened a clinic up there, the possibility of losing all those patients became quite real. So, I think that is when it kicked in. So it was out of necessity, out of competition basically."

"Batching": The Organization of Clinical Work for Mobility

These service mobilities influenced many aspects of the clinical procedures and organization. The procedure most conducive to a minimal—and mobile—medical specialist team is "batching," a term used to describe the practice of using hormone regimes to synchronize patients' menstrual cycles to allow for a cohort of women to undergo ART treatment within the period when the fertility specialists and embryologists are available.[1] As the term suggests, batching is a Fordist production-line practice allowing for efficient mass treatment, in this case for the extraction of eggs and transfer of embryos on an ART assembly line.[2] The term evokes food production lines, in contrast to bespoke cycles for individual patients governed by their own menstrual cycles and/or convenience or preferred timing. One embryologist, Peter, who travels regularly to a clinic in Namibia from South Africa, described the process:

> So patients are recruited, [local] doctors will do initially the first step. They will meet with the patient, do an initial consultation, send the patient for blood tests, do an ultrasound pelvic scan on them to see the baseline results for them. Then we will tell the patients the kind of treatment we are going to give them. . . . So they would see about fifteen, twenty, thirty patients, or maybe even more than that and then getting feedback from their patients—"Yes, doctor, I will be available in June"—so you collect all the patients who say they can be available in June . . . and then start putting them on treatment . . . to now navigate them to fall on those dates that we have planned for June.

In a technical field guide for IVF clinics, Baiju P. Ahemmed and Alex C. Varghese (2016: 27) note that, while "controversial" among specialists, batching allows for cost efficiency for clinics and patients and is usually associated with a shortage of well-trained, skilled, and experienced embryologists and lab technicians; those who are available may freelance for multiple clinics. Ahemmed and Varghese (2016) suggest that the main difficulty is maintaining high-quality clinical or embryological services while providing standardized treatment. The field guide provides lists of materials, logistic charts, timelines, and instructions on how to undertake and manage batched ARTs. It also notes the need to select patients discerningly for batching as ovarian stimulation protocols are standardized with limited variation in regimes, depending on individual factors, such as ovarian reserve. It suggests that patients with complex needs—who are poor responders; at risk of ovarian hyperstimulation syndrome (OHSS) (which is a strong response to injectable hormone medications that stimulate the development of eggs in the ovaries, causing the ovaries to swell and become painful, which may require emergency care); immunocompromised (which may be an issue in sub-Saharan Africa given the high prevalence of HIV); requiring more advanced technology for male-factor infertility; and faced with recurrent implantation failures—may need to travel to a better equipped clinic elsewhere (Ahemmed and Varghese 2016: 27).

Batching has advantages and disadvantages for clinics. It allows for a limited number of fertility specialists and embryologists to travel to a clinic and provide their services and expertise for a limited period of time. This makes treatments more cost effective for clinics. For example, two doctors from one clinic in South Africa alternate traveling to the Namibian satellite clinic, staying for seven to ten days to treat a batch of fifteen to twenty women. This means that a fertility specialist is present at the clinic in Namibia once every two months to do cycles and consultations. However, Peter noted the intensity of his workload during the periods in Namibia and elsewhere outside of South Africa: "I would say my biggest downside is that I am the only person that goes up, so I do everything. Instead of there being two or three people helping, there is only one person [in the lab]. . . . The workload is quite a lot for one person, so that is my biggest concern or challenge. But I cope and I still have all the correct thumb checking to make sure that I don't make mistakes and everything is in place."

Batching also carries several clinical disadvantages. The primary disadvantage noted by clinicians is the possibility of adverse side effects or outcomes, such as OHSS. Dr. Teo noted, "The other issue is if you have—which happens very rarely, thank God—a patient who after retrieval develops a bit of abdominal pain of concern, or whatever, and you've already left the country. We have to make sure that it's got back-up, a back-up there. So, we have one or two gynecologists that we work with, then you know—so, if I have a patient I'm worried about, then I'll phone them up and say, 'Look, listen, I'm going back to Cape Town, and I'm worried about this patient.'" FIFO doctors tend not to do surgeries as they are not available to monitor their patients' recoveries. At the clinics we visited, patients requiring surgeries must travel to South Africa. The need to rely upon rotating staff also means there is no provision of some services, such as the vitrification (freezing) of eggs. Moreover, all andrology services for male patients must be performed while the visiting embryologist is present or else require outsourcing.

Batching has implications for patients, too. Patients put on similar stimulation protocols to control the timing of their cycles may respond differently. Some women respond less favorably than others and thereby have lower chances of success. Peter explained:

> But both clinics [in Namibia] batch their cycles so we fit in a whole bunch of people into one week, and we only go up every now and then. . . . So unlike here (South Africa), where we don't force the patients into a cycle, we don't take control of their cycle that much, for batching up there we do, so that they all ovulate within one week. It also means that for any given patient, should they not respond well to those drugs, they may have a long wait in between cycles, or ultimately need to travel to South Africa anyway.

The lack of vitrification means that all cycles are fresh cycles and that a woman who experiences a failed cycle will have to undergo a repeat cycle of stimulation and egg retrieval. This may be problematic if there is no opportunity to modify the hormone protocol or create a bespoke cycle. Similarly, as the time is limited, there are few options for embryo transfer times; usually Day Two transfers are used due to the limited time of the embryologist.

One further disadvantage is that consumables, such as the culture media, must be timed to be fresh and available for each cohort of patients. This is not always straightforward in limited-resource settings. As another embryologist, Shawna, noted, supply chains for media can be unreliable, especially getting culture media and equipment across borders. It takes time for reliable "pathways" to import them. Shawna said, "But if a clinic in Africa is not within a big city, I think there might be problems getting media in." She always carries some culture media with her when she travels, just in case: "Here you cannot have your media go sour on you, then you can't do anything because by the time you actually get some media in, you are already starting patients the next day, and to try and organize something to fly in overnight quickly, with all the customs issues and stuff like that . . . it is not an easy thing. It is an easy way to run cycles cost effectively but should you run into problems, then you have got big problems." In addition, in batch IVF, there is always a risk of interruptions, such as laboratory issues, power failures,[3] or contamination, that could impact an entire cohort of patients in that cycle.

Furthermore, batching does not offer personalized care. If a patient fails to respond to the set stimulation protocol, there is no unique contingency plan, and patients may still need to travel to undergo surgery or access other medical services, such as vitrification. Dr. Klerk, a fertility specialist who was not involved in FIFO cross-border care, was critical of batching:

> I've been very much against that kind of batching system—not because of going there for a short time, but the fact that there's no follow-up. [Batching]'s a very lucrative thing to do for the doctor and the embryologist, because they go into a vulnerable community that doesn't have an IVF service. So, you walk in there and the patient thinks this is automatically going to be successful, so they'll happily come and spend their money there and stuff; and those people will make a ton of money for doing those twenty or thirty people, and then they'll leave. But that's a terrible service for the patient, because when they're gone and again there's no follow-up, you know, that patient really doesn't know what's going on. They've obviously often paid a lot more than they should even, because they're vulnerable and all that kind of thing. So, one has to be very careful with that whole batching story, that it's done in an ethical way and that there's proper follow-up.

The production logic of batching—efficient organization of staff, bodies, time, and resources—does not necessarily provide access and care to patients in locations with few facilities or specialists. This "one size fits all" approach compromises the ethos of personalized care most reproductive specialists aim to practice.

Moreover, while batching generates profit for the clinics and care providers, it does not necessarily translate into savings for the patient. This model generates profit through staffing savings; there is no walk-in facility that requires full-time staffing by specialists, and facilities provide a limited range of services that require less equipment. It also generates profit through its use of pharmaceuticals; medication left over from one patient may be used by another in the same cohort, minimizing waste.

While some patients, through this model, are able to save money by not traveling to other countries, such as India or South Africa, for care, many do not experience these financial benefits. As Dr. Klerk suggests, although some patients will succeed with pregnancies from batched IVF, others will pay much the same as they would have to receive more personalized care had they traveled. This procedure does not necessarily produce lower-cost IVF for all patients, but it does provide a means of cost savings for clinics.

Concerns over batching expressed by South African specialists mirror the controversies surrounding various interventions to introduce lower-cost IVF to African countries—how to maintain high-quality assisted reproductive services while increasing access. One fertility specialist suggested that it was a question tinged with colonialism: she maintained that no practices or standards should be acceptable in Africa that are not acceptable for First World women.

Conclusion

This chapter on FIFO clinicians and embryologists in sub-Saharan Africa offers insights into mobile reproductive labor—that is, modalities of value creation in a corporate model that relies on mobilities and intangible facets of worker collaboration. Rather than static entities, IVF clinics across sub-Saharan Africa need to be understood in terms of a reproscape of varying im/mobilities of patients, clinicians, technologies, human materials, resources, and ideas. The mobility of the staff is largely due to the paucity of skilled specialists in infertility and embryology and the reliance on outside consultants and capital.

This phenomenon draws attention to critical staffing shortages in sub-Saharan Africa and, in particular, the crucial role of a skilled embryologist in the success of IVF. In Africa, training for embryologists is currently only available in Egypt and South Africa (Ombelet and Onofre 2019). Embryologists are in high demand, and many are highly mobile. As a result, clinics in several parts of sub-Saharan Africa are organized around these FIFO mobilities of staff, with batching—from the perspective of clinic staff—as a means of efficiently and cost effectively undertaking IVF cycles, and a further example of how the new reproductive order manages infertility services in underresourced countries. However, so far little is known about the actual impact of batching practices on the women and men undergoing these treatments. How do they experience these practices grown out of shortages and efficiency reasons? How does batching affect their well-being and treatment outcomes?

For the medical staff we spoke to, the desire to help people to have families and have a very real impact upon their lives is combined with a desire to provide access to IVF services—to be "of assistance" in the reproductive quests of patients. This manifests in specialists' willingness to travel either in serial contracts with various clinics or through regular rotations of satellite clinics located outside reprohubs. At the same time, such movements also create value and profit for private-clinic shareholders, through efficiently increasing the turnover of standardized cycles in the expanded reach that travel allows.

Medical staff travel across borders and set up clinics abroad out of professional ambition and economic gain, but also inspired by genuine concern for the well-being of their patients. However, even with these satellite clinics and services, most patients in need will not be reached. Even for those patients who can mobilize enough capital to afford treatment, the type of care they receive, whether it is a mass batched service or a bespoke cycle, depends upon the form of "assistance" they receive. This reality highlights how current assistance for reproduction in sub-Saharan Africa remains an extractive industry, structured along lines of wealth, privilege, and mobilities.

NOTES

1 The term "batching" is also used within IVF to describe the division of oocytes produced by a single donor into smaller batches of eggs that can then be used for several recipients, thereby increasing the profits from any single donor. This chapter, however, refers to the term only when describing the organization of patient cycles into specific timed cohorts.

2 In sub-Saharan Africa, mass treatment of a cohort has its antecedents in programs treating prevalent diseases in poor settings, such as mass treatments of multidrug therapies for parasitic infections.

3 Power failures were a constant issue during our fieldwork in South Africa in 2022 during a period of constant load shedding. This was the result of aging infrastructure and lack of investment. Clinics used back-up generators, but embryologists noted their concerns that fluctuations could affect incubator functions and said they constantly had to monitor for temperature changes. To be successful, an IVF program needs standby generators and batteries to guarantee optimal laboratory conditions (Adageba et al. 2015).

REFERENCES

Adageba, Rudolph Kantum, Ernest Tei Maya, John Jude Kweku Annan, and F. J. Damalie. 2015. "Setting Up and Running a Successful IVF Program in Africa: Prospects and Challenges." *Journal of Obstetrics and Gynaecology of India* 65(3): 155–57.

Ahemmed, Baiju P., and Alex C. Varghese. 2016. "Batch IVF Programme in ART: Practical Considerations." In *Organization and Management of IVF Units*, ed. Steven D. Fleming and Alex C. Varghese, 27–50. New York: Springer International Publishing.

Allan, Sonia, Basak Balaban, Manish Banker, John Buster, Marcos Horton, Kathleen Miller, Edgar Mocanu, Steven J. Orly, Hirshikesh Pai, Sheryl van der Poel, and Fernando Zegers-Hochschild. 2019. "International Federation of Fertility Societies' Surveillance (IFFS) 2019: Global Trends in Reproductive Policy and Practice." *Global Reproductive Health* 4(1): 1–138.

Bochow, Astrid. 2015. "Ethics, Identities, and Agency: ART, Elites, and HIV/AIDS in Botswana." In *Assisted Reproductive Technologies in the Third Phase: Global Encounters and Emerging Moral Worlds*, eds. Kate Hampshire and Bob Simpson, 135–51. New York: Berghahn.

Botha, Barend, Delva Shamley, and Silke Dyer. 2018. "Availability, Effectiveness, and Safety of ART in Sub-Saharan Africa: A Systematic Review." *Human Reproduction Open* 2: hoy003.

Dyer, Silke, Paversan Archary, Liezel Potgieter, Inge Smit, Oladapo Ashiru, Ernestine Gwet Bell, and African Network. 2020. "Assisted Reproductive Technology in Africa: A 5-Year Trend Analysis from the African Network and Registry for ART." *Reproductive BioMedicine Online* 41(4): 604–15.

Gerrits, Trudie. 2016. "Assisted Reproductive Technologies in Ghana: Transnational Undertakings, Local Practices, and 'More Affordable' IVF." *Reproductive BioMedicine and Society Online* 2: 32–38.

———. 2018. "Reproductive Travel to Ghana: Testimonies, Transnational Relationships, and Stratified Reproduction." *Medical Anthropology* 37(2): 131–44.

Hörbst, Viola. 2016. "'You Cannot Do IVF in Africa as in Europe': The Making of IVF in Mali and Uganda." *Reproductive BioMedicine and Society Online* 2: 108–15.

Hörbst, Viola, and Trudie Gerrits. 2016a. "Assisted Reproductive Technologies in Private IVF Clinics in Ghana and Uganda: Local Responses to the Scarcity of Embryologists." In *Procréation Médicale et Mondialisation: Expériences Africaines*, eds. Doris Bonnet and Véronique Duchesne, 57–71. Paris: L'Harmattan.

———. 2016b. "Transnational Connections of Health Professionals: Medicoscapes and Assisted Reproduction in Ghana and Uganda." *Ethnicity & Health* 21(4): 357–74.

Inhorn, Marcia. C. 2015. *Cosmopolitan Conceptions: IVF Sojourns in Global Dubai*. Durham, NC: Duke University Press.

———. 2017. "Cosmopolitan Conceptions in Global Dubai." *Anthropology News* 58(1): e303–7.

Inhorn, Marcia C., and Pasquale Patrizio. 2015. "Infertility around the Globe: New Thinking on Gender, Reproductive Technologies, and Global Movements in the 21st Century." *Human Reproduction Update* 21(4): 411–26.

Moll, Tessa, Trudie Gerrits, Karin Hammarberg, Lenore Manderson, and Andrea Whittaker. 2022. "Reproductive Travel to, from, and within Sub-Saharan Africa: A Scoping Review." *Reproductive BioMedicine and Society Online* 14: 271–88.

Nahman, Michal. 2013. *Extractions: An Ethnography of Reproductive Tourism.* New York: Springer.

Ombelet, Willem, and Jaime Onofre. 2019. "IVF in Africa: What Is It All About?" *Facts, Views and Vision in Obstetrics and Gynecology* 11(2): 65–76.

Simpson, Bob. 2016. "IVF in Sri Lanka: A Concise History of Regulatory Impasse." *Reproductive BioMedicine and Society Online* 2: 8–15.

13

Motherworkers of Tbilisi

The Housewifization of Commercial
Surrogates in Post-Soviet Georgia

SIGRID VERTOMMEN

It's a warm spring day in Tbilisi, and Polina and I decided
to explore the city before commencing our fieldwork on
the Georgian surrogacy market. After climbing for a while,
we finally reach the top of the famous Sololaki hill, where
Mother Georgia awaits us, an impressive, twenty-meter-
high aluminum statue. Kartlis Deda is Georgia's most famous woman and also its national symbol. Since 1958, she
has been watching over the pearl of the South-Caucasus,
wearing a traditional garment with a glass of wine in her
left hand and a sword in her right. Welcoming but always
wary of new visitors, an understandable attitude given the
turbulent history of the former Soviet republic, with separat-
ist movements in Abkhazia and South Ossetia and constant
tensions with Russia.
—Fieldwork notes, May 10, 2018

Since the early 2000s, Mother Georgia has been receiving a new type of
visitor: intended parents with infertility issues who are looking for an
affordable and available surrogate to make their parenting dreams come
true. Surrogacy has been legal in Georgia since 1997, although the Georgian authorities recently announced a ban on commercial surrogacy for
foreign citizens, allowing it only on "the principle of altruism."[1] Because
of its permissive surrogacy legislation, cheap reproductive labor force,
and strategic location between Europe and Asia, Georgia is popular with
intended parents from all corners of the globe: Turkey, Spain, Saudi Ara-

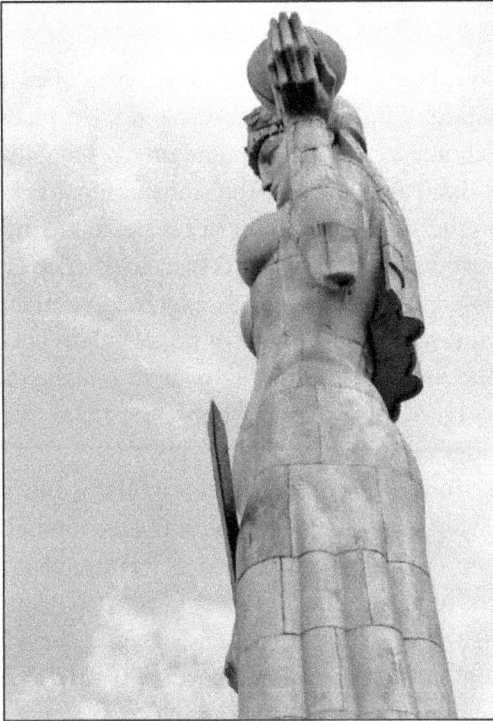

Figure 13.1. Kartlis Deda (Mother Georgia). Credit: Picture by Author

bia, Russia, the United States, and beyond. According to the Georgian Public Service Development Agency, approximately 80 percent of the children born through surrogacy in Georgia are from foreign couples, with Israel (34.42 percent) and China (9.20 percent) as the two countries with the highest demand for Georgian surrogates (Darchiashvili and Gavashelishvili 2023).[2] Georgia's capital of Tbilisi, and also other smaller cities such as Batumi and Kutaisi, have seen an impressive growth in private fertility clinics and surrogacy agencies, in what is portrayed in both national and international academic and journalistic accounts as an exploitative self-regulating industry (Channel 4 News 2021; Bowers, Politzer, and Lepapa 2022; Darchiashvili and Gavashelishvili 2023).

In line with this volume's emphasis on the comparative analysis of situated fertility transitions, this chapter examines how Georgia transformed into one of the main suppliers of gestational labor power on the global fertility market, especially after the closure of the Indian, Thai, Nepalese, and Mexican surrogacy markets for foreign couples. Drawing on the generative feminist work of the late Maria Mies (1982, 2014) on the housewifization of Indian lace makers and the capitalist divisions of re/productive labor, I argue that the popularity, profitability, and extractability of Georgian surrogates on the transnational surrogacy market partially rely on their hesitation or even refusal to identify and be identified as value-producing workers and their insistence on being identified as respectable mothers instead.[3] By exploring contemporary fertility changes from the vantage point of commercial surrogacy in Georgia, this chapter underlines the importance of analyzing the reconfigurations of fertility labor as a shifting dialectic between paid and unpaid forms of *motherwork* under capitalism.

The introduction of in vitro fertilization (IVF) in the late 1970s is widely seen as having contributed to both the technologization and the commercialization of reproduction and as having introduced the possibility of separating reproductive tissues (oocytes, wombs, embryos), processes (ovulation, gestation, parturition), and services that can be mobilized within and across national borders (Franklin and Lock 2003; Cooper and Waldby 2014; Winddance Twine 2015). In political economic terms, the expanding repro-economy has been both enabled and shaped by the development of what Marcia C. Inhorn (2015) famously describes as "reproflows" and "reproscapes," and what I, together with Michal Nahman and Vincenzo Pavone, term "global fertility chains" (Vertommen, Pavone, and Nahman 2022). Global fertility chains are what we call unevenly developed and highly gendered and racialized multi-actor networks of globalized fertility, in which the reproductive capacities, skills, bodies, biologies, and labors of oocyte vendors, surrogates, and tissue providers are increasingly deployed and marketized to fulfill the reproductive desires of intended parents and the capital accumulative needs of the fertility industry. According to recent estimates by market researchers, the fertility-services market is set to nearly double in value from $17 billion in 2021 to $32 billion by 2029, with surrogacy serving as one of its most lucrative flagship industries (Databridge Market Research 2022).

In dialogue with "newer" feminist science and technology studies (STS) and political economy accounts of the fertility industry that scrutinize socio-technical processes of datafication, financialization, automation, and platformization (Van de Wiel 2018), this chapter foregrounds a somewhat "old-school" feminist materialist analysis that emphasizes the embodied labor power of surrogates, in their capacity as both paid and unpaid *motherworkers*, as sites of value creation. While much research has approached surrogacy from a bio-ethical, legal, or cultural anthropological stance, Amrita Pande's (2014) ethnographic account of commercial surrogacy in Gujarat, India, was among the first to advance a comprehensive labor perspective. In analyzing how surrogacy is managed in the workplace, at home, and in the clinic, Pande noted how Indian surrogates were disciplined by professional medical teams and fertility agents through what she termed the "mother-worker paradigm." As a good mother, the surrogate was expected to care for herself and for the baby inside her without growing too attached, while as a good worker she was to be professional, submissive, healthy, and not too greedy when it came to discussing wages and labor conditions. When the surrogate dared to cross these carefully constructed boundaries, she was reprimanded. Pande (2014: 167) concluded that "the rhetoric of good motherhood is employed to restrain the surrogates as workers and the rhetoric of good workerhood to restrain them as mothers." Building on the inspiring scholarship of repro-scholars such as Pande (2014), Rudrappa (2015), Vora (2015), Nahman (2013), Cooper and Waldby (2014), and Lewis (2019), this chapter contributes to recent efforts to develop a labor theory of value (or a value theory of labor, as Diane Elson [1979] would rightfully call it) of the fertility industry. Relying on ethnographic accounts of how Georgian surrogates define their own reproductive labor as surrogates and mothers, and using Maria Mies's (1982) concept of "housewifization" as a reprolens, it foregrounds three interrelated questions: How is surrogates' labor productive of fertility value? What kind of fertility value does surrogate labor produce (and for whom)? And, how is the fertility value generated by surrogate labor situated within the wider economic calculus that determines global commodity, service, and market value?

Toward a Reproductive Worker's Inquiry of Surrogacy

This chapter is based on qualitative fieldwork conducted in Tbilisi and Batumi between May and July 2018 and in October 2022, as part of a larger research project on the political economy of the global fertility chain between Israel/Palestine and Georgia. The data consist of more than forty interviews with twenty Georgian surrogates, fertility agents, fertility doctors, representatives of governmental institutions, feminist organizations, and trade unions; (non)participatory observations in fertility clinics, agencies, and surrogacy fairs; and a close reading of policy documents on surrogacy in Georgia, surrogacy contracts, and promotional material and websites. The final fieldwork visit in October 2022 was dedicated to developing a surrogacy hotline and know-your-rights charter for surrogates in collaboration with the Solidarity Network, a union for precarious (health)care workers in Georgia.

This collaboration also gestures toward the methodological foundation of this research, which aims to further develop reproductive workers' inquiries (Vertommen 2021). A workers' inquiry is a method that was developed by Marx and later picked up by Marxists such as C. L. R. and Selma James and Mario Tronti to assess the labor conditions of the working class. The idea behind a workers' inquiry is that workers are not passive subjects to be researched, but the best-situated actors in describing and thus transforming their own conditions (James 1972; Woodcock 2017). While most of the workers' inquiries took the archetypical male factory worker as their methodological point of departure, Marxist feminists rightly argued that doing so overlooks most of the value-producing work performed by "women, nature and colonized subjects" in capitalist economies (James 1972; Mies 2014).

Drawing on Selma James's (1972) workers' inquiry of housewives, my research uses the experiences and perspectives of surrogates on their paid and unpaid reproductive work as a lens through which to view broader capitalist processes. The interviews with the surrogate mothers/workers therefore played a prominent role. There are methodological and ethical challenges in conducting a workers' inquiry of a practice that is not considered to be "real" work, in a workplace that is not perceived as a "real" site of labor, with participants who do not identify as "real" workers. This is precisely one of the main conceptual contributions of this chapter—namely, that the work of reproduction is naturalized and therefore in/visibilized and devalued, not only by the fertility doctors and surrogacy brokers but also by the motherworkers themselves (Vertommen and Barbagallo 2021).

Breadwinning Housewives: Post-ART Labor in Post-Soviet Georgia

Georgia became an independent republic in 1991, after almost seventy years of Soviet rule. Following a decade of civil conflicts and secessionist wars, the Rose Revolution led to the election of president Mikheil Saakashvili in 2003. Under his administration, Georgia pursued a strong pro-Western foreign policy, aimed at NATO and European Union integration, which resulted in a series of neoliberal reforms, including the deregulation of the labor market and the privatization of healthcare (Natsvlishvili, Kapanadze, and Japaridze 2022). In her research on contemporary logistics and labor regimes in Georgia, Evelina Gambino (2019: 8–9) explained how the government, in an attempt to attract foreign capital since the early 2000s, has been presenting Georgian workers as a "competitively priced workforce." There is no regulation on minimum wage and no effective system of labor inspections, or independent unions. Sopo Japaridze from the Solidarity Network added, "For female workers, the situation seems even worse. Most women are employed in the services sector, working long hours for low wages. Because of deeply ingrained gender stereotypes, these women are not only paid less than their male colleagues but have to take on all kinds of care work as well" (interview, Tbilisi, June 2, 2018).

In terms of reproductive politics, Georgia, like other post-Soviet societies, has experienced a remarkable revival of nationalist culture since 1991, emphasizing women's traditional roles within the household as mothers and housewives (Rener and Mirjana 1998: 121; Gal and Kligman 2000; Rekhviashvili 2010; Barkaia and Waterston 2018). A United Nations study on women's work reported that Georgian women spend on average forty-five hours per week on unpaid care work, compared to only fifteen hours for men (UN Women 2018). According to a survey by Caucasus Barometer, more than 80 percent of Georgians are convinced that men should be the only breadwinner in the family, and that women are more valued for their families than for successful careers. In reality, however, women are the main income providers in almost 40 percent of the Georgian households, with high numbers of male unemployment (Japaridze et al. 2014: 104).

During Soviet times, Georgian women were expected to partake in both the production and the reproduction of the socialist state and the nuclear family as "worker-mothers." Since the neoliberal turn, however, they are performing the same burdensome double shifts for both the national and the world market as "breadwinning housewives" (Paulovich 2016). Many Georgian women work in the so-called informal economy, with only 58 percent of the productive-aged women at work in the formal economy (UN Women 2018). The lack of accessible and affordable childcare and kindergartens is listed as one of the key factors preventing Georgian women from joining the labor market. Other factors that explain Georgian women's so-called economic inactivity are the disproportionate number of hours they spend on unpaid care work in the household and the discrimination they face at the workplace. With a gender pay gap of more than 40 percent, women's wages are often too low to be an incentive (UN Women 2018).

This is the postsocialist context in which Georgian women began to marketize some of their reproductive skills and capacities, which were previously exchanged outside of the cash nexus, within and between households. In her research on Georgian women's agency as workers and housewives, Paulovich (2016: 29) described how these women started utilizing their cooking skills for earning money, often as part of what she called "an underground economy." The inspirational oeuvre of the materialist ecofeminist scholar Maria Mies can also help shed light on the situation of Georgian women. In her early work, "Lace Makers of Narsapur: Indian Housewives Produce for the World Market," Mies (1982) provided a detailed ethnographic account of women's involvement in India's lace making industry. Expanding on Marx's crucial yet limited understanding of the working day, she meticulously described the endless work that the lace makers perform from their homes, and the sheer impossibility of distinguishing between production and reproduction relations. She also observed how the contributions of the lace makers were not considered as work that produced value to the capitalist economy but rather labeled as housework or subsistence work at most. She introduced the concept of "housewifization" to explain that, despite their full incorporation into a capitalist export-oriented production system as wage laborers, "the lace makers' integration was premised on their self-understanding as housewives who depend on the wage of the husband or breadwinner, although in reality their subsistence and income generating activities are work" (Mies 1982: 110). She added that housewives could be considered as capitalism's optimal labor force, contributing to capital accumulation but not identifying as workers, which is how their work became devalued. According to Mies, there is nothing necessarily "informal" or "underground" about Georgian women's contribution to the economy. It is simply the way capitalist economies operate.

The Housewifization of Georgian Surrogates

Housewifization is not a unique process for Indian lace makers, but it is viewed in Marxist feminist scholarship as a structural feature of capitalist economies, which reduces more and more types of labor, performed by both men and women, but especially by women, to housework (Vora 2019). In my own research on the Georgian surrogacy industry, I found housewifization a particularly useful concept for understanding processes of devaluation, naturalization, and invisibilization of surrogates' motherwork (Vora 2019; Vertommen and Barbagallo 2021; Vertommen 2021).[4]

As I have described elsewhere, some Georgian women are increasingly opting to perform gestational labor not only because it pays much better than conventional forms of employment but because it allows them to combine it with motherhood, in many cases single motherhood. Of the twenty surrogates I interviewed, sixteen were single mothers for whom the constant effort to generate enough income to support their families was a daily concern. Elena, for instance, a single mother eight months pregnant in her first surrogacy pregnancy, explained that she would have to work for three years as a laboratory assistant to earn the same amount—fifteen thousand dollars—as she does now while "doing nothing, except for being pregnant."[5] "Being" a surrogate also permitted Elena to stay at home to take care of her toddler, as she could not afford to pay for childcare when she worked outside of the house. However, when asked whether she considered surrogacy to be her job or profession, Elena adamantly answered "no." Despite all of the physical and emotional labor involved in gestating the fetus and the time spent on medical appointments, meetings with the fertility agents, and conversations with the intended parents, she refused to view surrogacy as her work. She clarified: "Pregnancy is an automatic thing; it's just happening on its own. I am just being a mother and a housewife, and I am doing this because I desperately need the money."

Nargiza, another surrogate whom I interviewed in the sixth month of her first surrogacy pregnancy, became annoyed by my question about whether she considered surrogacy work. She replied, "Pregnancy is just a state that you are in. It's not a good or a bad job. It's not a job. I chose to be a surrogate because I need to be a good mother. The well-being of my daughter means everything for me." Not only was "being" a good mother a crucial motivation for Elena and Nargiza to become surrogate motherworkers, but it was also a requirement for recruitment. As Elena's surrogacy agent had explained to her, only women who have already birthed their own child(ren) were accepted to become surrogates as this makes it less likely that the surrogate would want to keep the surrogacy baby after birth. It also proves that their gestational bodies and reproductive biologies are in good shape. While the Georgian surrogacy industry depends on the mutually formative work of motherhood, pregnancy, and surrogacy, for Elena and Nargiza, both the unwaged reproductive work of mothering and the paid reproductive work of gestating were viewed as an existential state of being, rather than as a performative state of laboring (Vertommen and Barbagallo 2021).

The naturalization of the reproductive labors of ovulation, gestation, and parturition is a common feature in capitalist economies. Even in the Georgian surrogacy industry, where surrogates are undeniably paid for their gestational services, fertility brokers still use the language of gift giving or altruism to promote their services (Ragoné 1994; Rudrappa 2015; Jacobson 2016; Lewis 2019). This means that Georgian surrogates are never given a salary or a wage, but rather a fee or compensation. Even when they are paid, they are not fully waged reproductive workers with labor contracts and rights protected by national labor codes (Rudrappa 2015). When asked about the costs of the surrogacy procedure, a famous Georgian surrogacy agent replied as follows:

> AGENT: The whole procedure costs $30,000, $36,000 with egg donation. The agency fee is $4,500. The whole process from the start until the end, the surrogate gets $15,000. During the pregnancy, she gets

$400 per month and then $11,400 after delivery; the egg donor
gets $1,000.

AUTHOR: Is the money for the surrogate considered as a salary?

AGENT: No, it's seen as a compensation.

AUTHOR: So, it's not seen as a job?

AGENT: No, it's like a financial help from the parents in return [for] the
thing they do.

This housewifization of surrogates, which transforms their work into
"a thing they do for financial help," is further enhanced by the fact that
they perform their gestational labor alone "at home." Contrary to Indian surrogates, for example, who were often grouped together by the
fertility agencies in so-called surrogacy hotels to avoid stigmatization in
their home communities, Georgian surrogates remain isolated, divided,
and invisible in the individual homeplace. Unlike the lace makers of
Narsapur, who also performed home-based labor, Georgian surrogates
often work not from their own homeplace but from a new house they
moved into in the third trimester of their pregnancy to avoid the judgment and interference of their neighbors, friends, and family. Although
surrogacy is legal in Georgia, it remains taboo in Georgia's patriarchal
society, where motherhood is placed strictly within the sphere of the
family (Sumbadze 2008). Surrogates are often judged for presumably
selling their own children. In 2014, Ilia II, Georgia's widely popular Orthodox patriarch, condemned surrogacy during his Christmas epistle
for bringing forth "problematic" children ("Abortion, Surrogacy" 2014).

The societal stigma surrounding surrogacy has forced many surrogates to remain as invisible as possible. Every time I met Elena, for instance, it was in the new flat she moved into during the seventh month
of her pregnancy, to avoid gossip from her neighbors. Even when I interviewed her during the day, the curtains of the apartment would be
closed, and she wore baggy clothes in order to hide her bump. Also,
Mariam, a single mother from Tbilisi who at the time of our interview
was pregnant with her third surrogacy baby, explained that she left her
neighborhood in the sixth month of her pregnancy "because the neighbors are nosy, and they talk and gossip a lot." After each time she gave
birth to the baby, she moved back: "Until the sixth month I was just pre-
tending that I gained weight to explain why I was chubbier than usual. I

mostly would hide, stay at home, and wouldn't leave my place so much. Whenever I had appointments, my father would drive me with the car that I bought for him with the money from my first surrogacy."

Nargiza quit her job as a barista because she did not want her colleagues to know she was a surrogate. During our interview, I noticed that she was wearing a wedding ring, so I asked her how her husband felt about the procedure. She laughed and replied, "Oh, I am not married. I wear this wedding ring as a tool to avoid glances and questions from people on the streets. The ring as such has no meaning for me, I don't care about being married or not; it's just not to get psychologically stressed with other people's opinion, judgment, and what not. I only wear it when I remember to do so, and there are times when I leave the house without it, but then I get those glances in the street."

Many of the surrogates I interviewed were single mothers, a status generally denigrated in Georgian society. Nogaideli (2012) noted that the resurgence of Georgian nationalism has politicized single motherhood as unsavory by viewing single mothers as women of loose behavior who lack respectability. For Georgian surrogacy brokers, respectability is therefore an important criterion in the selection and recruitment of Georgian surrogates, who, according to Darchiashvili and Gavashelishvili (2023), should be maternal and docile, not greedy and shameless. In their research on the surrogacy industry, they observed how Georgian fertility agencies and clinics opt for surrogates who fall into the category of "*tsesieri*," a Georgian word for a righteous and good woman. "Usually, a *tsesieri* Georgian woman is one who keeps her virginity before marriage and, after the marriage, becomes a devoted wife and a selfless mother" (Darchiashvili and Gavashelishvili 2023: 24). This is also the main reason why Nargiza was feigning conjugality, to pass as a proper *tsesieri* woman and garner respectability from her surroundings (Nogaideli 2012).

My interviews with Georgian surrogates illustrate that many sought to remain as invisible as possible to avoid being seen and shamed by nosy neighbors, to evade taxation by the state, and to protect themselves against the interference of intended parents or surrogacy agents. However, this invisibility is also structurally enforced by society and one of the reasons why surrogates do not easily identify as workers

(Vertommen and Barbagallo 2021). The hesitation or even refusal of a workers' consciousness and identity in turn deepens practices of hyperexploitation in the fertility industry. Elena, along with several other interlocutor surrogates, explained that she has no control over many aspects of the surrogacy procedure, including the number of embryos that are transferred to her womb, how to give birth, whether to perform a fetal reduction or abortion, and whether to breastfeed. The surrogacy contract stipulates that these reproductive decisions are first and foremost made by the intended parents in consultation with the surrogacy agencies and the doctors, in what is mostly a self-regulating industry that faces very few governmental restrictions. During our interview, Elena mentioned, "The intended parents do ask me, but I think my opinion counts for like two percent of the choice, because the genetic material is theirs. I am just the womb." Georgian fertility doctors explained that, depending on the quality of the embryos, usually two, but sometimes up to four embryos are transferred to the womb of the surrogate, as a way of supposedly enhancing the chances of a successful pregnancy. This means that Georgian surrogates often carry twins or even triplets, which in turn poses more risks during the pregnancy. Elena will also remain invisible on the birth certificate of the surrogacy baby, which will only mention the commissioning parents, another reason why Georgia is such a popular surrogacy hub.

Furthermore, surrogates in Georgia do not have access to adequate medical and life insurance. Medical complications due to the surrogacy pregnancy are not seen as work accidents. Mariam, for instance, mentioned during our interview, "I had a C-section, and it was written in the contract that I was entitled to medical check-ups until I felt 100 percent, but nobody remembered that contract. After the birth, they just counted down the money, gave it to me, and it was finished. So, the medical care I needed after the C-section, I had to cover that myself."

Lastly, when a Georgian surrogate suffers a miscarriage, she often receives only part of the payment, depending on whether the doctors decided it was her "fault" or not. A recent report also suggested that some surrogacy agencies even forced women to give birth early in order to deny them full remuneration, leading to serious mental and physical health complications (Gabritchidze 2023).

Surrogates of the World, Unite!

Because of continued reports of abusive and fraudulent practices in the surrogacy industry, and fears that surrogacy babies, in contravention of Georgian law, were ending up with same-sex couples, the Georgian authorities announced in June 2023 a prohibition on surrogacy and IVF services for foreign citizens starting in January 2024. While surrogacy would remain available to Georgian citizens, Health Minister Zurab Azarashvili announced that it would only be permitted on an altruistic rather than commercial basis, stating that "a Georgian citizen who wants to be a donor or surrogate must act within the altruism principle" (quoted in Gabritchidze 2023). But by March 2024, the new bill on assisted reproduction had not been adopted by the Georgian Parliament.

While (more) state regulation could help ensure the safety and well-being of surrogates and surrogacy babies, it is less likely that surrogacy bans will be effective in mitigating the powers of the global fertility industry, which—whether we like it or not—is not about to disappear anytime soon. As with previous national bans on commercial surrogacy issued in Thailand, India, Nepal, Mexico, or Cambodia, surrogacy companies and clinics tend to look for legal loopholes across the globe in moving their businesses to another "mother destination." When I asked a Georgian surrogacy agent who was present at the latest European Society of Human Reproduction and Embryology conference in Copenhagen in June 2023 how the new legal restrictions would affect transnational surrogacy arrangements, she reassured me that their agency had already opened a new proxy clinic and agency in Romania. Albania and Kazakhstan have also emerged as new potential destinations for transnational surrogacy by Georgian agencies. However, beyond the practical limitations of national regulatory initiatives, banning commercial surrogacy while keeping the door open for altruistic forms of surrogacy fundamentally assumes that women's gestational labor should always be performed for free as an expression of motherly love or a gift of life. It furthermore strips commercial surrogates of their (survival) income without offering them any alternative (Rudrappa and Collins 2015).

Another strategy to curb unethical practices in the fertility industry while guaranteeing the well-being of surrogates could be for them to organize as what I call *motherworkers* through unions or cooperatives. To date, I have not come across any official union of surrogates or other assisted reproductive technology (ART) workers, despite the global scale and popularity of transactional fertility. In the United States, Canada, Israel, and India, surrogates mainly organize via informal social media networks where they exchange information and advice on the medical, logistical, and financial aspects of the surrogacy procedure. While these social media groups are useful for connecting dispersed surrogates and offering support, they are often created and controlled by the fertility agents and clinics, which limits participants' ability to organize collectively in ways that might be perceived as against the interests of the fertility industry. Moreover, labor unions have shown little interest in organizing with surrogates and other paid or unpaid reproductive workers. Dorothy Sue Cobble (2010: 282) referred to the limitations of the "factory paradigm of labor organizing" in which labor unions take the "archetypical male proletariat toiling away on the mass production assembly line" as their privileged subject of collective organizing. Also, Mies (2014) noted a lack of interest from trade unions in organizing with the lace makers, who were identified as home-based housewives. "Housewives are atomized and isolated, their work organization makes the awareness of common interests, of the whole process of production very difficult. Their horizons remain limited by the family" (Mies 2014: 116).

This is certainly the case in Georgia, where, according to Gambino (2019: 8–9), unions are failing to organize the majority of workers, who slip through the mazes of labor categories: day laborers, informal laborers, and an expanding number of precarious service sector workers. This is paired with a distrust of institutional unions, dating from Soviet times, when trade unions were seen as an extension of the ruling party. Newer so-called social movement labor unions, like the Tbilisi-based Solidarity Network, are trying to fill these gaps by organizing with precarious workers, often women working in healthcare and other care industries, including nurses and psychologists.

In October 2022, I collaborated with Sopo Japaridze and Revaz Telia Karanadze from the Solidarity Network in setting up a surrogate hotline, which surrogates can contact, through its Facebook and other social media pages, for more information about their rights when entering a surrogacy agreement. Based on close readings of surrogacy contracts and follow-up interviews with surrogates, oocyte providers, and other fertility industry workers, we compiled a know-your-rights document that was translated into Georgian. The document addresses various matters, including health and life insurance, wages, reproductive decision making, and legal representation of surrogates. Three issues were crucial for us when assembling this reproductive-union initiative. First, we refrained from using moralizing rescue narratives in our communication with (potential) surrogates. Rather than dissuading them from entering a surrogacy agreement or convincing them to look for other, more acceptable means of income, we wanted to provide them with some basic and independent medical and legal insights about the surrogacy procedure, allowing them to negotiate—either individually or collectively—for better working conditions. Second, we were adamant in approaching the surrogates as "motherworkers" and looking at the dis/continuities between their reluctant workers' identification as paid surrogates and unpaid mothers. Rather than viewing Georgian women's family-oriented subjectivity as a sign of conservative backwardness or as a hurdle for their emancipation as "real workers," we aimed to draw the connections between their gendered conditions of work at home and in the fertility clinic and surrogacy agency. Third, we were keen to build connections and solidarities between surrogates and other un/paid reproductive workers, including nurses, mothers, domestic workers, egg providers, and cleaners, to see whether and how their working conditions share elements of invisibilization, precaritization, and devalorization.

Conclusion

The surrogacy hotline is still at the starting block. Given that this was not a bottom-up initiative from surrogates, but instead was introduced by activists and/or scholars, it remains to be seen whether the unionizing strategy is effective and sustainable in reaching (potential) surrogates and ameliorating their work and life conditions. Moreover, with the regulatory ban on surrogacy announced in early 2024, the future of the Georgian surrogacy industry was placed in limbo.

However, I have a humble "optimism of the will," to use Gramsci's (1975) famous phrase concerning the political significance of a

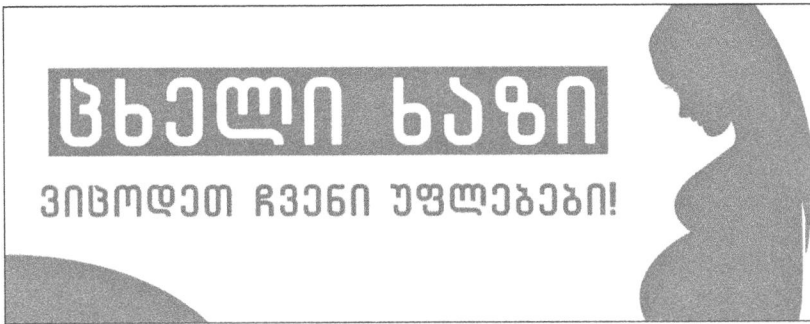

Figure 13.2. Hotline—Know Our Rights Facebook Page. Credit: Solidarity Network

surrogate union, which could potentially serve as a good practice in other surrogacy hubs. Following Cobble's (2010) plea for more "intimate unions" and drawing on decades-old union experiences of sex workers, cleaners, and domestic workers, I propose that we urgently need more reproductive unions as sites where contemporary fertility changes are collectively negotiated and bargained, and where capitalist contradictions between production and reproduction, home and the workplace, motherhood and work can be challenged and transcended.

NOTES

Dr. Polina Vlasenko and I collaborated during my first fieldwork trip to Georgia in May/June 2018, as we both share an interest in fertility markets in former Soviet countries. Vlasenko conducts research on oocyte markets in Ukraine, while my postdoctoral research focused on the global surrogacy chain between Israel/Palestine and Georgia. Vlasenko assisted during some of the interviews with surrogates, fertility agents, and doctors that were conducted in Russian. She also transcribed some of the interviews.

1 Surrogacy is regulated in Georgia through the Health Protection Law, which states, "In vitro fertilization shall be allowed (a) to treat infertility, if there is a risk of transmitting a genetic disease from the wife or the husband to the child, using the gametes or embryo of the couple or a donor, if a written consent of the couple has been obtained; (b) if a woman does not have a uterus, by transferring the embryo obtained as a result of fertilization to the uterus of other women (surrogate mother) and growing it there; obtaining a written consent of the couple shall be obligatory" (Law on Health Protection, Chapter XXIII—Family Planning, Article 143, 1997). The Georgian government has announced that it intends to pass legislation that would prohibit surrogacy for foreigners starting January 1, 2024.

2 For a more in-depth analysis of the global surrogacy chain between Israel/Palestine and Georgia, and the emergence of its demand and supply side, see Vertommen and Reyns (2019) and Vertommen and Barbagallo (2021).

3 Parts of this chapter on the Georgian surrogacy industry are included in earlier publications: Vertommen and Reyns (2019), Vertommen and Barbagallo (2021), and Vertommen (2021).

4 Some ethnographic accounts in this section are also included and discussed in Vertommen and Barbagallo (2021) and Vertommen (2021).

5 In 2018, the average annual income for women was $1,830 USD (GEL 4.517) compared to $3,110 USD for men (UN Women 2018).

REFERENCES

"Abortion, Surrogacy, and Artificial Insemination in Christmas Epistle of Ilia II." 2014. *Georgian Journal*, January 7. Video. https://georgianjournal.ge.

Barkaia, Maia, and Alisse Waterston. 2018. *Gender in Georgia: Feminist Perspectives on Culture, Nation, and History in the South Caucasus*. New York: Berghahn.

Bowers, Simon, Malia Politzer, and Naipanoi Lepapa. 2022. "The Baby Broker Project: Inside the World's Leading Low-Cost Surrogacy Agency." *Finance Uncovered*, December 18. www.financeuncovered.org.

Channel 4 News. 2021. "Selling Wombs for Hire in Georgia." Unreported World, October 24. Video, 00:23:57, www.youtube.com.

Cobble, Dorothy Sue. 2010. "More Intimate Unions." In *Intimate Labors: Cultures, Technologies, and the Politics of Care*, eds. Eileen Boris and Rhacel Salazar Parreñas, 280–95. Stanford, CA: Stanford University Press.

Cooper, Melinda, and Catherine Waldby. 2014. *Clinical Labor: Tissue Donors and Research Subjects in the Global Bioeconomy*. Durham, NC: Duke University Press.

Darchiashvili, Mariam, and Elene Gavashelishvili. 2023. "Entanglement of the Formal and Informal in Everyday Surrogacy Negotiations: The Case of Georgia." *Studies of Transition States and Societies* 15(1): 18–31.

Databridge Market Research. 2022. "Global Fertility Services Market: Industry Trends and Forecast to 2029." www.databridgemarketresearch.com.

Elson, Diane, ed. 1979. *Value: The Representation of Labour in Capitalism*. London: Verso.

Franklin, Sarah, and Margaret Lock, eds. 2003. *Remaking Life and Death: Toward an Anthropology of the Biosciences*. Sante Fe, NM: SAR Press.

Gabritchidze, Nini. 2023. "Georgia to Ban Surrogacy for Foreigners." *Eurasia Net*, June 13. https://eurasianet.org.

Gal, Susan, and Gail Kligman. 2000. *The Politics of Gender after Socialism: A Comparative Historical Essay*. Princeton, NJ: Princeton University Press.

Gambino, Evelina. 2019. "The Georgian Logistics Revolution: Questioning Seamlessness across the New Silk Road." *Work Organisation, Labour & Globalisation* 1: 190–206.

Gramsci, Antonio. 1975. *Letters from Prison*. Selected, translated from the Italian, and introduced by Lynne Lawner. London: Harper Colophone Books.

Inhorn, Marcia C. 2015. *Cosmopolitan Conceptions: IVF Sojourns in Global Dubai*. Durham, NC: Duke University Press.

Jacobson, Heather. 2016. *Labor of Love: Gestational Surrogacy and the Work of Making Babies*. New Brunswick, NJ: Rutgers University Press.

James, Selma. 1972. "A Woman's Place." In *The Power of Women and the Subversion of the Community: A Mariarosa Dalla Costa Reader*, ed. Camille Barbagallo, 57–79. London: Falling Wall Press.

Japaridze, Elena, Maia Barkaia, Nina Zhghenti, and Mariam Amashukeli. 2014. *The Study of Georgian Youth's Awareness, Perceptions, and Attitudes of Gender Equality*. Tbilisi, Georgia: Center for Social Sciences.

Lewis, Sophie. 2019. *Full Surrogacy Now: Feminism against Family*. London: Verso Books.

Mies, Maria. 1982. *The Lace Makers of Narsapur: Indian Housewives Produce for the World Market*. London: Zed Press.

———. 2014. *Patriarchy and Accumulation on a World Scale: Women in the International Division of Labour*. London: Zed Books.

Nahman, Michal. 2013. *Extractions: An Ethnography of Reproductive Tourism*. Hampshire, UK: Palgrave Macmillan.

Natsvlishvili, Beka, Nodar Kapanadze, and Sopo Japaridze. 2022. "Social Consequences of Privatization of Healthcare." *Friedrich-Ebert-Stiftung*, Tbilisi Office.

Nogaideli, Eter. 2012. *Single Mothers: Un-Respectable Others of Georgian Nationalism; Production of Subjectivities through Nesting Respectability*. Unpublished master's thesis, Gender Studies, Central European University, Budapest, Hungary.

Pande, Amrita. 2014. *Wombs in Labor: Transnational Commercial Surrogacy in India*. New York: Columbia University Press.

Paulovich, Natallia. 2016. "A Breadwinner or a Housewife? Agency in the Everyday Image of the Georgian Woman." *Anthropology of the Contemporary Middle East and Central Eurasia* 3(2): 24–44.

Ragoné, Helena. 1994. *Surrogate Motherhood: Conceptions of the Heart*. Boulder, CO: Westview Press.

Rekhviashvili, Ana. 2010. *Nationalism and Motherhood in Contemporary Georgia*. Unpublished master's thesis, Central European University, Budapest, Hungary.

Rener, Tanja, and Ule Mirjana. 1998. "Back to the Future: Nationalism and Gender in Post-Socialist Societies." In *Women, Ethnicity, and Nationalism: The Politics of Transition*, eds. Robert E. Miller and Rick Wilford, 120–32. London: Routledge.

Rudrappa, Sharmila. 2015. *Discounted Life: The Price of Global Surrogacy in India*. New York: New York University Press.

Rudrappa, Sharmila, and Caitlyn Collins. 2015. "Altruistic Agencies and Compassionate Consumers: Moral Framing of Transnational Surrogacy." *Gender and Society* 29(6): 937–59.

Sumbadze, Nana. 2008. *Gender and Society: Georgia.* Tbilisi, Georgia: United Nations Development Programme.

UN Women. 2018. "Women's Economic Inactivity and Engagement in the Informal Sector in Georgia: Causes and Consequences." Tbilisi, Georgia: UN Women Georgia Office.

Van de Wiel, Lucy. 2018. "Prenatal Imaging: Egg Freezing, Embryo Selection, and the Visual Politics of Reproductive Time." *Catalyst* 4(2): 1–35.

Vertommen, Sigrid. 2021. "Marx in Utero: A Workers' Inquiry of the In/Visible Labours of Reproduction in the Surrogacy Industry." In *Marx in the Field*, ed. Alessandra Mezzadri, 189–202. London: Anthem Press.

Vertommen, Sigrid, and Camille Barbagallo. 2021. "The Invisible Wombs of the Market: Waged and Unwaged Reproductive Labor in the Global Surrogacy Industry." *Review of International Political Economy* 29(6): 1945–66.

Vertommen, Sigrid, Vincenzo Pavone, and Michal Nahman. 2022. "Global Fertility Chains: An Integrative Political Economy Approach to Understanding the Reproductive Bioeconomy." *Science, Technology & Human Values* 47(1): 112–45.

Vertommen, Sigrid, and Ailien Reyns. 2019. "Van Vraagouder tot Draagmoeder: De Babybusiness Tussen Israël en Georgië en de Babybusiness Boom" [From Intended Parent to Surrogate Mother: The Baby Business between Israel and Georgia]. *Mo* Magazine*. Mo Papers, December, 1–12.

Vlasenko, Polina. 2015. "Desirable Bodies/Precarious Laborers: Ukrainian Egg Donors in Context of Transnational Fertility." In *(In)Fertile Citizens: Anthropological and Legal Challenges of Assisted Reproduction Technologies*, ed. Venetia Kantsa, Giulia Zanini, and Lina Papadopoulou, 197–216. (In)FERCIT: Lab of Family and Kinship Studies, Department of Social Anthropology and History, University of the Aegean, Mytilene, Greece.

Vora, Kalindi. 2015. *Life Support: Biocapital and the New History of Outsourced Labor.* Minneapolis: University of Minnesota Press.

———. 2019. "After the Housewife: Surrogacy, Labour, and Human Reproduction." *Radical Philosophy* 20(4): 42–46.

Winddance Twine, France. 2015. *Outsourcing the Womb: Race, Class, and Gestational Surrogacy in a Global Market.* New York: Taylor and Francis.

Woodcock, Jamie. 2017. *Working the Phones: Control and Resistance in the Call Centres.* London: Pluto Press.

14

Haunted Data "Goldmine"

Repropolitical Anxieties and Injustice in Finland

MWENZA BLELL AND RIIKKA HOMANEN

In this chapter, we closely examine the production of Finnish population databases, asking whether this area of high-tech development in Finland can be considered a form of "reproductive politics" (Briggs 2018). We fix our attention on Finland's famed Nordic data "goldmine" (Kongsholm et al. 2018), referring to the exceptionally valuable national data resources originating from historical practices of keeping population-level registers rather than relying on census data. These registers include personal identity codes for all Finnish residents (Alastalo and Helén 2022) so that personal data about them can be easily linked, thus allowing for Finnish practices of large-scale personal data collection to emerge. We also show the ways these data-collection regimes are an archive of long-standing and continuing repropolitical anxieties in Finland, as well as a direct method of control of Finland's population and reproduction landscape. Moreover, the fame and value of this store of data obscure the various forms of violence they both represent and produce.

Today, fertility rates are falling across the globe, including in Nordic countries. In Finland, the fertility rate hit an "ultra-low" point of 1.32 children per woman (Statistics Finland 2023), causing a great deal of public concern, as similar trends do in many other countries (e.g., De Zordo, Marre, and Smietana 2022). However, over several decades and even before ultra-low fertility arose, collective affects in the form of repropolitical anxieties have been deployed to focus concerns on national futures, especially economic futures (Homanen and Meskus 2023). In Finland, repropolitical anxieties have revolved around white, middle-class Finns' declining fertility rates and reproductive behavior for many decades. Research on the genealogy of the biopolitics of populations in

Finland demonstrates a prevailing historical tendency to link together fertility, reproduction more broadly, and the vitality of the nation as a way of making policy (Homanen and Meskus 2023).

We describe these as *repropolitical anxieties*, rather than using alternative terms like "demographic anxieties" (De Zordo, Marre, and Smietana 2022; Mattalucci and De Zordo 2022) or "population anxieties" (Homanen and Meskus 2023), to avoid euphemistic connotations of demography or population and to highlight the reproductive politics at the heart of these affects. Further, we use the term *repropolitical* in this chapter to avoid the grammatical awkwardness of turning "reproductive politics" into an adjective and also to playfully hint at a relationship between the necropolitical and repropolitical.

In this chapter, we show how several factors crucial to the making of these data, including residency and citizenship status, are obscured for political and ideological reasons. In contrast to the narrative of a data "goldmine," we reveal data about the Finnish population to be haunted by the missing drivers of demographic change they obscure. We link this process to the work of several scholars, including Avery Gordon (2008) and Laura Briggs (2018), and suggest that Finland's data goldmine is haunted by the reproductive injustices that it represents. For us, reproductive justice is a framework that centers on the human right to maintain personal bodily autonomy, have children, not have children, and parent the children we have in safe and sustainable communities and environments.

This chapter is based on research that we have undertaken in the past and are performing now. In our ongoing research, we explore reproductive technologies in Finland (Blell and Homanen 2023; Sudenkaarne and Blell 2022). Our previous research (Homanen and Alastalo 2018, 2025; Alastalo and Homanen 2015, 2018; Homanen and Meskus 2023) on population and fertility policy and state knowledge production is retheorized in this chapter through our lens of repropolitics to show how data are used to promote certain ideas about Finnishness to both affect fertility and market the data, or market Finland as a whole. The research material of the original studies includes ethnographic materials, such as observation and interviews, as well as documentary sources, including policy documents, newspaper articles, and official websites.

While we have been doing this research, Gordon's (2008) unique theorization of haunting, which is entirely distinct from that, for example, of Derrida (Gordon 2011), has felt increasingly salient. This concept has a power of affective evocation that is inseparable from its power of explanation. According to Gordon, something is haunted when social violence has been suppressed and hidden but is very much alive, troubling, and eerie. Haunting describes just those "experiences to which the fixed forms do not speak at all, which . . . they do not recognize" (Gordon 2008: 130), and yet haunting "makes everything we do see just as it is, charged with the occluded and forgotten past" (195). We take Gordon's concept of haunting and turn our gaze to the marginalized and the denied in the past and today, those whose fertility and family making are or have been allegedly in need of violent control and technological governance in a Nordic welfare state that, in the name of social equality and universality, is not supposed to allow such things. We suggest that when one looks past the golden glow of imagined profit, the data of the historical registers of Finland demonstrate repetitive instances of injustice wrought by the state that are uncomfortable and eerily unfamiliar for those invested in the status quo and denial of wrongdoing. As we show, Finland's data, including population-register data, healthcare data, birth-register data, and assisted-fertility-treatment data, contrary to the way they are celebrated and marketed, are all haunted records of unjust exclusions and of the level of effectiveness of policies of exclusion, just as the registers are both a tangible, haunted record of, and were a way to measure the effectiveness of, eugenic policies.

The Finnish Data Landscape and (New) Nordic Welfare State Citizenship

Data can be considered a defining feature of our times. Tremendous value, financial and otherwise, is tied to data. Even though the most powerful data actors are transnational companies like Amazon and Alphabet, which draw personal information from all over the globe, "Data-driven digital economy issues are increasingly considered to be national matters" (UNCTAD 2021: 99). This is the case because of concerns about sovereignty and privacy, as well as many countries' desires to benefit from the data economy.

As Hepp, Jarke, and Kramp (2022) note, there is a concentration of data availability in specific regions of the world, such as the Nordic region, which leads to potential concentrations of power in those regions. Nordic countries, including Finland, are actively seeking to gain a place in the European and global health-data economy (Tupasela, Snell, and Tarkkala 2020; Tupasela 2021)—in the quest for economic growth, national competitiveness, and private business development.

Finland has been marketed as a place in which the Nordic welfare state has created exceptionally valuable data resources. The possibility of accessing broad and combinable data on a population without discontinuities is, from a scientific perspective, an important competitive advantage, since researchers would not have to account for bias or holes in data (Tupasela 2021: 116; Snell, Tarkkala, and Tupasela 2023). Population data (register, genomic, and healthcare data) and human biological samples are seen as attracting innovation and business development, which are key to producing wealth, health, and services in this socio-technical vision for the future (Snell, Tarkkala, and Tupasela 2023). A well-functioning data ecosystem is part of the imaginary of Finland as a tech-savvy nation providing a lucrative environment where use of data and samples is politically and economically supported. Finnish datasets of its populations, in turn, are described as socioeconomically broad, but overall, highly educated, without inequalities, and without blind spots and discontinuities—perfect for pharmaceutical and health research, and biotechnical innovation (Snell, Tarkkala, and Tupasela 2023; Tarkkala 2018).

In marketing materials, Finland's data are presented as desirable precisely as a byproduct of the welfare state having created a homogeneous and highly equal society, offering "socioeconomically non-biased data" because of a lack of socioeconomic differences, supposedly with "nationwide, equal access to healthcare," whose companies and officials can be trusted ("ranked first in ethical behavior of companies" and "ranked third least corrupted country"), and whose population is characterized by "genetic isolation," "trust in authorities," and high levels of education ("ranked first in health and primary education") and is "tech savvy" (Sitra 2015; see also Tarkkala 2018). Such marketing seems to suggest an ethical claim, in addition to the more pragmatic scientific one, about the quantity and quality of linked data. Core to this argument is the claim that data from a society so described must be ethical itself, seemingly because the population is willing, is not vulnerable, and thus is not being exploited. Thus, in many ways, "It is Finland as a whole, the whole history of data collection, that is being sold and marketed" (Tarkkala and Snell 2022: 6).

Presenting Finnish people as a "willing population" is also a common rhetoric in promoting Finnish data, referring to engaged (read: educated) public support for sharing data and participation in biobanking. The welfare state data ecosystem is premised on an implicit social contract within which values such as solidarity, social equality, universality, and reciprocity are linked to a model of reciprocity via generous and universal welfare provision (Snell, Tarkkala, and Tupasela 2023). This idea of social reciprocity, coupled with the image of Finnish citizens as comparatively well educated, supportive of their welfare state, and trusting toward the medical and scientific professions, enhances the image of the country as a source of good, reliable, and abundant biodata. The suggestion that Finns are a "willing population" has been appropriated to bolster the abandonment of any attempt to gain informed consent for data usage. According to this argument, as the majority of Finns report positive feelings about biobanks, biobanks need not obtain formal consent; instead, a retroactive opt-out option is sufficient (Snell and Tarkkala 2019). The claim of standing out from other countries by being exceptionally ethical, while moving away from clear hallmarks of ethics such as consent, and simply declaring the population willing, is noteworthy. Such a notion of ethics may be haunted by a history of actors empowered by the state to carry out actions on behalf of the nation, for the good of the nation, against the will of individuals (Sudenkaarne and Blell 2022).

Relatedly, several legislative changes introduced over the past ten years have facilitated the streamlining of access to data and samples and reduced ethical and legal constraints (Tupasela 2021; Snell, Tarkkala, and Tupasela 2023) as part of efforts to secure Finland a position as market leader. In this context, the commercialization of Finnish data has been promoted as providing diagnostic, preventive, and treatment tools as well as partially funding public healthcare (Snell, Tarkkala, and Tupasela 2023; Tupasela 2021: 117). However, Snell, Tarkkala, and Tupasela (2023: 5–6) point out that the benefits for sharing data to international commercial actors can only be realized through growth and market mechanisms, via, for example, health technology directly sold to citizen-customers. This does not accord with the original welfare state data regime's rhetoric in which data were supposedly collected and shared to directly improve the health and welfare of the citizen and the public in the nation-state context (Snell, Tarkkala, and Tupasela 2023: 10). Yet Finnish people are supposed to keep contributing to the national welfare project of data gathering in the name of solidarity, despite the change in context: from welfare state to global health data economy (Snell 2019; Snell, Tarkkala, and Tupasela 2023).

This apparent paradox can be understood by reference to the fact that, underpinning the rhetoric of benefit from welfare state data, there has always been structural (reproductive) injustice being forcefully enacted on behalf of white, middle-class, ethnic Finns, the group that is still most likely to benefit from the data-driven health technologies of the future. This is an example of the haunted quality to Finnish data politics; injustice is repeating and yet it seems to be confusing and unfamiliar to those watching it unfold. It is one of those "repetitive instances when home becomes unfamiliar . . . when what's been in your blind spot comes into view" (Gordon 2008: xvi). In the following section we will start to unpack this genealogically.

Whence the Goldmine? Finland's Haunted Eugenic Past

The idea that fertility rates in Finland were too low entered loudly into political and policy discourse during the 1930s (Bergenheim and Klockar Linder 2020), at which point civil society, politicians, and government officials started demanding political measures to support population growth (Jutikkala 1997). However, these pronatalist anxieties over the future of the nation differentiated the population according to lives considered more and less valuable to national development when a politically powerful nongovernmental organization, the Family Federation of Finland, supported the implementation of "racial hygiene" (as eugenics was called in the Nordic context) to "protect the future generations" from what were regarded as inferior hereditary traits (Homanen and Meskus 2023). In this same period, routine population data practices, such as the gathering of data to population registers, were established that endure today (Alastalo 2009; Bauer 2014).

During this period, Finland's public policies were influenced by eugenic imperatives to improve the quality of the population by targeting those deemed undesirable: the poor, the working class, the disabled, and populations minoritized by ethnicity, including the indigenous Sámi people (Sudenkaarne and Blell 2022). This approach was premised on the idea that the survival of the desired middle-class, supposedly morally and physically superior, (white) ethnic Finns was threatened by the fertility of all others, and so pressure needed to be exerted to encourage the former to reproduce and discourage the latter. Thus, as has been pointed out by historians, for much of Finnish history, "Population policy, eugenics, public health and family policy have been more or less the same thing" (Bergenheim 2017: 12).

Finland enacted a host of eugenic policies, including the denial of social benefits, banned marriage, and compulsory eugenic abortions and forced sterilizations (Sudenkaarne and Blell 2022), in the name of the good of the nation. In many ways, Finnish doctors were given a frontline eugenic role, as important and particularly powerful civil servants in the context of the welfare state, tasked with the protection of state interests through medical procedures (Blell and Homanen 2023).

The effectiveness of eugenic interventions required evaluation as well. The establishment of registers and data-collection practices and infrastructures dates back to this period, from the 1930s to the 1970s (Alastalo 2009; Bauer 2014). These are the foundation stones of Finland's impressive data landscape, particularly the famed Finnish registers, which continue to amass data day in and day out in Finland; they are a record of Finland's eugenics-informed repropolitical anxieties and an indication of how entangled these are with the practice of medicine. This is most evident in the following registers (although evident in the logic or practices associated with others as well), which indicate repropolitical anxieties:

- The Register of Congenital Malformations (established in 1963) is based on the eugenic notion of hereditary hygiene (*perintöhygienia*) (Sudenkaarne and Blell 2022).

- The Register on Induced Abortions and Sterilizations (formerly the Register of Induced Abortions, established in 1950, and the Register of Sterilizations, established in 1939), records sterilizations that, from 1935 until 1970, were performed for eugenic reasons, with the number of such sterilizations peaking in the period 1956–1963 (Bergenheim 2017; Mattila 2003). In addition, between 1950 and 1970, abortions were performed on eugenic grounds (Mattila 1999), and access to abortion during this period was conditional upon sterilization (Hemminki, Rasimus, and Forssas 1997).
- The Register on Infectious Diseases (encompassing what was formerly the Register of New Cases of Sexually Transmitted Diseases, established in 1958) records data on sexually transmitted infections, collected because eugenicists saw these conditions as a threat to the nation (Bergenheim 2018).

The registers served as a tool for evaluating the effectiveness of eugenic policies established in response to repropolitical anxieties; they remain entangled in such anxieties in multiple ways.

The Repropolitical Anxieties of Finnish Fertility

One key ongoing anxiety that feeds into the way in which Finnish population data are both used and generated is that of an inadequate fertility rate, with the "vitality of the nation" depicted as under threat (Homanen and Meskus 2023). For example, the Family Federation of Finland, founded in 1940, was a key pro-eugenics force in the era of (explicit) eugenics and continues to be influential in population and reproduction conversations in Finland; its data analyses continue to circulate, fueling repropolitical anxieties that drive policy decisions (Homanen and Meskus 2023). During the years of building the welfare state, except for the brief period after World War II, during the postwar baby boom, population concerns continued to focus on the fertility rate. In 1947, the overall fertility rate reached 3.5. After this, the rate started to decline again. In 1973, the fertility rate stood at 1.5. It then increased and remained almost unchanged until the first decade of the new millennium (Statistics Finland 2007). Finland was not alone in these demographic developments, as many European countries experienced a new phase of population decline, with birth rates turning downward between 1965 and 1975 (Brown 2019).

The fertility rate reached 1.87 in 2010; since then, it has declined, reaching an all-time historical low of 1.32 in 2022. Since the turn of the millennium, population concerns have centered on how to ensure what was considered beneficial population development, with a new source of population anxiety emerging alongside that of a very low birth rate: "greying Finland" (Miettinen et al. 1998: 88; Homanen and Meskus 2023). These continued anxieties have fueled haunted repetitions, most notably when in 2017 Prime Minister Antti Rinne suggested that women engage in a "birthing bee" (*synnytystalkoot*), a term that drew upon both traditions of help for neighbors and nationalist slogans of reproducing "for the nation" (Sudenkaarne and Blell 2022). While some who were outraged identified this as Nazi sloganeering, what seemed harder for commentators to recognize was that it drew from Family Federation of Finland's propaganda from the postwar period (Sudenkaarne and Blell 2022).

In recent years, migration has increased population growth (Statistics Finland 2007; Sudenkaarne and Blell 2022). But many in Finland view migration as a threat, not an asset (Blell and Homanen 2023). As in many places around the world, decreasing fertility rates are used by right-wing politicians to fuel xenophobic sentiments (e.g., De Zordo, Marre, and Smietana 2022; Mattalucci and De Zordo 2022). Data from the Medical Birth Register, which includes birthing parents' nationality information, is used by the right-wing populist Finns Party to represent relatively high immigrant fertility rates as a political threat to Finland (Blell and Homanen 2023). More generally, Finnish xenophobic anxieties about migration are vocal and draw on ideas about the quality of population that is seen as tarnished by "low-quality" migrants, most of whom are from racialized groups.

Finnish Homogeneity, Data, and Politics

It is often said that the Finnish population is and always has been especially homogeneous and isolated. Indeed, the political importance of this idea would be difficult to overstate. Much social science work has explored the powerful myth of historical and contemporary sociocultural, racial, and population homogeneity in Nordic countries, showing

how widespread the perception of the Nordic countries as exceptionally homogeneous is in administrative, public, as well as academic
discussions (Alghasi and Eriksen 2009; Keskinen et al. 2009). This
misunderstanding is ubiquitous despite the fact that diversity is documented in historical research on multiculturalism of the area (Kivisto
and Wahlbeck 2013). Normative understandings of homogeneity neglect
and silence histories of transnational migration and both recent and
long-standing communities minoritized by ethnicity within the Nordic
national regions, including the presence of Tatar and Roma populations
in Finland for hundreds of years.

Yet the idea of homogeneity has served as a selling point in the marketing of Finland's data (Sitra 2015). Finland has laid claim to genetic
homogeneity and traceability in its population history, which is thought
to help scientists generate enough statistical power to identify specific
disease-causing genes (Tarkkala and Tupasela 2018). Tupasela (2021)
traces this branding of the Finnish population in Finland back to the
1960s and 1970s, when rare-disease researchers studied the mechanisms
underpinning hereditary diseases overrepresented in Finland. Ultimately,
their explanation for this was translated into a national characteristic and
genetic origin story—an isolated and insulated, yet European, population
marketed for research (Tupasela 2021; see also Oikkonen 2018).

Yet, the political importance of concluding that Finland is homogeneous and isolated seems to distort even the conclusions drawn from
genetic evidence because the genetic data about Finnish people could be
used to describe the population in an entirely different way than homogeneous and isolated. Indeed, it has been widely publicized within Finland that people from eastern Finland and those from western Finland
are considered genetically so different that it is questionable whether
these two groups can be considered homogeneous at all (Lappalainen et
al. 2006; Palo et al. 2009). Moreover, on the basis of nuclear DNA, non-
Sámi, aka ethnic/white Finns, have been described as closer to other
"Europeans" than to the Finnish Sámi (Lahermo et al. 1996), indicating
a lack of homogeneity between two groups that have long lived in the
country, the indigenous Sámi and historically self-described white settlers, the white Finnish population.

As Tarkkala (2018: 72) has noted, "The crucial point is the sampling:
Who will be chosen to represent Finns in a study design?" Indeed, in

this process, only certain people are deemed to represent the population (Tupasela and Tamminen 2015). The sampling protocols for different projects include exclusion criteria, which exert a great influence over the resulting sample's homogeneity. Later rhetoric will deem this selective sample to be the same as the population and thus consider it proof of the population's homogeneity.

These processes of reinforcing the myth of homogeneity are crucial because mythic white homogeneity is linked to understandings of the basis for the welfare state's societal security and support, which, in turn, has been perceived as dependent on the experience of social cohesiveness and togetherness, legitimizing the welfare state and white homogeneity (Sudenkaarne and Blell 2022). It has been a powerful repropolitical tool to naturalize and legitimize exclusion and discrimination in the Nordic welfare state, including through access to reproductive technologies (Blell and Homanen 2023; Sudenkaarne and Blell 2022). At the same time, the myth of white homogeneity also acts to conceal ongoing and past violence and dispossession of indigenous peoples of the European Arctic like the Sámi and Kven, including colonial appropriation of land and assimilation policies toward the indigenous groups who were represented as threats to the modern state (Keskinen 2019). This Nordic settler-colonial history has also involved forced sterilization of indigenous people and adoption of Sámi children.

The way the myth of homogeneity continues to reassert itself and silence other histories, even Finland's more widely acknowledged historical ethno-class struggle involving ethnic Finns and Karelians (in the east) and Swedish-speaking Finns (who live more in the west), has a haunted quality. This "tangled exchange of noisy silences and seething absences" (Gordon 2008: 200) is a characteristic of haunting. Specifically, the data's haunted inheritance of Finnish repropolitics reflects these silenced histories, which are loud to anyone willing to listen.

Reproductive Injustice in Finland Today

In the Nordic welfare system with "universal" welfare services, such as free healthcare and other social benefits like parental leave, the state still has an apparent desire to identify specifically what it deems to be its own welfare subjects to ensure that obligations and rights are correctly assigned. In addition to this administrative function on the individual level, the register data have for many decades been an integral part of health and social care, governance, research, and policymaking (e.g., Finland's famed pronatalist policies) in the Nordic welfare states (Desrosières 1998).

The population register, specifically, contains basic information about all Finnish citizens and foreign nationals residing permanently or temporarily in Finland and is thus used practically everywhere in public administration and widely in private businesses. Each individual resident is issued a personal identity code that links their data across all registers (Alastalo and Helén 2022); this allows for the systematic surveillance of the public health of the entire resident population over time and in real time, without a separate census.

Moreover, by law, the register data are to be considered publicly reliable, so the public authorities make decisions about an individual's eligibility for social rights, services, and benefits, including access to reproductive healthcare, on the basis of register entries (Alastalo and Homanen 2018). This constitutes a form of "everyday bordering" within national borders that is pervasive in life in Finland (Tervonen, Pellander, and Yuval-Davis 2018), with important implications for reproductive justice. Those who cannot access public reproductive care (including abortion and assisted reproductive technologies), free and low-cost childcare for those on lower incomes, or Finland's widely celebrated free, high-quality public education system, exist outside the "universality" of the welfare state's pronatalism. Family-relation entries in the population register are as important to migrants as permanent-residency entries, because they determine social rights linked to family life, such as child home care allowances and maternity grants (known also as "the baby box").

Thus, any homogeneity Finnish data may show is partially an accomplishment of the policing of access to the Finnish welfare state at borders, via the rejection of documents that would aid in family reunification or registration of family relationships, and the state's denial of access to the welfare state and its institutions for migrant families. Furthermore, everyday bordering occurs in reproductive healthcare, and in yet more subtle forms of racial, ableist, and class steering in clinical contexts (Sudenkaarne and Blell 2022). However, the data are not used as a means to evaluate what unjust exclusions are being wrought by Finland's systems.

In a haunting irony, the family relationships missing from the register due to the rejection of "unreliable" foreign documents, often from Arab countries from which many migrants in the asylum system hail, are suddenly made visible and reorganized in the official statistics, created according to the nuclear family model, from inferred marital-status information and coresidence (Homanen and Alastalo 2025). These "reassembled" families are not officially recognized by the Finnish administrative authorities, although they are visible to the state through statistical practices of inference. The practice of inference does not mean that the families visible in the state statistics are de facto families, because the system does not recognize, for example, the extended families that are important in Arab cultures (Homanen and Alastalo 2018, 2025). Through this contingent and arbitrary, but strategic, data politics, a haunted repropolitics that aims to know all, to control repropolitical threats, and to care for some more than others, is perpetuated.

Conclusion

In this chapter, we have explored this volume's key question of how perceptions of fertility influence and determine fertility change by closely examining Finnish population databases. We fixed our attention on Finland's famed data "goldmine," showing that, far from being ethical, it is a record of the eugenic "racial hygiene" policy of the early years of nation building and ongoing exclusion of many migrants in order to refuse them family life in the safety net of the Nordic welfare system. By following the data, we have shown how several factors crucial to the making of these registers are obscured and hidden for political reasons. In contrast to the narrative of data goldmine, we revealed Finnish population data to be haunted by the missing drivers of demographic change they obscure, particularly the work done to maintain myths of white homogeneity and the innocent, ethical Finnish society. We have shown that even the seemingly unrelated politics of data and datacentric technologies may indeed be reproductive politics, supporting Briggs's (2018) argument.

Linked to the theme of this volume, we have shown that reproductive politics constitute both cause and effect of the data economy in Finland. Relatedly, we showed that the stories surrounding the data goldmine, what it conveys, why it is valuable and desirable, and how it will secure positive futures contain confusing tensions and contradictions. The repetitive reverberation of violence across time is part of haunting, a repetition that leads to confusion when the official story does not acknowledge that violence. Through this analysis we revealed issues blocked from view, such as the violence that repropolitical anxieties have wrought and continue to wreak, including in cases where the state's "oppressive nature is continuously denied" (Gordon 2008: 181), such as immigration policies and practices that disrupt the reproductive lives of migrants. This is the only way to facilitate change and end the cycle of violence.

REFERENCES

Alastalo, Marja. 2009. "Viranomaistiedosta Tilastoksi: Rekisteriperustaisen Tilasto-järjestelmän Muodostaminen Suomessa" [From Administrative Knowledge to Statistics: The Formation of a Register-Based Statistics System in Finland]. *Sosiologia* 46(3): 173–89.

Alastalo, Marja, and Ilpo Helén. 2022. "A Code for Care and Control: The PIN as an Operator of Interoperability in the Nordic Welfare State." *History of the Human Sciences* 35(1): 242–65.

Alastalo, Marja, and Riikka Homanen. 2015. "Hyvinvointivaltion Rajankäyntiä Maistraatissa: Maahanmuuttajien Rekisteröintikäytännöt Erilaisten Statusten ja Tiedon Lähteenä" [Enacting Borders for the Welfare State at the Register Offices: Migrant Registration Practices as a Source of Status and Knowledge]. *Yhteiskuntapolitiikka* 2: 147–59.

———. 2018. "Yksilöfaktaa ja Väestötietoa: Väestökirjanpito Ulkomaalaisten Hallinnan ja Tietämisen Teknologiana" [Facts about Individuals and Knowledge about Populations: Population Bookkeeping as a Technology of Governance and Knowledge Production]. *Sosiologia* 55(2): 147–66.

Alghasi, Sharam, and Thomas Hylland Eriksen. 2009. *Paradoxes of Cultural Recognition: Perspectives from Northern Europe*. London: Routledge.

Bauer, Susanne. 2014. "From Administrative Infrastructure to Biomedical Resource: Danish Population Registries, the 'Scandinavian Laboratory,' and the 'Epidemiologist's Dream.'" *Science in Context* 27(2): 187–213.

Bergenheim, Sophy Maria Cecilia. 2017. "'The Population Question Is, in Short, a Question of Our People's Survival': Reframing Population Policy in 1940s Finland." In *Reformer Og Ressourcer = Reforms and Resources: Rapporter Til Det 29. Nordiske*

Historikermøde, Vol. 2, eds. Martin Dackling, Poul Duedahl, and Bo Poulsen, 109–42. Aalborg: Aalborg University Press.

———. 2018. "Cherishing the Health of the People: Finnish Non-Governmental Expert Organisations as Constructors of Public Health and the 'People.'" In *Conceptualising Public Health: Historical and Contemporary Struggles over Key Concepts,* eds. Johannes Kananen, Sophy Bergenheim, and Merle Wessel, 101–18. London: Routledge.

Bergenheim, Sophy Maria Cecilia, and My Klockar Linder. 2020. "Pursuing Pronatalism: Non-Governmental Organisations and Population and Family Policy in Sweden and Finland, 1940s–1950s." *History of the Family* 25(4): 671–703.

Blell, Mwenza, and Riikka Homanen. 2023. "Reproductive Justice and Assisted Reproduction in Finland: Capitalism and the Myth of Homogeneity in a Nordic Welfare State." *Travail Genre et Sociétés* 4: 79–95.

Briggs, Laura. 2018. *How All Politics Became Reproductive Politics: From Welfare Reform to Foreclosure to Trump.* Oakland: University of California Press.

Brown, Jenny. 2019. *Birth Strike: The Hidden Fight over Women's Work.* Oakland, CA: PM Press.

Desrosières, Alain. 1998. *The Politics of Large Numbers: A History of Statistical Reasoning.* Trans. Camille Naish. Cambridge, MA: Harvard University Press.

De Zordo, Silvia, Diana Marre, and Marcin Smietana. 2022. "Demographic Anxieties in the Age of Fertility Decline." *Medical Anthropology* 41(6–7): 591–99.

Gordon, Avery F. 2008. *Ghostly Matters: Haunting and the Sociological Imagination,* 2nd ed. Minneapolis: University of Minnesota Press.

———. 2011. "Some Thoughts on Haunting and Futurity." *Borderlands* 10(2): 1–21.

Hemminki, Elina, Anja Rasimus, and Erja Forssas. 1997. "Sterilization in Finland: From Eugenics to Contraception." *Social Science & Medicine* 45(12): 1875–84.

Hepp, Andreas, Juliane Jarke, and Leif Kramp. 2022. "New Perspectives in Critical Data Studies: The Ambivalences of Data Power—an Introduction." In *New Perspectives in Critical Data Studies: The Ambivalences of Data Power,* eds. Andreas Hepp, Juliane Jarke, and Leif Kramp. London: Palgrave Macmillan.

Homanen, Riikka, and Marja Alastalo. 2018. "Perhesuhteet Ulkomaalaisten Rekisteröinnissä ja Tilastoinnissa" [Family Relations in Migrant Registration and Population Statistics]. In *Maahanmuutto, palvelut ja hyvinvointi. Kohtaamisissa kehittyviä käytäntöjä,* eds. Johanna Hiitola, Merja Anis, and Kati Turtiainen, 76–97. Tampere, Finland: Vastapaino.

———. 2025. "Making and Unmaking Migrants' Family Relations in Finland: A Study of Nordic Welfare State Population Registration and Statistics Production." *Nordic Journal of Migration Research* 15 (1).

Homanen, Riikka, and Mianna Meskus. 2023. "Population Anxieties in Constituting Nordic Welfare State Futures: Affective Biopolitics in the Age of Environmental Crises." *BioSocieties.* Online First.

Jutikkala, Eino. 1997. "Väestöpolitiikan ja Väestöprognoosien Historiaa" [The History of Population Policy and Prognosis]. In *Väheneekö Väki—Paranevatko Pidot?*

Väestöntutkimuslaitos 50 Vuotta, eds. Paula Alkio, Mika Takoja, and Ismo Söderling, 31–41. Helsinki: Väestöntutkimuslaitos.

Keskinen, Suvi. 2019. "Intra-Nordic Differences, Colonial/Racial Histories, and National Narratives: Rewriting Finnish History." *Scandinavian Studies* 91(1–2): 163–81.

Keskinen, Suvi, Salla Tuori, Sari Irni, and Diana Mulinari, eds. 2009. *Complying with Colonialism: Gender, Race, and Ethnicity in the Nordic Region*. Farnham, UK: Ashgate.

Kivisto, Peter, and Östen Wahlbeck, eds. 2013. *Debating Multiculturalism in the Nordic Welfare States*. Basingstoke, UK: Palgrave Macmillan.

Kongsholm, Nana Cecilie Halmsted, Søren Tvorup Christensen, Janne Rothmar Hermann, Lars Allan Larsen, Timo Minssen, Lotte Bang Pedersen, Neethu Rajam, Niels Tommerup, Aaro Tupasela, and Jens Schovsbo. 2018. "Challenges for the Sustainability of University-Run Biobanks." *Biopreservation and Biobanking* 16(4): 312–21.

Lahermo, P., A. Sajantila, P. Sistonen, M. Lukka, P. Aula, L. Peltonen, and M. L. Savontau. 1996. "The Genetic Relationship between the Finns and the Finnish Saami (Lapps): Analysis of Nuclear DNA and mtDNA." *American Journal of Human Genetics* 58(6): 1309–22.

Lappalainen, Tuuli, Satu Koivumäki, Elina Salmela, Kirsi Huoponen, Pertti Sistonen, Marja-Liisa Savontaus, and Päivi Lahermo. 2006. "Regional Differences among the Finns: A Y-chromosomal Perspective." *Gene* 376(2): 207–15.

Mattalucci, Claudia, and Silvia De Zordo 2022. "Demographic Anxiety and Abortion: Italian Pro-Life Volunteers' and Gynecologists' Perspectives." *Medical Anthropology* 41(6–7): 674–88.

Mattila, Markku. 1999. "Kansamme Parhaaksi: Rotuhygienia Suomessa Vuoden 1935 Sterilointilakiin Asti" [For the Best of Our Nation: Racial Hygiene in Finland until the 1935 Sterilization Law]. PhD Thesis, Helsinki University.

———. 2003. "Rotuhygienia Ja Kansalaisuus" [Racial Hygiene and Citizenship]. In *Kansalaisuus Ja Kansanterveys*, eds. Ilpo Helen and M. Jauho, 109–42. Helsinki: Gaudeamus.

Miettinen, Anneli, Ismo Söderling, Antti Ehrnrooth, Elli Heikkilä, Reino Hjerppe, Tuija Martelin, Mauri Nieminen, and Riikka Shemeikka. 1998. *Suomen Väestö 2031: Miten, Mistä ja Kuinka Paljon? Väestöpoliittinen Raportti Suomen Väestön Kehityksestä Vuoteen 2030* [Finnish Population 2031: How, Where from, and How Many? Population Political Report on the Development of the Finnish Population until the Year 2030]. Helsinki: Väestöliitto. www.eduskunta.fi.

Oikkonen, Venla. 2018. *Population Genetics and Belonging: A Cultural Analysis of Genetic Ancestry*. London: Palgrave Macmillan.

Palo, Jukka U., Ismo Ulmanen, Matti Lukka, Pekka Ellonen, and Antti Sajantila. 2009. "Genetic Markers and Population History: Finland Revisited." *European Journal of Human Genetics* 17(10): 1336–46.

Sitra. 2015. "Finland: Your Testbed for Next Generation Research & Innovation." Slideshare, December 3. www.slideshare.net.

Snell, Karoliina. 2019. "Health as the Moral Principle of Post-Genomic Society: Data-Driven Arguments against Privacy and Autonomy." *CQ: Cambridge Quarterly of Healthcare Ethics: The International Journal for Healthcare Ethics Committees* 28(2): 201–14.

Snell, Karoliina, and Heta Tarkkala 2019. "Questioning the Rhetoric of a 'Willing Population' in Finnish Biobanking." *Life Sciences, Society, and Policy* 15(4): 1–11.

Snell, Karoliina, Heta Tarkkala, and Aaro Tupasela. 2023. "A Solidarity Paradox: Welfare State Data in Global Health Data Economy." *Health: An Interdisciplinary Journal for the Social Study of Health* 27(5): 664–80.

Statistics Finland. 2007. "Population Development in Independent Finland: Greying Baby Boomers." Helsinki. December 5. www.stat.fi.

———. 2023. "Preliminary Population Statistics 2022." Helsinki. www.stat.fi.

Sudenkaarne, Tiia, and Mwenza Blell. 2022. "Reproductive Justice for the Haunted Nordic Welfare State: Race, Racism, and Queer Bioethics in Finland." *Bioethics* 36(3): 328–35.

Tarkkala, Heta. 2018. "Reorganizing Biomedical Research Biobanks as Conditions of Possibility for Personalized Medicine." PhD thesis. Helsinki: University of Helsinki.

Tarkkala, Heta, and Karoliina Snell. 2022. "'The Window of Opportunity Is Closing': Advocating Urgency and Unity." *Humanities and Social Sciences Communications* 9(1): 1–9.

Tarkkala, Heta, and Aaro Tupasela. 2018. "Shortcut to Success? Negotiating Genetic Uniqueness in Global Biomedicine." *Social Studies of Science* 48(5): 740–61.

Tervonen, Miika, Saara Pellander, and Nira Yuval-Davis. 2018. "Everyday Bordering in the Nordic Countries." *Nordic Journal of Migration Research* 8(3): 139–42.

Tupasela, Aaro. 2021. *Populations as Brands: Marketing National Resources for Global Data Markets.* London: Palgrave Macmillan.

Tupasela, Aaro, Karoliina Snell, and Heta Tarkkala. 2020. "The Nordic Data Imaginary." *Big Data & Society* 7(1): 1-13.

Tupasela, Aaro, and Sakari Tamminen. 2015. "Authentic, Original, and Valuable: Stabilizing the Genetic Identity in Non/human and Human Populations in Finland." *Studies in Ethnicity and Nationalism* 15(3): 411–31.

UNCTAD. 2021. "Digital Economy Report 2021." Development. New York. September 29. https://unctad.org.

PART IV

In-Fertile Environments

The chapters in this final section provocatively document the extent to which in-fertilities have increasingly come to represent a shared multi-species condition, linking plants, animals, and human beings amid rising concerns about the environment, climate change, and the deteriorating health of the planet. The direct links between in-fertility and a host of environmental concerns—including soil erosion, mining extraction, pesticide overuse, water toxicity, air pollution, rising sea levels, overfishing, species extinction, earthquakes, and other natural disasters—represent alarming demonstrations, both literal and symbolic, of an altered chain of reproductive cause and effect. Yet, the existential questions surrounding these rapidly emerging in-fertile environments have given rise to new forms of activism, protest, and environmental stewardship.

Concerns about environmental degradation in the new world order are evident in many countries around the world, including in Peru, where "reproductive extractivism" vis-à-vis an unregulated mining industry has sapped the reproductive vitality of various living communities. However, peasant protestors are actively fighting back, invoking provocative "reproductive grammars" that question the deaths of their animals and the pollution of their rivers in a standoff with the mining industry (chapter 15). In Japan, a tectonic nation of frequent earthquakes, courageous women managed to give birth during the devastating March 2011 Fukushima earthquake and the nuclear accident that followed. However, they experienced feelings of "moral vulnerability" about the "maternal environment," in which children are brought into an uncertain world where the border between natural and human-made disasters is increasingly blurred (chapter 16). In the hills of southern India, the parallel worlds of plants, animals, insects, and emerging human diseases intersect in the story of a family's colonial-era coffee plantation, one in which monocropping with pesticides has led to "landscapes of infertility" and family conflict (chapter 17). In contrast, in parts of the

United Kingdom, growing concerns about loss of agricultural land, reduced biodiversity of plant species, and food insecurity in urban and rural communities have led to vibrant activist movements. In London, individuals who save and trade heritage seeds are attempting to generate "heterotopian ecologies," whereby increased biodiversity among plant species can lead to better conditions of food production in small urban garden spaces (chapter 18). Similarly, in England, a countrywide movement to restore old orchards is generating "fruitility activism" on the part of local communities, as they reimagine "veteran" disused apple trees as the source of fruitility value (chapter 19). All of the chapters in this section demonstrate important new interdisciplinary connections between reproductive studies and environmental anthropology and sociology. They also provide powerful lessons about the ways in which in-fertility awareness is being mobilized to restore the planet's threatened ecosystems and to create a truly *multispecies reproductive justice framework* in the Anthropocene.

15

Reproductive Extractivism

*Mining and the Reproductive Grammar
of Multispecies Destruction in Peru*

JULIETA CHAPARRO-BUITRAGO

On a three-hour journey from Cajamarca city to Bambamarca in the Hualgayoq province of northern Peru, our route meanders along a serpentine road, navigating alternating paved and unpaved sections. I am traveling with a group from DEMUS–Women's Rights Advocacy Group, a feminist nongovernmental organization based in Lima. They are visiting Bambamarca for a capacity-building workshop with Peasant women leaders.[1] As we leave the city behind, the horizon reveals mountains draped in various shades of green beneath a pristine blue sky. The roadside is adorned with small restaurants, a quaint gas station covered with a tin roof, and a picturesque ensemble of cows, alpacas, and sheep.

Approximately twenty minutes into the ride, a flat-capped hill interrupts the scenic view, marking our approach to the Yanacocha mine. The once-vibrant tapestry of green transforms into an arid mountain, the color palette shifting to the earthy tones of yellow, reddish, and gray. Our driver, Fredy, apprises us of our proximity to the mining site.

The dramatic change in the landscape produced by almost three decades of mining activities in Yanacocha leaves me perplexed and saddened. As we continue, the green tapestry slowly reappears, occasionally revealing the sight of cows, sheep, or alpacas. About forty minutes later, another imposing hill of a piercing gray color obstructs the view. It is the Cerro Corona mine, located forty kilometers north of the Yanacocha mine and just minutes away from the Hualgayoq district. As we traverse the steep streets of Hualgayoq and its outskirts, a new municipal stadium and a bullring stand by the side of the road. Fredy explains that the mining company constructed these facilities in recent years. Yet, despite such infrastructure improvements, the local people lack access to water. Instead, a tank truck dispatched by the company delivers potable water to Hualgayoq's residents.

The impact of extensive mining activities in Cajamarca becomes evident not only during the car ride but also in daily conversations with people in the region. Many lament the environmental damage wrought by the extractive industries, while others laud the efforts of the *rondas campesinas*, or Peasant patrols, in thwarting the Minas Conga project in 2012. Under the rallying cry, "*Agua si, oro no!*" (Water yes, gold no!), protestors vehemently opposed the construction of another pit for gold and copper extraction, slated to replace four lagoons supplying fresh water to neighboring communities (Li and Paredes Peñafiel 2019). The project would have required draining the lagoons to replace them with artificial reservoirs, but communities opposed it, illustrating how people in the region understand water not as a resource to be managed but as a flowing source of vitality (Li and Paredes Peñafiel 2019; Paredes Peñafiel and Li 2019).

Cajamarquinos were already familiar with the consequences of draining water bodies for mining activities; the construction of Yanacocha in 1992 necessitated draining its namesake lagoon, leading to subsequent complaints about water shortages, contamination, and a devastating fish die-off in Granja Porcon's fish farm (Franco 2016). In response to the proposed expansion through the Conga Project, protests erupted, and Peasant patrols organized marches, roadblocks, and *rondas* around the lagoons to prevent the construction of the mine (Boudewijn 2020: 189). Clashes with the armed forces left five people dead (Boudewijn 2020), immortalized as fallen heroes in the collective memory of the uprising.

People's concerns about environmental damage find expression through what I term a *reproductive grammar*—not the rules of a language but a reproductive vocabulary, the words people use to account for the factors that shape their reproductive experiences, expanding our understanding of what reproduction is and what can be studied through it (Franklin and McKinnon 2001; Gunnarsson Payne 2016). Peasants express their concerns about toxic exposure and its repercussions on childrearing, animal welfare, and land fertility, bringing together a constellation of minerals, living beings, soil, and humans. They voice concerns about feeding children and animals given the dwindling land productivity and the sickening effects of contaminated water. This reproductive grammar emerges against the backdrop of three decades of industrial mega-mining, threatening life's perpetuity in extractive zones. The heightened perception of life's fragility underscores the awareness that environmental damage jeopardizes the reproduction of all life forms, as evidence of what this book terms "new fertility vernaculars" (Franklin, chapter 19). These vernaculars, articulated around environmental tropes such as biodiversity loss, signify a planetary interconnected consciousness, a theme explored further in subsequent sections of this chapter.

My awareness of this reproductive grammar rose during research I conducted research on the aftermath of a state-mandated sterilization program in Peru. Survivors recount a sense of debility that left them unable to work, which constitutes in their life stories one of the main harms caused by reproductive violence (Chaparro-Buitrago 2022). The coexistence of these reproductive grammars lays the groundwork for understanding a new reproductive order, where fertility precarity is indexical of various forms of extraction of vital (re)productive cycles, spanning human reproduction, labor power, and the continuation of life amid environmental devastation.

In this chapter, I introduce the framework of *reproductive extractivism* to highlight two important aspects. First, what is extracted goes beyond "raw" materials like gold or copper, to include the reproductive vitality of diverse living communities, emphasizing the need to examine reproduction in a multispecies register. Second, extractivism is itself a reproductive process. Reproductive extractivism sheds light on the interdependence between human reproduction and that of other living communities. The coexistence of these two reproductive grammars highlights the salience of reproduction not only in the most explicit cases, like forced sterilization, but also when addressing environmental degradation (Dow 2016; Wahlberg 2018; Lamoreaux 2023) and the impact of extractive industries. Reproduction is not simply a biological process but an entry point to understanding larger socioeconomic processes, in this case, industrial mining. This chapter reflects on the centrality of reproduction in the laments of affected communities, asking critical questions about the intersections of reproduction and extractivism.

The opening vignette, while rooted in Cajamarca, transcends its geographical confines. Peru, South America's second-largest mining economy and one of the world's top twenty mining countries, is emblematic of global mining challenges. In 2019, seventeen of Peru's twenty-four departments had mining activities (GPAE 2019), indicating the ubiquity of mining across the country. My exploration of the concept of reproductive extractivism in Peru began in 2020, coinciding with the onset of the COVID-19 pandemic, which, unfortunately, hindered ethnographic fieldwork. I did not think it was appropriate to put an extra burden on Peasant families with my presence at a moment of global uncertainty. Additionally, the connectivity gap in Peru, a condition shared with other Latin American countries, also limited the possibilities of conducting interviews via Zoom or other online platforms. Unlike other forms of research that continued online during the COVID-19 pandemic, the lack of computers or smartphones and Internet connection, paired with unreliable energy supply in rural areas in the Andean region (Anaya, Montalvo, and Arispe 2021), made remote ethnography unlikely.

This chapter exemplifies Günel, Varma, and Watanabe's (2020) proposal of "patchwork ethnography," which uses "fragmentary yet rigorous data" to expand "what we consider acceptable material, tools, and objects of our analyses." I assembled a patchwork of data, including ethnographic vignettes, a phone interview with the former president of the women's Peasant patrol in Bambamarca, Facebook posts, and journalistic reports on extractive industries in Peru. These journalistic reports often include statements from Peasants whose communities were affected by mining activities in Cajamarca and other locations like Puno and Huancavelica, which also suffer the impacts of environmental destruction. Despite its fragmented nature, this material illustrates the concept of reproductive extractivism, offering a nuanced perspective on the intricate interplay among reproduction, environmental degradation, and the repercussions of extractive industries.

Mining in Peru

With a historical lineage dating back to colonial times, Peru has long embraced its association with mining practices. In contemporary times, it has branded itself as a *"pais minero,"* a mining country, underscoring its deep roots in mining and positioning itself as an alluring hub for mining investments. This narrative gained prominence following the economic liberalization in 1990, a period marked by foreign capital dominating the industry (Bury 2005; Boudewijn 2020; Li and Paredes Peñafiel 2019). The inauguration of the Yanacocha gold mine in 1993, during the first presidency of Alberto Fujimoru, marked the start of a new era of neoliberal extractivism. Yanacocha, the largest gold mine in the world at the time, and currently the fourth-largest worldwide, altered the economic landscape of Cajamarca. Previously dominated by agriculture and animal husbandry, the region saw mining ascend as its primary economic sector, steadily climbing from 3.6 percent in 1987 to 40 percent in 2005. Despite this transformation, rapid economic growth did not translate into widespread local prosperity, rendering Cajamarca one of the country's poorest departments, mirroring the trend observed in other resource-rich areas (Franco 2016).

The designation "*pais minero*" is not a mere moniker; mining is indeed a cornerstone of Peru's economy. It represents 9 percent of Peru's gross domestic product and 60 percent of national exports; globally, Peru is one of the top-ranked countries in the extraction of metals (GPAE 2019). In Peru's northern region, especially in the departments of Cajamarca and La Libertad, mining activities account for 25 percent of gold extraction (GPAE 2019). The central region is home to sixty-three mining units, the largest in Peru, while the southern region contains the fewest (GPAE 2019).

When Yanacocha was inaugurated three decades ago in Cajamarca, it promised "clean mining," allegedly possible through cutting-edge technologies (Cuevas Valenzuela and Vejar 2016; Li 2015; Li and Paredes Peñafiel 2019), distinguishing itself from the perceived "old" mining practices of the Central Andean region, often associated with La Oroya mine (Li 2015). Yanacocha pledged to employ, instead of a smelter, "chemical processes, powerful machinery, and sophisticated laboratories" (Li 2015: 19) to mitigate environmental impacts. Modern open-pit mines are often characterized as *mega mineria* to describe their large-scale operations and the "huge imprint of areas that overlapped with Peasant communities, pastures, and agricultural land" (Li 2015).

The reality has starkly contradicted the promise of "clean mining." Communities, animals, and land have endured persistent exposure to hazardous chemicals, including cyanide and mercury, resulting from metal spills and contamination of water sources. The most infamous accidents occurred in Choropampa, Cajamarca, in 2000, when a truck transporting liquid mercury, a residue of mining activities, derailed and spilled 151 kilograms on the main road. This environmental catastrophe mobilized Peasant social unrest. Despite the community's resistance, the spill inflicted severe harm on livestock and agriculture—two vital economic activities in the region—and on the bodies of Peasants, who report an array of symptoms, from headaches to skin rashes, bone pain, and joint aches (Li 2015).

Birthing Gold: Reproductive Metaphors in Mining Processes

Reproductive grammars extend beyond the concerns voiced by Peasant women impacted by extractive industries; they are engrained in the description of the process of extracting precious metals from the ground. This is evident in the language employed by mine engineers to describe heap leaching, a mining technique utilizing chemical reactions to absorb specific metals and separate them from the ore. T. J. Manning and D. W. Kappes's (2016) chapter in the handbook *Gold Ore Processing* offers a glimpse into this process, serving as a guide for professionals in the gold industry, including metallurgists, geologists, chemists, and mine engineers.

The mining process starts with the perforation of the earth. Then an explosive solution is introduced into the holes, which generates a significant amount of fragmented rock. In Yanacocha, the mineralization of the terrain, "characterized by extremely fine-grained disseminated gold" (Arehart 1996: 384), necessitates the removal of substantial rock to make extraction profitable. For example, approximately three tons of rock must be taken for every ton of gold. The "metal-bearing ore" is separated from "waste" rock and transported by large trucks capable of carrying up to 250 tons of soil to a lixiviation pad—a large, stepped pyramid structure atop a waterproof geomembrane—where the heap leaching process unfolds over an extended period of time. The process is described as follows: "In the simplistic sense, heap leaching involves [the] stacking of metal-bearing ore into a heap on an impermeable pad, irrigating the ore for an extended period of time (weeks, months, or years) with a chemical solution to dissolve the sought-after metals, and collecting the leachant (*pregnant solution*) as it percolates from the base of the heap" (Manning and Kappes 2016: 413, emphasis added).

Reproductive tropes are fundamental to the description of the entire process—"metal-bearing," "pregnant solution." The chemical solution, a mixture of cyanide and water, metaphorically becomes a life-giving substance that becomes "pregnant" as it drips down the pad. The cyanide dissolves the gold particles, washing them down to the heap's base, where the "offspring" are collected in a leaching pit. The pregnant solution is then pumped to a processing plant where, through methods like ADR or Merrill-Crowe, gold is separated from the cyanide solution by precipitation in an oxygen-deprived environment or filtered in tanks with activated coal. The remaining dilute cyanide solution and rock transform into a "barren solution," stripped from its vitality and commodity-making capacity.

As I describe the process, it is hard not to think of Emily Martin's (2001: xxiv) *Woman in the Body: A Cultural Analysis of Reproduction*, where she describes the "metaphors of production [that] inform medical descriptions of female bodies." Extractivism, inverting the order of the relationship between production and reproduction, uses reproductive metaphors to describe the process of production. According to Martin, the metaphors of production used for explaining human reproduction, seated in gendered descriptions of female and male reproduction, give shape to grammar hierarchies in which women's reproduction is often described as wasteful, pathological, and failed production. The reproductive metaphor to describe resource extraction is illuminated through the framework of reproductive extractivism. Extractivism is not simply about removing metals from underground; a million micro-gold particles are not valuable per se. For them to become a commodity that circulates in the capitalist economy, gold is birthed through a reproductive cycle that is invisibilized as the process is often thought of as exclusively productive and profit generating. The framework of reproductive extractivism, using Emily Martin's words (1991: 501), "wake[s] up sleeping metaphors" in the descriptions of the extractive process, revealing the centrality of reproduction to it.[2]

The process mirrors female reproductive cycles, from fertilization to pregnancy and infertility, repeating as long as the mine's productive cycle allows. The argument here aligns with social reproduction theory's refusal to take for granted "what seems to be like a visible, finished entity" (Bhattacharya 2017: 2). Asserting that extractivism is a reproductive process brings to light how nature has been commodified to "unearth" the reproductive processes at the core of extractivism. Just as the reproductive labor that is required to "produce and sustain the worker" (Bhattacharya 2017: 2) is invisibilized, the reproductive cycle of resource extraction has equally been buried into "non-existence" (Bhattacharya 2017: 2).

The production of gold requires not only the commodification of minerals but also the earth's capacity to bear them, emphasizing a multispecies approach. In essence, resource extraction is not merely about removing raw materials; it involves a reproductive process that contributes to the commodification of both human and nonhuman capacities.

The River Is Dead: Reproduction in a Multispecies Register

The birthing of gold has caused significant reproductive damage to the environment, with extractive industries wreaking havoc on rivers, soil, and living beings. The grievances and pleas of Peasants mark a threshold of livability, a point where different conditions make a place unsuitable for habitation. Once that threshold is crossed, the effects of this break manifest as wildlife die-offs and adverse health conditions in humans. In the context of severe environmental damage, reproduction emerges in its dual character, both as a longing for life making and as signaling the realities of death and sterility, not only as human qualities but as conditions shared with other living beings.

In Roberth Orihuela Quequezana's (2022) report, *Pasivos Ambientales: Los Residuos de la Minería que Nadie Quiere Asumir* (Environmental Liabilities: The Mining Waste That No One Wants to Take Responsibility For), Estanislao Muña, a villager of Villaqollo Quilca in the department of Puno, declares that the Ramis River is dead:

> This river has been seriously polluted for many years. This pollution affects all of us who live along the river. Weeks ago, the river was murky, murky, but recently, it has cleared up a little. The river is still polluted despite years of so many claims, strikes, and strikes. The biggest problem

is that our animals die. I have lost two cows that drank the river water. So, we do not know when we will continue to be contaminated because this river affects us a lot. Now, as we see in this river, there are no seagulls, ducklings, toads, or fish. It is absolutely a dead river. (Orihuela Quequezana 2022)

In Muña's account, the river is dead because of the disappearance of its living communities; therefore, the river as a living being refers not simply to an inherent characteristic but is determined in relation to biodiversity. The absence of seagulls, toads, and ducks, coupled with the death of his own animals after consuming the water from the river, is a testament to the river's demise. Flora Rivera from the community of Catuyo Grande depicts a similar scenario: "The animals drink the water, get diarrhea, and then die. Even if we give them medicine, they don't survive. My alpacas, my best cows, also died, even pregnant. There is no medicine to cure them. We are sad in the countryside" (Orihuela Quequezana 2022).

These two vignettes echo Katharine Dow's (2016: 5) assertion that "the endangerment and extinction of species are ultimately a reproductive failure, the inability to produce future generations." Peasants, witnessing the devastation of rivers, land, and animals due to mining activities, without access to compensation or remedies from state or private actors, share a collective sense of grief, constituting what anthropologist Meztli Rodríguez-Aguilera (2021: 2) calls "grieving geographies" as "spaces of complex collective loss due to interconnected forms of violence."

The life-making capacity of the river is stifled by mining activities as heavy metals and waste are dumped into it, or when environmental liabilities such as leaching heaps or tailings ponds overflow during the rainy season and the water that carries toxic residues merges with the river (Orihuela Quequezana 2022). Peru's National Water Agency measured the Rami River's water quality and found alarming levels of acidity, dissolved oxygen, and substances like aluminum, copper, iron, manganese, and even sulfates and nitrites, that exceed the maximum levels allowed for human health and animal consumption (Orihuela Quequezana 2022). These metals pose severe health risks to humans, including kidney problems, liver and brain damage, and heart failure, and to fish populations, particularly trout, a crucial component of the Puneños' natives' diet.

Communities linked closely to water bodies constitute what anthropologist Kimberly Theidon (2022: 74) calls a "circle of care," where water is the connector of all life forms that depend on it: "The river itself was part of a circle of care in an interdependent world, with that interdependence understood as a condition that made river lifeways possible. Now the land was poisoned, the river polluted, the fish depleted. Nostalgia is not a strong enough word to describe this" (Theidon 2022: 74).

Viewing extractivism through a reproductive lens brings this circle of life and care into sharp focus. In a multispecies register, reproductive concerns transcend the exclusive domain of human life. This perspective aligns with this book's central theme on the changing perceptions of in-fertility. The multispecies reproductive grammar signals concerns about the possibility of sustaining life on a planet ravaged by extractive industries. These industries will only expand as the energy transition continues to depend on metals such as cobalt and lithium to produce solar panels and rechargeable batteries for electric cars. Infertility, miscarriage, fetal malformation, and facets of reproductive failure are discussed in the context of both human and nonhuman life.

During a phone conversation with Tatiana, the former president of Bambamarca's women's Peasant patrol, she describes the increasing reproductive challenges among some women in her community who experience difficulties getting pregnant or persistent miscarriages, attributing them to extractive activities. Pablo Soncco, a nurse at the San Isidro Health Center in the Department of Puno, whose testimony is also part of Orihuela Quiquiezana's (2022) report, also refers to premature deaths and congenital malformations in children, some of whom "were born without nostrils, another without an eye, one without a mouth and two years ago a mermaid baby, with its lower limbs fused" (Orihuela Quequezana 2022).

Similar reproductive outcomes are observed in animals, leading to abortions, birth defects, and deaths that impact families' livelihoods. Peasant communities relying on dairy or animal products as sources of income face significant setbacks. Rosa Huamanlazo's case exemplifies this struggle. Living in a rural area in the Huancavelica department,

Rosa raises alpacas and llamas. Between 2020 and 2022, she lost about a dozen animals to illnesses attributed to contamination from the Corihuarmi mine. The creek, Shutoc, where their animals drink, originates near Corihuarmi mine and has suffered from acid water spills containing zinc, arsenic, and cadmium, all known carcinogens (Mitma 2022) and responsible for other health conditions, including skin lesions, diabetes, asthma-like allergies, and heart problems. Alpacas are a source of wool, an important raw material for export, which families like the Huamanlazos sell to countries such as Italy, China, and Korea, constituting about 70 to 80 percent of the family income (Mitma 2022). Considering these numbers, the death of an alpaca is a significant loss for the family (Mitma 2022). Environmental degradation has not only resulted in economic losses but also forced Peasant families to seek work elsewhere to compensate for financial setbacks.

Reproductive extractivism compounds the detrimental effects on agricultural practices in the Andean world. Farmlands are contaminated, leading to a decline in potato production. In the San Isidro community in the Puno Department, where *chuño*—or dehydrated potato—is a staple food, lower agricultural yields heightened the risk of food insecurity (Orihuela Quequezana 2022). *Chuño* is an important part of the diet in the highlands of the Andean region and relies on water for its preparation. Moraya, or white *chuño*, must be soaked in running water for long periods of time and then "freeze-dried to assure long-term storability and consequent availability of food during scarcity. . . . *Chuño* can be stored for up to ten years and is generally prepared as a food by just boiling the freeze-dried tubers" (De Haan et al. 2010: 217). As a result of environmental contamination, not only has potato production declined, but the water needed for *chuño* has become unavailable. Contamination hampers the *chuño* production process, forcing community members to seek alternative water holes where only small batches can be processed (Orihuela Quequezana 2022). The ramifications extend beyond economic losses to a rupture in kin relations, as potatoes in the Andean region "do not feature as food to be passively ingested [but] rather as kin imbued with intentionality and affectivity" (Potato Poetry 2021). In other words, kin relations are also being severed by reproductive extractivism.

Conclusion

Reproductive extractivism emerges as a pivotal framework for comprehending the intricate interplay between human reproduction and the broader socioeconomic dynamics catalyzed by the advent of "modern mining" within a neoliberalized economy. This framework not only serves as a comprehensive analytic model but also functions as a compelling ethnographic guide and lens for everyday perception. The reproductive grammar of Peasants becomes a potent indicator of shifting perceptions of infertility, intricately linked to environmental degradation and extractive economies.

Considering the theoretical foundations laid out in this book, reproductive extractivism wields substantial political power and analytical capacity to dissect interconnected reproductivities across human, animal, and plant dimensions. Extractivism, as a cornerstone of the capitalist economy, exerts profound influences on human, animal, and land reproduction, fundamentally altering life's organizational structure (Gilberthorpe and Rajak 2017; Valladares and Boelens 2017). This impact jeopardizes one of life's fundamental imperatives—reproduction (Murphy 2017).

While literature on environmental justice recognizes the interdependence of humans, animals, and ecologies (Ford 2020; Hoover 2018; Sturgeon 2010; Di Chiro 2010), this synergy is not yet mirrored in the discourse on reproduction (Dow and Chaparro-Buitrago 2023). The framework of reproductive extractivism proposes a comprehensive exploration of human reproduction's reliance on other nonhuman communities, highlighting their co-constitutive reproductive capacity and vitality for the sustenance of life.

The Peruvian case is a poignant illustration of challenges faced by Indigenous and Peasant communities globally, echoing concerns about the interlinked impacts of extractive industries on landscapes, water health, animal life, and nearby communities. It delineates a shifting fertility consciousness that transcends individual decision making, encompassing a myriad of actors and their co-constitutive reproductive capacities vital for our world's survival. These reproductive grammars exemplify this evolving fertility consciousness, symbolizing novel connections among various reproductive beings (Franklin and McKinnon 2001).

Reproductive extractivism also illuminates the systemic nature of extraction, underscoring its disproportionate effects on Indigenous, Black, and Peasant communities. This reveals the racialized and classed distribution of vulnerabilities to chemical exposure, highlighting the racial and economic disparities in the impact of toxic environments (Hoover 2018; Lappé, Hein, and Landecker 2019; Goldstein 2020; Nelson 2013; Rodriguez-Aguilera 2021).

In the context of severe environmental damage and reproductive precarity, the reproductive extractivism framework proposes an exploration of how two principles of reproductive justice—the right to have children and the right to parent them in dignified conditions—extend beyond human relations. Well-being and care encompass animals and land, integral elements in the intricate web supporting life's reproduction. This framework underscores the importance of Peasant mobilization in fostering a different fertility consciousness, prioritizing water and life over gold.

Reproductive extractivism invites scholars to document life-making practices amid environmental degradation, recognizing Peasant mobilization as a crucial force in shaping a distinct fertility consciousness around environmental damage. To envision a livable world, both in reproductive terms and beyond extractivism, entails an awareness of a broader circle of life. In essence, reproductive extractivism lays bare that what is "extracted" transcends raw materials—it encompasses the strength and vitality of all its living communities.

Acknowledgments

I would like to extend my heartfelt gratitude to Wellcome Trust Grant 225597/Z/22/Z and to Sarah Franklin and Marcia C. Inhorn for their invaluable contributions to the Changing (In)Fertilities Project. Their dedicated efforts not only facilitated the collaboration of a remarkable group of reproductive-studies scholars but also played a pivotal role in orchestrating the compilation of this volume. This work stands as a significant and lasting contribution to our field, and I am deeply appreciative of their leadership and commitment. Additionally, I want to express my sincere thanks to the people in Cajamarca with whom I engaged in insightful conversations on extractivism. These discussions opened a new perspective that I introduce in this chapter.

306 | REPRODUCTIVE EXTRACTIVISM IN PERU

NOTES

1 In this chapter, "Peasant" is capitalized, following writing conventions that capitalize "Black" and "Indigenous" to identify a group of people who share a sense of community and belonging.

2 An intriguing parallel emerges when one examines these reproductive metaphors in Spanish content about heap leaching. The pregnant solution is labeled "rich," a transposition of a reproductive/gendered and class grammar.

REFERENCES

Anaya, Tania, Jorge Montalvo, and Claudia Arispe. 2021. "Escuelas Rurales en el Perú: Factores que Acentúan las Brechas Digitales en Tiempos de Pandemia (COVID-19) y Recomendaciones para Reducirlas" [Rural Schools in Peru: Factors That Accentuate the Digital Divide in Times of Pandemic (COVID-19) and Recommendations to Reduce Them]. *Educación* 30(58): 11–33.

Arehart, Greg B. 1996. "Characteristics and Origins of Sediment-Hosted Disseminated Gold Deposits: A Review." *Ore Geology Reviews* 11: 383–403.

Bhattacharya, Tithi. 2017. "Introduction: Mapping Social Reproduction Theory." In *Social Reproduction Theory: Remapping Class, Recentering Oppression*, ed. Tithi Bhattacharya, 1–20. London: Pluto Press.

Boudewijn, Inge. 2020. "Negotiating Belonging and Place: An Exploration of Mestiza Women's Everyday Resistance in Cajamarca, Peru." *Human Geography* 13(1): 40–48.

Bury, Jeffrey. 2005. "Mining Mountains: Neoliberalism, Land Tenure, Livelihoods, and the New Peruvian Mining Industry in Cajamarca." *Environment and Planning* 37: 221–39.

Chaparro-Buitrago, Julieta. 2022. "Debilitated Lifeworlds: Women's Narratives of Forced Sterilization and Delinking from Reproductive Rights." *Medical Anthropology Quarterly* 36(3): 295–311.

Cuevas Valenzuela, Hernán, and Dasten Julián Vejar. 2016. "Extractivismo y Teoria Social en America Latina. Una Entrevista a Eduardo Gudynas" [Extractivism and Social Theory in Latin America: An Interview with Eduardo Gudynas]. *Pléyade* 18: 269–88.

De Haan, Stef, Gabriela Burgos, Jesus Arcos, Raul Ccanto, Maria Scurrah, Elisa Salas, and Merideth Bonierbale. 2010. "Traditional Processing of Black and White Chuño in the Peruvian Andes: Regional Variants and Effect on the Mineral Content of Native Potato Cultivars." *Economic Botany* 64(3): 217–34.

Di Chiro, Giovanna. 2010. "Polluted Politics? Confronting Toxic Discourse, Sex Panic, and Eco-Normativity." In *Queer Ecologies: Sex, Nature, Politics, Desire*, eds. Catriona Mortimer-Sandilands and Bruce Erickson, 199–203. Bloomington: Indiana University Press.

Dow, Katharine. 2016. *Making a Good Life: An Ethnography of Nature, Ethics, and Reproduction*. Princeton, NJ: Princeton University Press.

Dow, Katharine, and Julieta Chaparro-Buitrago. 2023. "Toward Environmental Reproductive Justice." *Companion to the Anthropology of Reproductive Medicine and*

Technology, eds. Cecilia van Hollen and Nayantara Sheoran Appleton, 266–82, NJ: Wiley Blackwell.

Ford, Andrea. 2020. "Purity Is Not the Point: Chemical Toxicity, Childbearing, and Consumer Politics as Care." *Catalyst: Feminist Theory, Technoscience* 6(1): 1–25.

Franco, Pedro P. 2016. "Project Conga: An Unresolved Social License." In *Corporate Social Performance in the Age of Irresponsibility: Cross National Perspective*, ed. Agata Stachowicz-Stanusch, 209–36. Charlotte, NC: Information Age Publishing.

Franklin, Sarah, and Susan McKinnon. 2001. "Introduction." In *Relative Values: Reconfiguring Kinship Studies*, eds. Sarah Franklin and Susan McKinnon, 1–28. Durham, NC: Duke University Press.

Gilberthorpe, Emma, and Dinah Rajak. 2017. "The Anthropology of Extraction: Critical Perspectives on the Resource Curse." *Journal of Development Studies* 53(2): 186–204.

Goldstein, Ruth. 2020. "Mercury's Toxic Touch." *Anthropology News*, October 2.

GPAE. 2019. *Reporte de Analisis Economico Sector Minería* [Sectoral Economic Analysis Report, Mining Sector] 8(12). www.osinergmin.gob.pe.

Günel, Gökçe, Saiba Varma, and Chika Watanabe. 2020. "A Manifesto for Patchwork Ethnography." Society for Cultural Anthropology, June 9. https://culanth.org.

Gunnarsson Payne, Jenny. 2016. "Grammars of Kinship: Biological Motherhood and Assisted Reproduction in the Age of Epigenetics." *Signs: Journal of Women in Culture and Society* 41(3): 483–506.

Hoover, Elizabeth. 2018. "Environmental Reproductive Justice: Intersections in an American Indian Community Impacted by Environmental Contamination." *Environmental Sociology* 4(1): 8–21.

Lamoreaux, Janelle. 2023. *Infertile Environments: Epigenetic Toxicology and the Reproductive Health of Chinese Men*. Durham, NC: Duke University Press.

Lappé, Martine, Robbin Jeffries Hein, and Hannah Landecker. 2019. "Environmental Politics of Reproduction." *Annual Review of Anthropology* 48: 133–50.

Li, Fabiana. 2015. *Unearthing Conflict: Corporate Mining, Activism, and Expertise in Peru*. Durham, NC: Duke University Press.

Li, Fabiana, and Adriana Paila Paredes Peñafiel. 2019. "Stories of Resistance: Translating Nature, Indigeneity, and Place in Mining Activism." In *Indigenous Life Projects and Extractivism: Ethnographies from South America*, eds. Cecilie Ødegaard and Juan Javier Rivera Andía, 219–43. Cham, UK: Palgrave Macmillan.

Manning, T. J., and D. W. Kappes. 2016. "Heap Leaching of Gold and Silver Ores." In *Gold Ore Processing: Project Development and Operations*, ed. Mike Adams, 413–28. Amsterdam: Elsevier.

Martin, Emily. 2001. *The Woman in the Body: A Cultural Analysis of Reproduction*, 2nd ed. Boston: Beacon Press.

Mitma, Daniel. 2022. "Hay un Pueblo que se Extingue al Pie de una Mina de Oro" [There Is a Town That Is Becoming Extinguished at the Foot of a Gold Mine]. *Salud con Lupa*, July 21. https://saludconlupa.com.

Murphy, Michelle. 2017. *The Economization of Life*. Durham, NC: Duke University Press.

Nelson, Diane. 2013. "Yes to Life = No to Mining: Counting as Biotechnology in Life (Ltd) Guatemala." *S&F Online* 11(3).

Orihuela Quequezana, Roberth. 2022. "Pasivos Ambientales: Los Residuos de la Mineria que Nadie Quiere Asumir" [Environmental Liabilities: The Mining Waste No One Wants to Be Responsible For]. *La Republica, Connectas*, August 21. www.connectas.org.

Paredes Peñafiel, Adriana Paola, and Fabiana Li. 2019. "Nourishing Relations: Controversy over the Conga Project in Northern Peru." *Ethnos* 84(2): 301–22.

Potato Poetry. 2021. "Tuberous Respect after Progress: Praising Verses and Potato Flourishing in the Andean Highlands." After Progress. https://potatopoetry.org.

Rodriguez-Aguilera, Meztli. 2021. "Grieving Geographies, Mourning Waters: Life, Death, and Environmental Gendered Racialized Struggles in Mexico." *Feminist Anthropology* 3(1): 28–43.

Sturgeon, Noël. 2010. "Penguin Family Values: The Nature of Planetary Environmental Reproductive Justice." In *Queer Ecologies: Sex, Nature, Politics, Desire*, eds. Catriona Mortimer-Sandilands and Bruce Erickson, 102–33. Bloomington: Indiana University Press.

Theidon, Kimberly. 2022. *Legacies of War: Violence, Ecologies, and Kin*. Durham, NC: Duke University Press.

Valladares, Carolina, and Rutgerd Boelens. 2017. "Extractivism and the Rights of Nature: Governmentality, 'Convenient Communities,' and Epistemic Pacts in Ecuador." *Environmental Politics* 26(6): 1015–34.

Wahlberg, Ayo. 2018. "Exposed Biologies and the Banking of Reproductive Vitality in China." *Science, Technology, and Society* 23(2): 307–23.

16

Maternity amid Disaster

Childbearing and Moral Vulnerabilities in Tectonic Japan

TSIPY IVRY

Japan is a tectonic nation, intermittently shaken by the movement of the earth's crust. On New Year's Day, 2024, a 7.6-magnitude earthquake hit the western coastline of Japan, killing more than two hundred people and moving the coastline more than eight hundred feet in the north-central Noto Peninsula. This "New Year's Earthquake," as it has come to be called, nonetheless paled in comparison to the earthquake that hit Japan on March 11, 2011. Unprecedented in magnitude, it shook the eastern coast of Japan, followed by a tsunami that wiped out whole communities along the northeastern shore and caused an accident in the nuclear power plant at Fukushima.

Amid the images of destruction that flooded the local and international media, the new babies born on March 11, 2011—or "that day," "*sono hi*," as it is often referred to by the Japanese—were celebrated as beacons of hope and harbingers of the restoration of Tohoku, the northeastern region of Honshu, which had been suffering from dire population decline (even in Japanese terms) for decades preceding the earthquake. Indeed, Japan's shaky tectonics exacerbated a long-standing economic recession and a shrinking birth rate in the country as a whole, which eventually reached a record low of 1.26 in 2022 and persists today despite policies to improve childcare services, enlarge financial support for families, and subsidize assisted reproductive technologies (ARTs) for the purposes of family making (Ministry of Health, Labour, and Welfare 2022).

Disasters, as scholars argue, are "revealers" of societies' long-standing relations with their environment and technological infrastructures, and particularly of "who has been made most vulnerable" (Hoffman 2005: 19).

In post-disaster humanitarian-aid discourses around the globe, children have often emerged as potent signifiers of both survival and hope (Borland and Schencking 2020). Perhaps not surprisingly, then, in Japan, the media became abundantly interested in the reproductive experiences of mothers whose babies were born on March 11, 2011, particularly stories that occurred during the intense moments of the earthquake and the ensuing nuclear disaster that followed (e.g., Namikawa and Kobayashi 2012; NHK 2014). This chapter thus seeks to understand what disasters might tell us about the new reproductive order in societies such as Japan, which are prone to both environmental and human-made disasters. Specifically, what do Japanese women's stories of pregnancy, childbirth, and childcare during March 11 and its aftermath reveal about material and metaphorical relations with environmental-cum-technological infrastructures and their ensuing vulnerabilities? Such stories of maternity amid disaster have relevance well beyond Japan, given a twenty-first-century new reproductive order in which devastating earthquakes have occurred in the Indian Ocean, Haiti, China, Kashmir, Turkey, Syria, Morocco, and Afghanistan, affecting women and children in their wake.

In this chapter I take a close look at the childbirth accounts of the mothers of the celebrated babies born on that day of disaster in Japan, also touching on issues of pregnancy and childcare. I argue that the configurations of the mothers' maternal responsibilities under tectonic pressures (amid disorder) illuminate tensions woven deep into the matrix of maternal responsibilities underpinning the Japanese reproductive order. My focus is threefold. First, I examine the reproductive labor involved in prospective revivals: the intense, embodied-experience–cum–emotional-moral work involved in pregnancy, birth, and childcare. Second, I pay heed to the kinds of vulnerabilities that these childbirth stories reveal and the implicit relations of maternal embodiment with the environment at play. I draw on Butler, Gambetti, and Sabsay's (2016) reframing of vulnerability as the state of being affected rather than simply weak and on Cheryl Mattingly's (2014) "moral vulnerability," which is, she insists, much more than moral subjugation. These scholars use vulnerability to capture amalgamations of power and fragility: for Butler, Gambetti, and Sabsay (2016), vulnerability can become a resource for resistance, while Mattingly (2014: 120) shows how it is precisely a dedicated "super strong black mother" of a child with severe sickle cell anemia who faces "moral perils." With this amalgamation in mind, Oomachi's account of childbirth on March 11 haunted me.[1]

Oomachi's Birth Story

In the late afternoon of March 11, 2011, Oomachi, age thirty-two, was lying on a hospital bed experiencing labor contractions and waiting for epidural anesthesia to take effect when she felt the earth start to move. At first, her husband and sister, who had accompanied her, told her that the shaking was merely an aftershock of a quake they had experienced the previous day. Quakes always present interpretive challenges; not every movement of the earth becomes an actual earthquake. It might, in addition, be difficult to recognize at first whether one is experiencing an inner body sensation or there is a tectonic movement outside in the world. However, on March 11, 2011, the shaking intensified, and Oomachi felt an urge to disconnect herself from the IV and run outside. Oomachi's husband and sister rushed to cover her with their bodies to protect her and the unborn baby should the building collapse. After six long minutes, the shaking subsided somewhat, but the emergency sirens—the soundscape of earthquakes in Japan—lingered. Oomachi looked out of the hospital window. Snow was falling on the debris from a gray sky: "I was sure," she told me, "that the world had come to an end." "Please," she pleaded with the midwife, "I want to stop the birth."

Fast forward to the moment of the birth of a healthy baby boy, and Oomachi was tearful: "But these were not tears of gratitude to the baby for being born healthy [a sentiment often expressed by new mothers in Japan] but tears of grief and regret. . . . I couldn't stop apologizing to the baby. In my heart I told him, 'I am so sorry that I gave birth to you at such a time' . . . a time when one cannot see ahead."

This was not the first or last time that I encountered Japanese women apologizing to their unborn or newborn babies (Ivry, Ogawa, and Murotsuki 2023). However, this time, the sheer scope of responsibility that a human mother was taking for the earth's violence felt overwhelming. Could Oomachi possibly be blaming herself for the timing of her birth or for the massive environmental disruption into which her baby arrived? When I protested Oomachi's self-accusations, suggesting that she should, instead, be proud of herself for giving birth safely to a healthy baby against all odds, she insisted, "You must understand; I panicked, and I did not think about the baby."

Oomachi was relating to a particular maternal morality in Japan with its three commitments: first, securing a safe material environment in which to welcome a child; second, staying composed regardless of the circumstances; and third, maintaining awareness of the birthing baby throughout the birth. Yet, she articulated an extended version of this long-standing morality, which culminates in a moral panic around panic and the inversion of causality: the mother, not the earth, is responsible for the timing of the birth. Thus, the delivery of a healthy baby amid disaster becomes both an agentic moment of culpability and a statement of maternal power.

Living along the Tohoku coastline is risky. As scholars studying the political economy of disasters note, placing population centers close to the seashore in spite of a long history of recurrent earthquakes and tsunamis is a social decision that endangers these populations (Fortun and Frickel 2012). Likewise, building a nuclear power plant so close to the shore and on such shaky ground and leaving the residents of an already-vulnerable periphery to cope with radioactive leaks reveal a sociopolitical disposition toward relying on technological systems despite their unavoidable risks (Fortun and Frickel 2012; Hoffman 2005; Numazaki 2012). Such sociopolitical decisions and dispositions rendered Tohoku's residents physically vulnerable. Here, however, I focus on a different kind of vulnerability.

I listened attentively to Oomachi's accounts of her birth and postpartum experiences and to the stories of sixty other parents, parents-to-be, and maternity and obstetrics healthcare providers during and in the aftermath of March 11. My research was designed to explore the impact of the disaster on maternity care and experiences of pregnancy, birth, and childcare. Fieldwork stints took place in February and March of 2014 through 2017, as well as 2020. From this research, I suggest that *moral vulnerabilities*—namely, the predisposition to experience the failure to rise to the moral imperatives embedded in the matrix of maternal responsibilities—are key to understanding these individuals' feelings of a ruptured *maternal environment* amid a tectonic disaster. As discussed below, maternal-child connectedness, as both an embodied moral imperative and a causality system of child health and illness, were pushed to the forefront of public debates in Japan over the course of disaster recovery.

The Ecosystem Model of Maternity: The Reproductive Order before March 11

One way to make sense of Oomachi's apology to her newborn baby is to see her as a citizen of the Japanese "political ecology of procreative labor" (Ivry 2015: 285), and particularly as a "graduate" of Japanese prenatal care's authoritative conceptualization of pregnant women as "environments" in and of themselves, as the ecosystems of their in-utero "babies," and as fully fledged "mothers" (Ivry 2009). Medical care providers, women, and their supporters in Japan do not distinguish between fetuses and babies: they often use "*akachan*" (baby) to convey both. Henceforth, I use "baby" in the context of pregnancy to convey the emic term used by my informants.

The medical professionals I met during four fieldwork stints conducted during the 2000s made wide use of metaphors relating to the ecosystem to explain the physiological development of pregnancy and birth.[2] An OB/GYN physician I met in 2002 explained, "If you want to grow nice flowers, you need good soil . . . Pregnancy is the same thing. The earth is the womb. The womb is [in] the mother's body. . . . [Just as one has to] till the earth, water, and nourish it to grow nice flowers, so the mother's body has to be cultivated. . . . The mother has to create a proper environment for the baby" (Ivry 2009: 94–95).

OB/GYN physicians and pregnant women used the ecosystem metaphor to emphasize the impact of myriad aspects of the pregnant woman's health on fetal health and to reiterate the importance of pregnant women, including those in "normal," "low-risk" pregnancies, taking responsibility for monitoring and managing their daily lives according to detailed medical instructions.[3] Maternity healthcare providers were particularly authoritative in imparting dietary restrictions and monitoring weight gain:[4] "From one visit to the next the mother should check how much she has gained and correct her daily conduct. . . . It's not good to live an idle life," said an OB/GYN physician who, back in 2002, believed unequivocally that it is the woman's quality of self-care during pregnancy that determines whether the birth is *anzan* (a safe birth) or *nanzan* (a complicated birth). Women took these monitoring endeavors seriously even if they were critical of them, some meticulously noting everything they ate and some dreading the prospective weighing at each checkup.

But weight gain was only one element of the maternal environment that both the women and the doctors chose to monitor. *Kankyō* (physical environment) is a formal set of categories for monitoring the woman's pregnancy in her medical pregnancy record. Under the heading "Pregnant Woman's Occupation and Environment," the pregnant woman is required to answer a detailed survey mapping the physical conditions of her daily life (which, as discussed below, are also indexes of the woman's mental state): With whom does she live, in what type of accommodation? If she lives in an apartment building, on which floor, is it quiet or noisy, and does it have an elevator? Questions surrounding her work conditions are central to monitoring her environment: Does she work outside the home and how many hours? How does she commute, how long does it take, and is it during rush hour? Does she take breaks at work, and how long are they? The woman's responses are registered in the pregnancy record and were often discussed in the prenatal checkups that I observed. OB/GYN physicians often insisted that these aspects both influence women's well-being and affect the quality of the fetus's intrauterine environment. The way the mechanisms of influence work, however, was open to creative interpretations, as detailed below.

I found that women were expected to take responsibility for managing various aspects of their daily lives as mothers and not as "mothers-to-be" or "expectant mothers." Whereas the pregnant women with whom I spoke did not necessarily feel they had become mothers upon conception, the medical bureaucratic management of pregnancy stretches the formal definition of motherhood way back to the initial stages of pregnancy. For example, the medical monitoring card obtained from the local National Health Insurance Center on diagnosing pregnancy is called the "Mother and Child Health Handbook." Indeed, OB/GYN physicians were often concerned about the mental well-being of their patients, assuming that these women were already fully fledged mothers who were deeply bonded to their babies. They considered the pregnant woman's mental state in terms of the emotional environment (*shinkyō*) of the baby and thus expressed concern for the woman's own welfare and the emotional environment she provided for the baby. During the first stages of my fieldwork, I thought that practitioners were just joking when they recommended listening to good music and relaxing or when they cautioned that "the baby will not develop if you [and your husband] fight." But I came to realize that the efforts to enhance pregnant women's emotional well-being (or *anshin*, emotional safety), prevent distress, and relieve their worries shaped important aspects of medical care while, at the same time, introducing tensions.

Protecting women's *shinkyō* is the logic behind the way in which Japanese OB/GYN physicians provide medical information, particularly about reproductive technologies. Technologies to diagnose fetal anomalies in utero have been available in Japanese medical institutions since the 1960s (Ivry, Ogawa, and Murotsuki 2023; Tsuge 2015) but do not appear in the pregnancy record. Japanese physicians have been cautious about using them as explicit tools of fetal diagnosis (Ivry 2006, 2009; Ivry, Ogawa, and Murotsuki 2023). I found them particularly reluctant to discuss technologies that explicitly diagnose fetal anomalies, such as amniocentesis (Ivry 2006; Ivry, Ogawa, and Murotsuki 2023).[5] Doctors attributed this reluctance to the idea that pregnant mothers (who had presumably already bonded with their babies) would feel guilty for contemplating a diagnostic test that implies termination if the baby is diagnosed with an anomaly.

Working outside of the home was regarded as the archetypical stressor, and some professionals were openly critical. In 2007, a respected member of the Japan Society of Obstetrics and Gynecology (JSOG) told me that he used to persuade women to stay home and devote themselves to maintaining a proper physical and emotional environment for the sake of their baby's health: "You will only carry a baby for about two years out of eighty, so devote yourself to the baby; the other seventy-eight are your freedom" (Ivry 2009: 103).

These opinions reflected both the gendered division of paid labor in Japan in the decades before the earthquake and the declining birth rate that has been a focus of national concern since the 1960s. The M curve of women's employment during the 2000s, which shows a sharp decrease in paid labor during a woman's childbearing years, suggests that women tended to devote far more than two years of their lives to childcare.[6] Indeed, many of my interlocutors quit their jobs soon after learning that they were pregnant—or even soon after deciding they wanted to conceive—and only returned to the workforce many years later. Yet, regardless of whether women quit their jobs or continued working, tensions emerged in the navigation between their responsibilities for maximizing the physical health of the unborn baby and their commitment to providing an emotional environment that is as calm as possible.

The pregnant women explained what they saw as their own transgressions of medical or pseudo-medical prohibitions using the same theory of interconnectedness: "If I stay home all day I'll be anxious; I'm better going out to work" or "I actually think that if I don't drink coffee, my child will be more anxious because I will get more and more anxious, so I guess it's better to drink coffee and relax for the sake of my child." Even occasional smoking could be explained by drawing on maternal-fetal connectedness: "It's better for the baby that I smoke one cigarette and relax" (Ivry 2009: 167).

The maternal-fetal bond is a dominant cultural notion in Japan that lends itself to various uses. The use that most surprised me was made by birth educators who, as part of their instructions on breathing techniques and methods to avoid bodily tension, suggested that the woman think about the efforts that the *baby* is making to get born. In the notes that one of my informants took during a birthing class she wrote, "When it hurts, it is because the baby is descending. In my heart, I should say 'Baby, hold on, *gambare* (fight)' and help cheer it along." When I spoke to her after the birth, she said that the idea that she was not the only one making an effort "strengthened her heart."

The Moral Panic around Panic in the Aftermath of March 11

"Strengthening the heart" certainly became a challenge during and after March 11. Mothers said they sometimes managed to use their consciousness of maternal-fetal connectedness to transcend earthquake anxieties. Yamada, a woman in her late thirties reaching the end of her second pregnancy, was alone in a taxi on her way to the hospital when the earthquake started. She recalled that her head hit the taxi's ceiling several times but insisted, "I didn't panic at all." Yamada described talking to her baby throughout, telling him that all was okay and that she was protecting him. She explained that she was able to keep calm due to her certainty that her four-year-old daughter, parents, and husband were safe and far away from the coast.

But Suki, who was six months pregnant when the earthquake hit, told me she had been terrified. She was on a train platform with a friend and, as the shaking intensified, "we crawled under a bench and held hands." Throughout the earthquake she worried about how the baby was doing and prayed for its safety. Suki's daughter was born safely at term but was, she reported, exceptionally sensitive and difficult to calm down. Suki wondered whether her own anxiety during the earthquake had caused her daughter's nervous disposition and was still haunted by this causality theory when I met her three years later.

Anxieties and their manifestation emerged as a focus of intensive and recurrent reflection in the accounts of parents, parents-to-be, pregnant women, and those whom the earthquake caught in the middle of labor. The long-standing moral imperative of maternal-fetal connectedness was now to be maintained in the face of anxiety, whose expression became a moral issue in and of itself in the aftermath of March 11. In other words, the implicit tensions that lurked beneath the double commitment to secure both the physical and the emotional environment of fetuses and children became explicit and amplified. Anxiety management, namely, whether one expresses anxiety and how, emerged as an index of connectedness. Keeping anxiety at bay or claiming, like Yamada, not to feel anxious at all is associated with effective human connectedness (with the unborn baby and other family members). In contrast, the inability to stave off one's anxieties is associated with impaired connectedness. Oomachi, for example, did not think about the baby, while others, like Suki, might think about the baby and still feel anxious, remaining trapped in concerns about the damage their anxiety may have caused the baby. Indeed, notions of the harmful effects of parents' anxieties on fetal and children's health were explicit and prevalent at the time.

Attempts to eliminate expressions of anxiety from their interactions with their children were foremost in parents' consciousness both during and after the earthquake. Many explained that children, when uninterrupted by adult anxieties, can cope well with earthquakes and disasters and interpret them in surprisingly positive ways. Koike, for example, said that her four-year-old enjoyed the feeling of shaking and being at the evacuation center with other children. Other parents said their young children had slept through the earthquake and only started crying when they woke them up to flee the building. One mother of a two-year-old toddler and a nine-month-old baby had been nursing when the earthquake struck: "I remember when the earth started moving, I couldn't make up my mind whether or not to stop nursing the baby, wake my elder child, and run outside. I didn't want to upset them." She continued nursing.

The cessation of shaking was followed by a chain of catastrophes. A tsunami of unprecedented height, which swept inland as far as ten kilometers, took the lives of around 15,895 people, left 6,156 severely injured and 2,539 missing, and caused an accident at the Fukushima nuclear power plant. People living in proximity to the plant were ordered to evacuate—a radius that expanded from three to twenty kilometers within the first hours after the explosion and that was negotiated and contested for months after.[7]

On March 15, 2011, JSOG advised pregnant and nursing women to go far away from Fukushima "to avoid KI treatment and radiation" but to undergo potassium iodide (KI) treatment in cases of more than fifty thousand microSv exposure to reduce risk of thyroid cancers. Worsening radioactive fallout caused low-dose contamination of tap water in Tokyo (210 Beq/Kg),[8] and mothers were warned not to use it to feed their babies (Japan Society of Obstetrics and Gynecology 2011). Agricultural and sea products were soon deemed risky.

On April 1, 2011, with escalating public anxieties, the Japanese Ministry of Health, Labour, and Welfare issued a pamphlet entitled "We Respond to the Radiation Concerns of Pregnant Women and Mothers of Small Children." The pamphlet, which was distributed to three million pregnant women and mothers, asserted that, outside the restricted zones announced by the government, the food, water, and breast milk were all safe and within the government's provisional standards. It stated, "We beg you to refrain from excessive worry for the sake of your to-be-born baby and yourself and to continue monitoring your health as usual." The statement clearly builds on the assumption that pregnant women are already engaged in self-monitoring (of their nutrition and weight, etc.) and are required only to enlarge the scope of their monitoring to include the extra-somatic environment outside of their pregnant bodies. A more detailed pamphlet by the Ministry of Education addressed to both educators and parents and called "Understanding Radioactivity Correctly" stated that "parents' depression and anxieties lead to emotional instability in children. It is important that parents have accurate knowledge about radiation problems and do not worry too much. . . . Worry and stress damage the health of the mind and the body. . . . The mind and body are connected" (Ministry of Education, Culture, Sports, Science and Technology 2011: 35–37). How much worry is "too much" and what makes knowledge "accurate" remained unclear and often contestable for many parents and parents-to-be.

Such public government statements explicitly marked anxiety as a health risk factor and formulated a causal relation between parental, specifically maternal, anxieties and damage to their (born or unborn) children's health. Controlling anxieties about radioactivity, loss, and economic challenges, among other concerns, for the sake of one's dependents became a moral imperative.

Scientists and healthcare providers were pushed to the front line of the effort to eliminate anxieties through the provision of technology-based assessments of exposure to radioactivity and the production of accessible explanatory materials about radioactivity risks. The idea was that people could be taught to "fear correctly," the English translation of the title *Tadashiku Kowagaru*, a book by Shunichi Yamashita (2012), a renowned international expert on the health effects of radioactivity. Accordingly, understanding how to monitor the environment for radioactivity, how to interpret measurements and translate them into a risk assessment, and how to infer adequate behavior (e.g., whether to stay indoors or go outside) would reduce people's anxieties. Indeed, many healthcare professionals with whom I spoke who came from Sendai to provide support for the affected areas insisted, in a quasi-reversal of cause and effect, that anxiety rather than the low radioactivity risk was the "real" problem of the disaster-stricken areas.

Yamashita, the son of survivors of the Nagasaki atomic bomb, conducted longitudinal research on the health impact of the Chernobyl accident on child and adult health (e.g., Takamura and Yamashita 2012). Soon after the Fukushima accident, he embarked on a series of lectures in local community centers. He invoked findings from his research on Chernobyl and Nagasaki to persuade Fukushima residents that, if they heed his instructions, "there is no need to worry so much" and to reassure them about the process of restoration. However, Yamashita angered many of the residents of the affected areas, who accused him of irresponsibly minimizing the dangers posed to the local population on the basis of false premises. In a conversation with Yamashita, he intimated that, of those whose worries are difficult to assuage, "mothers are the worst."

Indeed, parents went a long way (often literally, by being evacuated to shelters or moving far from their homes) to ensure safe physical and mental environments for their children. However, the tension between the imperative to monitor the environment and to govern their anxieties heightened. Mothers, particularly those living in the districts around the power plant and beyond, became dedicated to monitoring radiation levels and soon demanded that the government provide clear information about radioactivity measurements (Morioka 2013; Slater, Morioka, and Danzuka 2014). The contents of school lunches, for example, became a conflict zone between mothers and local governments, and the Safe Lunch Box Movement was started by Katsuma Yoriko when the school dismissed her request not to use food ingredients from affected areas in its lunches. The information about the ingredients she received after repeated requests contained blacked-out columns, and further investigation revealed that the school served beef that was contaminated with a radioactive isotope of cesium, a hazardous chemical (Kimura 2016). Mothers (and grandmothers), in line with Butler, Gambetti, and Sabsay (2016), transformed their affectedness into resistance and led the protest in the name of maternal responsibility for their children's environments, demanding that the government take responsibility for ensuring their children's safety. In a paradoxical reversal, however, these mothers became the target of public pressure calling on them to refrain from spreading rumors and panic and were thus reprimanded for fulfilling the maternal responsibilities entrusted to them by long-standing national gender ideologies. Both the official appeals for mothers to control their anxieties and the mothers' protests against the government's failure to take responsibility for securing the environment draw on interpretations of the same matrix of maternal responsibility for children. Maternal-child connectedness was pushed to the center of debates over navigating ruptured environments.

The model of an all-powerful maternal ecosystem, its tension-ridden commitment to securing both the physical and emotional environments of unborn babies and children, and its intensification under tectonic pressures echoes Butler, Gambetti, and Sabsay's (2016) and Mattingly's (2014) use of vulnerability and moral vulnerability, respectively, to understand the merging of power and fragility. It might help explain why Oomachi referred to feeling responsible for her anxiety and the timing of her birth when recalling giving birth during the earthquake. Yet, the same matrix of commitments underlying her wish to stop the birth worked to bring Oomachi back into the birth process. She said that when she panicked and cried that she wanted to stop the birth, her husband and sister tried to calm her down, and the nurses assured her that the building was earthquake-proof. But it was only when the midwife invoked the baby's dependence on her that Oomachi managed to pull herself together: "Your baby is fighting to be born," said the midwife. "The baby is perfectly fine; he needs you in order to be born." Rather than serving as an accomplice in a national project to control anxiety, the midwife called on the mother's responsibility toward her baby to restore Oomachi's will to fight for both of their lives. Oomachi's apology to her newborn child—"I am so sorry that I gave birth to you at such a time"—was repentance for her temporary disconnection and a manifestation of the renewal of her full commitment to him once he was born. Guilt emerges as a constructive emotion in this context. Nonetheless, Oomachi had no more children.

Conclusion

Anthropological studies of reproductive labor during and after disasters are surprisingly scant.[9] Particularly for societies along the so-called Ring of Fire (such as Japan), disasters are recurrent events rather than departures from the norm. Yet, calamities, as disaster scholars explain, lurk beneath modernity itself (Fortun and Frickel 2012). Hypertechnological societies like Japan are prone to the catastrophes that develop in industrial societies at the intersection between their environments and their technological infrastructures. I suggest, on the basis of my findings, that explorations of reproductive experiences in the midst of disaster can benefit attempts to understand the new reproductive order with its environmental-cum-technological infrastructure and its accompanying vulnerabilities. Moreover, importantly, the stories included here give a sense of what is at stake for those involved in pregnancy, birth, and childcare when disaster strikes.

Feminist anthropologists have critiqued public depictions of reproduction as processes that can be governed through rational, "informed" choices and controlled through reproductive technologies. However, this chapter's stories transcend reproductive disruptions at the individual somatic level, drawing attention to mega environmental disruption.[10] They remind us of the unforeseeable environmental, sociopolitical, and economic chaos that those engaged in reproductive labor might encounter. While mothers and mothers-to-be exercise no choice or control over the eruption of chaos, they are in no way exempt from, nor do they exempt themselves from, responsibility for their children. On the contrary, their reproductive responsibilities may expand to the point of making them culpable in both the public eye and their own eyes. Becoming a mother makes women susceptible to guilt in constructive and disruptive ways.

The local formulation of reproductive responsibilities—namely, how women are expected to exercise their responsibilities, which aspects of their own health are understood to impact their children's health, at which point in the preconception-conception-gestation-childbirth-childcare timeline they are responsible,[11] which causal theories about health and illness underlie these expectations, and which notions of the environment are at play—emerge as key to understanding how a reproductive order is embodied and how "political ecologies of procreative labor" (Ivry 2015: 285) are constituted.

The March 11 disasters intensified the inner tensions and paradoxes underlying the matrix of maternal responsibilities, particularly the tensions between two kinds of environments. The stories of Oomachi, Yamada, Suki, and others who were engaged in reproductive labor in the midst of these disasters illuminate how far the implications of commitments to such a matrix of maternal responsibilities might reach. Although the stories here did not include maternal or child loss, they show how vulnerable—both physically and morally fragile and strong—women can become when governed by the notion of the all-powerful maternal environment and how taxing the matrix of maternal responsibilities can be. Why, we might ask, would a mother apologize for the earth's violence? Stories from Japan during the March 11 earthquake provide a poignant reminder of both reproductive and environmental vulnerabilities and their intimate connection. Amid the recent upsurge of media coverage of pregnant and childbearing women during "natural" and human-made disasters around the globe,[12] we might also ask to what extent, within the new world order, these images become articulations of existential and environmental precarity.

NOTES

1 Except for Oomachi's, all the names mentioned here are pseudonyms.

2 The research was designed as a comparative ethnography of pregnancy and prenatal care in Japan and Israel. Fieldwork included over one hundred formal interviews with pregnant women and OB/GYN physicians in Japan and Israel, as well as countless informal conversations and observations of clinical encounters in maternity checkups and birth-preparation courses in Japanese and Israeli institutions (Ivry 2009).

3 Ecosystem-oriented theories of children's health can be traced back to population policies that attempted to bind women's reproductive capacities to national reproductive goals soon after the forced opening of Japan to the West in 1854, the "gynocentric" eugenic policies of the first half of the twentieth century, and the valorization of women as mothers throughout Japan's modern history.

4 OB/GYN physicians explained that since the width of the pelvic bone is proportional to height, and since Japanese women tend to be relatively short, limiting the weight of the baby at birth is crucial to ensure a safe birth (Ivry 2009: 267).

5 Elsewhere I map the complex reproductive politics and disability-rights politics, as well as the history of state-sponsored eugenics, that underly their reluctance (Ivry 2009; Ivry, Ogawa, and Murotsuki 2023).

6 The rate of working mothers before the earthquake was 61.9 percent; since the 1970s, women's employment rates have followed an M-curve, indicating a dip in employment during childbearing years, while men's employment rates have remained largely unchanged (Japan Institute for Labour Policy and Training 2023).

7 For a conclusive review of the challenges in the aftermath of the Tohoku disaster, see Gill, Slater, and Steger (2015).

8 Sievert (Sv) is a unit used for measuring ionizing radiation in terms of the potential for causing harm to tissues and organs. Becquerel per Kg (Bq/Kg) is a unit for measuring radioactive substances in foodstuffs or water. "Ionizing Radiation and Health Effects: Key Facts," World Health Organization, July 27, 2023. https://www.who.int.

9 Exceptions include Petryna's (2003) account of mothers' radiation concerns in the aftermath of the Chernobyl disaster, Brunson's (2017) account of maternal, newborn, and child health after the 2015 Nepalese earthquake, and Wick and Hassan's (2012) account of childbirth in the midst of the Israeli attack on Gaza.

10 Indeed, accounts of childbirth during March 11 reveal that the earthquake often rendered obstetrical technologies unusable (Ivry, Takaki-Einy, and Murotsuki 2019).

11 Interestingly it is through the *ninkatsu* (active pursuit of pregnancy) discourse, which stretches reproductive responsibilities to cultivate a "suitable environment" for "babies" to develop back to women's early teens, that Japanese policymakers and reproductive health professionals have attempted to combat the birth crisis (see Gagné, chapter 2).

12 Examples from the February 2023 earthquake in Turkey include a baby being born ("A Newborn Delivered" 2023), a baby being reunited with its mother ("Baby Pulled" 2023), and thousands of pregnant women needing urgent help (Goodyear 2023). There was similar coverage from the war in Ukraine and the August 2023 earthquake in Morocco.

REFERENCES

"Baby Pulled from Turkey Earthquake Rubble Reunited with Mother." 2023. *CBS Evening News*, April 3. Video, 00:00:24, www.youtube.com.

Borland, Janet, and J. Charles Schencking. 2020. "Objects of Concern, Ambassadors of Gratitude: Children, Humanitarianism, and Transpacific Diplomacy Following Japan's 1923 Great Kantō Earthquake." *Journal of the History of Childhood and Youth* 13(2): 195–225.

Brunson, Jan. 2017. "Maternal, Newborn, and Child Health after the 2015 Nepal Earthquakes: An Investigation of the Long-Term Gendered Impacts of Disasters." *Maternal and Child Health Journal* 21: 2267–73.

Butler, Judith, Zeynep Gambetti, and Leticia Sabsay, eds. 2016. *Vulnerability in Resistance*. Durham, NC: Duke University Press.

Fortun, Kim, and Scott Frickel. 2012. "Making a Case for Disaster Science and Technology Studies." Post to online forum, *An STS Forum on Fukushima*. https://fukushimaforum.wordpress.com.

Gill, Tom, David H. Slater, and Brigitte Steger, eds. 2015. *Japan Copes with Calamity*. Oxford: Peter Lang.

Goodyear, Sheena. 2023 "Hundreds of Thousands of Pregnant Women Need Help in Earthquake-Torn Turkey, Syria." *CBC*, February 20. www.cbc.ca.

Hoffman, Susanna M. 2005. "Katrina and Rita: A Disaster Anthropologist's Thoughts." *Anthropology News* 46(8): 19.

Ivry, Tsipy. 2006. "At the Back Stage of Prenatal Care: Japanese Ob-Gyns Negotiating Prenatal Diagnosis." *Medical Anthropology Quarterly* 20(4): 441–68.

———. 2009. *Embodying Culture: Pregnancy in Japan and Israel*. New Brunswick, NJ: Rutgers University Press.

——. 2015. "The Pregnancy Manifesto: Notes on How to Extract Reproduction from the Petri Dish." *Medical Anthropology* 34(3): 274–89.

Ivry, Tsipy, Maki Ogawa, and Jun Murotsuki. 2023. "Virtuous Indecisiveness: Structural Moral Ambivalence and the Tentative Implementation of Non-Invasive Prenatal Testing in Japan." *Cultural Anthropology* 38(2): 171–97.

Ivry, Tsipy, Rika Takaki-Einy, and Jun Murotsuki. 2019. "What Disasters Can Reveal about Techno-Medical Birth: Japanese Women's Stories of Childbirth during the 11 March, 2011 Earthquake." *Health, Risk & Society* 21(3–4): 164–84.

Japan Institute for Labour Policy and Training. 2023. "Figure 3–2: Labour Force Participation Rate by Age Group." April 4. www.jil.go.jp. [In Japanese.]

Japan Society of Obstetrics and Gynecology. 2011. "Suidōsui ni Tsuite Shinpai Shiteorareru Ninshin: Junyūchū Josei he no Goannnai" [Guidance to Pregnant and Nursing Women Who Are Worried about Tap Water]. March 24. www.jsog.or.jp.

Kimura, Aya Hirata. 2016. *Radiation Brain Moms and Citizen Scientists: The Gender Politics of Food Contamination after Fukushima.* Durham, NC: Duke University Press.

Mattingly, Cheryl. 2014. "The Moral Perils of a Superstrong Black Mother." *Ethos* 42(1): 119–38.

Ministry of Education, Culture, Sports, Science, and Technology. 2011. *Hōshanō wo tadashiku rikai suru tameni* [Understanding Radioactivity Correctly]. www.mext.go.jp.

Ministry of Health, Labor, and Welfare. 2011. *Ninshin no Kata, Chiisana Okosan wo Motsu Okaasan no Hōshasen he no Goshinpai ni Okotaeshimasu* [We Respond to the Radiation Concerns of Pregnant Women and Mothers of Small Children]. www.mhlw.go.jp.

——. 2022 *Jinkō Dōtai Tōkeigeppō Nenkei (Gaisū) no Gaikyō* [Overview of Vital Statistics Monthly Report Annual Total (Approximate Number)]. www.mhlw.go.jp.

Morioka, Rika. 2013. "Mother Courage: Women as Activists between a Passive Populace and a Paralyzed Government." In *Japan Copes with Calamity: Ethnographies of the Earthquake, Tsunami, and Nuclear Disasters of March 2011*, eds. Tom Gill, Brigitte Steger, and David H. Slater, 177–200. Oxford: Peter Lang.

Namikawa, Shin, and Kiyohara Kobayashi. 2012. *Happy Birthday 3.11: Ano hi Shinsaichi de Umareta Kodomotachi to Kazoku no Monogatari* [Happy Birthday 3.11: The Stories of the Children Who Were Born on That Day and Their Families]. Tokyo: Asukashinsa.

"A Newborn Delivered in the Rubble of Turkey's Earthquake Is Adopted by Her Relatives." 2023. *NPR*, February 21. www.npr.org.

NHK. 2014. *Ano hi Umareta Inochi (110 nin ijō)* [The Lives Born on That Day (More Than 110)]. Documentary broadcast on NHK, March 11. www.dailymotion.com.

Numazaki, Ichiro. 2012. "Too Wide, Too Big, Too Complicated to Comprehend: A Personal Reflection on the Disaster That Started on March 11, 2011." *Asian Anthropology* 11(1): 27–38.

Petryna, Adriana. 2003. *Life Exposed: Biological Citizens after Chernobyl.* Princeton, NJ: Princeton University Press.

Slater, David H., Rika Morioka, and Haruka Danzuka. 2014. "Micro-Politics of Radiation: Young Mothers Looking for a Voice in Post-3.11 Fukushima." *Critical Asian Studies* 46(3): 485–508.

Takamura, Noboru, and Shunichi Yamashita. 2012. "Lessons from Chernobyl." *Fukushima Journal of Medical Science* 57(2): 81–85.

Tsuge, Azumi. 2015. "Considering the Social Background of Prenatal Tests in Japan." *Meiji Gakuin Sociology and Social Welfare Review* 145: 137–64.

Wick, Laura, and Sahar Hassan. 2012. "No Safe Place for Childbirth: Women and Midwives Bearing Witness, Gaza 2008–09." *Reproductive Health Matters* 20(40): 7–15.

Yamashita, Shunichi. 2012. *Tadashiku Kowagaru: Hoshanou no Hanashi 100 no Gimon.* [Fearing Correctly: Talking about Radioactivity, 100 Questions]. Nagasaki: Bunkensha.

17

Landscapes of Infertility

The Afterlives of Colonialism in Indian Plantation Economies

SHARMILA RUDRAPPA

In my book on reproductive medical markets in India, *Discounted Life: The Price of Global Surrogacy in India* (Rudrappa 2015), I describe how women's overdetermined and messy lives are converted into undifferentiated biomass bases of egg donors and surrogate mothers. The particularities of the lives, hopes, and desires of women, once they become potential surrogate mothers, do not matter as long as these women can successfully gestate and emotionally separate themselves from the infants extracted out of their bodies through cesarean surgeries. The women are not workers anymore; instead, much like the lands they lived on, they have been converted to substrate that creates social and surplus value, their fertility producing the infants that intended parents could not, or did not, want to germinate. They are an emergent labor market of clinical laborers (Waldby and Cooper 2014), who offer up their bodies to extract rent for themselves and their families, while repro-travelers (Inhorn and Patrizio 2015; Gerrits 2018; Whittaker, Inhorn, and Shenfield 2019), clinics, brokers, and banks accrue both social value and profits.

Much of the work on surrogacy, including mine, explains how working-class women's reproductive capacities are harnessed even as their lifeworlds are denied. The fetuses in the surrogate mothers' wombs become superordinate beings imbued with family resemblances, personalities, even family histories, and are imagined as fully formed children ensconced within middle-class families. Simultaneously, the surrogate mothers themselves are effaced; their desires for themselves, their children, and their families in working-class neighborhoods must necessarily be erased to make intended parents and their surrogated child an ideal dyad in a nuclear family (Rudrappa 2016).

As a slow ethnographer (Grandia 2015) of southern Karnataka around the megalopolis of Bangalore, I have observed that working-class women and agricultural land have a shared genealogy in the region's bioeconomic development. Women and land occupy specific locations in Indian techno-pastoral imaginaries as the nation-state recalibrates profits that can be harvested from the regenerative capacities of life itself, selling life as product to supplement the injuries of global infertilities (Rudrappa 2018).

Yet, despite these ethnographic explorations on reproductive markets embedded in southern Karnataka, where my extended family lives and where I come from, I have kept myself outside the grist of the mill of sociological speculation. In this chapter, I address this omission. Through an autoethnography, I locate myself in the techno-pastoral imaginaries of the Indian nation-state in its aspirations for orderly, hierarchical landscapes where the earth, plants, beasts, bugs, and viruses are managed through technocratic expertise to generate profits (Rudrappa 2018). Focusing on my visceral sense of belonging and abiding love for the coffee-growing hills of Malnad, southern India, where I grew up, and my eventual exile from there to my current home in Austin, Texas, this chapter describes the parallel worlds of plants, animals, insects, and diseases that weave in and out of the narratives of human reproduction, which are deeply imbued with ideas of family, belonging, inheritance, and private property. As a sociologist studying reproduction, through this personal narrative, I ask, What must be carefully nurtured and what must be exterminated in order to render life as we know it possible? Just as surrogate mothers are erased in order to make nuclear families complete, my own very loving, middle-class family, too, is forged through obliterations. The practices embedded in the ownership of private property and in the pursuit of profit in coffee plantations must necessarily erase other peoples, plants, and forms of life.

The connections between human populations and the environment have been studied and racially politicized from economist Thomas Robert Malthus's (1798) *Essay on the Principle of Population* to the more contemporary accounts in biologists Paul Ehrlich and Anne Ehrlich's (1968) sensationalist *Population Bomb*. Feminist scholars have adeptly disproven these deeply racist, antiwomen, antipoor overpopulation anxieties (Collins 1988; Roberts 1998; Bashford 2014; Clark and Haraway 2018). In this chapter I invoke human reproduction and the environment together, but I move attention away from the vilified figure of the Third World child and her parents, conjured up time and again as desperately hungry mouths ransacking an already ravaged planet. The other extreme, as seen in some repro-scholarship, portrays the idealized figure of the child (Castañeda 2002) who embodies hope. Instead, through narrating my disinheritance and what I perceive as exile from the carefully managed and beautifully manicured coffee plantations of Malnad, which used to be home, to my eventual settlement in Texas with its own problematic histories of occupation, forcible removal, and slavery, I map the *landscapes of infertility* that necessarily accompany familial human reproduction embedded in private property. I organize the rest of the chapter into three sections—delusions, disintegrations, and disarticulations—to map stories of familial belonging and exiles, where plants, mosquitoes, viruses, fungi, and humans commingle in ways that might allow for reparative futurities.

Delusions

In December 2018, for five months, I returned from Texas to southern India, which I had always considered home. This longer stay meant I could begin doing what I had dreamed of doing since I had arrived in the US Midwest in 1989 as a graduate student: I could return to those lush, green coffee plantations on the Western Ghats of Karnataka that are home to generations of my extended family. Growing up, I had spent every summer and winter vacation there, visiting aunts and grandmothers and, with my cousins, hiking through coffee bushes and splashing in rivers that ran thick during the monsoons. It was here that I truly felt home, loved and nurtured by my mother, her sisters, and my paternal grandmother. When I visited, my grandmother took me on long walks through the coffee bushes, pointing to fruit trees my grandfather had planted decades ago and to other medicinal herbs and their cures. When she died, she said, she wanted her ashes scattered on that land. During winter vacations away from school, and in the evenings during the coffee-picking season, older cousins encouraged us younger

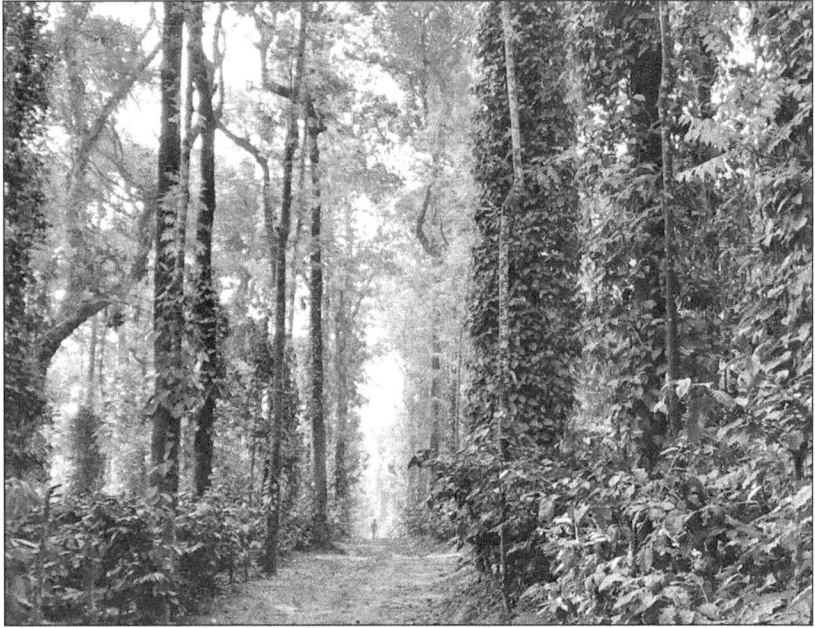

Figure 17.1. Part of Forty Acres of Robusta Coffee (*Coffea canephora*) under Thinned Silver Oak (*Grevillea robusta*) with Black Pepper Vines (*Piper nigrum*) Trained on the Silver Oak, Sakleshpur, South India, December 2018. Credit: Picture by Author

ones to strip down to our underwear and jump into the pulped coffee beans, laughing, playing, and sliding along the coolness of fermented and just-pulped, wet, underprocessed coffee beans. When I close my eyes, I can still feel the slippery beans against my skin. To say that I feel part of that land, and that that land is a part of me, is no exaggeration. Returning in December 2018, I claimed the forty acres of coffee that my father had always said was mine. Figure 17.1 is a photograph I took of part of this land.

My dream, I happily shared with my father, was to reimagine a different kind of plantation that grew coffee but that also made space for the creatures that have always lived there: the snails, insects, birds, civets, pangolins, and elephants. I wanted to return every summer and winter to be in that land. I excitedly proposed alternative methods of land management, halting the heavy sprayings of weedicides and pesticides. I wanted to see what would grow in the absence of chemicals. I expected that the insurgent weeds, which competed with *Coffea* for space, light, and nutrients, would thrive once again, and perhaps prevent soil erosion. I hoped that, protected by a multitude of plant species, frogs, insects, and the birds that fed on them would return, seeking refuge from the chemical deluges unleashed on the lands around them. Coffee monocultures had erased what I imagined to be a complex vitality, and through imagining a different type of coffee plantation, I hoped to reanimate, or re-produce what had been destroyed.

My father fell silent. A few days later, he sat me down and explained that I had misunderstood him. The land was mine in deed, but not in reality. He told me there was other property in Bangalore and Mysore that could be mine, but not this particular piece of land, because this tract belonged to my brother. If, and when, this piece of property was sold, I would receive the money.

I was devastated. Over time I have come to realize that it was not just my gender and his calculations on bloodlines that led to his decision. Instead, he worried about my disloyalties to plantation cultures. His anxieties were about me being that dreaded figure, the absentee landlord who is driven by ideals and not grounded in the everyday rhythms of being there, rooted in the land, and answerable to the communities of coffee planters, nursing the delicate, recalcitrant, and often remunerative *Coffea* on their small holdings. All of this was exacerbated when I professed contrarian ideas on how to manage land that were guaranteed to interfere with the cadences inherent to the cultures of plantation life.

Almost in perfect synchrony, my father and his neighbors employed plantation laborers to weed the land two or three times a year. During the monsoon season weeds were slashed with a machete, and after monsoons, mostly women workers manually pulled weeds (figure 17.2). Or, the land was treated with weedicides such as Paraquat-di-chloride or Glyphosate. Fertilizers were applied when the coffee bushes blossomed in February/March every year, before the monsoons in May/June, after the monsoons in August, and a fourth time in October, as the berries ripened to be picked in December. Every few years soil needed to be amended to carefully maintain a pH closer to 6.1. If the soils became more acidic, agricultural lime or dolomite was added to the soil to make it more alkaline. If the pH rose above 6.2, acid-forming

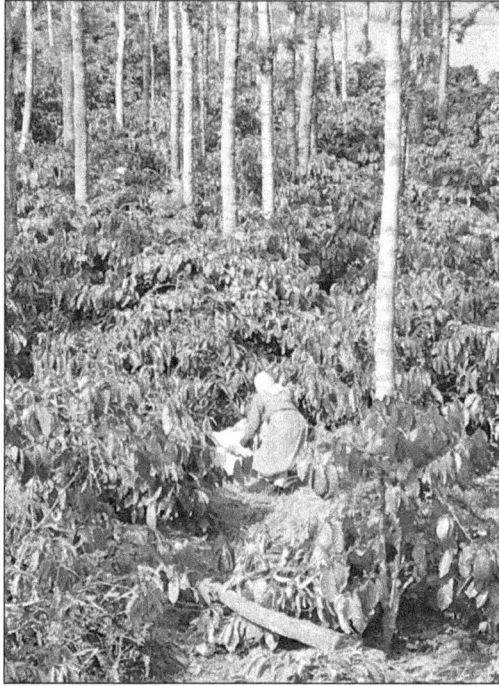

Figure 17.2. Woman Worker in Field of Robusta Coffee under Thinned Stands of Silver Oak Trees (*Grevillia robusta*), Sakleshpur, South India, January 2019. Credit: Picture by Author

fertilizers were applied. The fertility of coffee plantations depends on these chemical rebalances.

The various species of ants that nurtured mutualistic relationships with mealy bugs needed to be controlled through regular applications of pesticide (Vinod Kumar et al. 2016). If ant populations were not suppressed, they would foster colonies of mealy bugs, which then sucked the sap out of coffee plants and weakened them, making the plants more vulnerable to diseases. Fungi, such as powdery mildews and leaf rust, that always threatened to invade the fragile *Coffea*, had to be minimized through three to four sprayings of fungicide every year, preferably before the rains washed away the chemicals from the leaves of plants, but before the berries ripened. And, coffee berry borers (see figure 17.3) needed to be controlled by burning or burying leftover or off-season coffee berries.

I imagined a radically different kind of land-management regime, the polar opposite from what my father and his neighbors knew and practiced. Just one landowner like me, who did not adhere to collective practices, could spell disaster for everyone. Such "mismanagement" would make my land a safe haven for weeds, pests, and microflora and fauna that would eventually migrate to neighboring properties with repercussions far beyond just forty acres of land, because contrary to the boundaries established by the decrees of private property, mildews, coffee leaf miners, and berry borer beetles know no human boundaries. From the sanctuary of forty acres of land free of chemicals, they could launch a million mutinies across the carefully manicured landscape.

My desires for other kinds of fertilities, my father feared, would bring discord between him and his kin. Would I antagonize them through

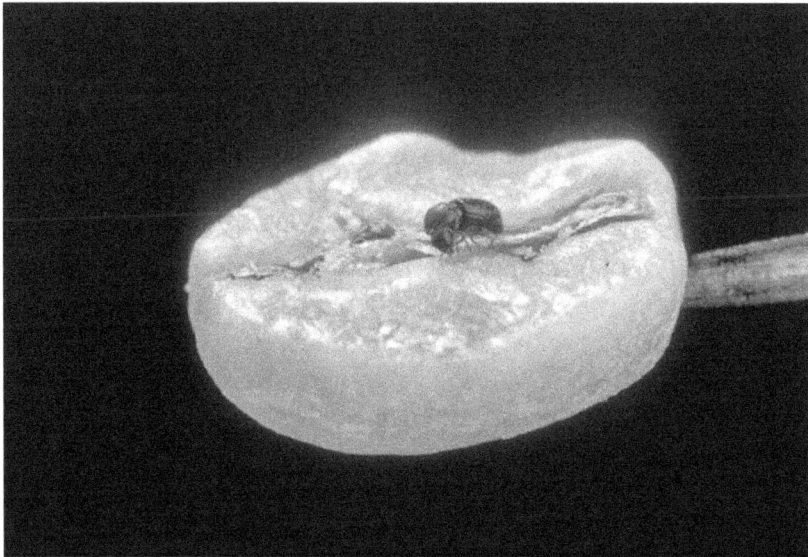

Figure 17.3. The tiny coffee berry borer, the female *Hypothenemus hampei*, lays between thirty-five and fifty eggs within the berry. Credit: Gattuso (2019)

"mismanaging" the land I inherited from him? And would they be upset with him for permitting me to deviate from the practice of coffee monocultures? The reproduction of plantation culture, where my childhood and my nostalgia are rooted, was a coordinated, concerted effort by neighboring landowners to minimize the proliferation of life in order to grow manicured gardens of *Coffea* bushes that bloomed in synchrony every February/March after the gentle blossom rains, and trimmed just so that the beans that ripened by the year's end could be picked by women laborers working in groups. My dreams for that piece of land were antithetical to plantation culture and threatened to upset that coordinated labor effort across space and time, a menacing break in a seamless, collective effort.

Pierre Bourdieu's (2013) concept of "doxa" best explains the implicit beliefs that were taken for granted in Malnad's plantation communities. Common sense and conventional wisdoms were etchings onto the subconscious, rather than mindful practices. The erasure of life in order to proliferate coffee was so deeply entrenched that to think otherwise was deemed delusional.

In theorizing delusions that come with schizophrenia, Miyazono and Salice note that delusions are commonly defined as individual psychological orientations characterized by "epistemic defects . . . with respect to evidence, reasoning, judgment" (2021: 1831). As "fixed beliefs that are not amenable to change in light of conflicting evidence," delusions are understood to be ideas "based on incorrect inference about external reality" and "firmly held despite what almost everyone else believes and despite what constitutes incontrovertible and obvious proof or evidence to the contrary" (American Psychiatric Association 2013, cited in Miyazono and Salice 2021: 1832). Instead of understanding delusions as individual experiences, Miyazono and Salice (2021) suggest that delusions are social phenomena. Fundamentally, they seek to understand why people under schizophrenic delusions believe what they believe in spite of what they see, and what they are told. They note that groupthink is central to the acceptance of social truths; that is, when persons self-categorize as similar to others in a group, as a social self, they engage in collaborative endeavors. In their understanding of delusions, schizophrenic individuals are unable to group identify and regard the information they receive as insincere, and perhaps false. Similarly, if individuals feel a fundamental difference from others—what Miyazono and Salice (2021) call "ontological dissimilarity"—they do not share notions of a common sense, and they act in ways that are deemed delusional.

In Salice and Miyazano's formulations, then, I become the schizophrenic individual, acknowledging the bees, annelids, and pill-millipedes of the *Arthrosphaera* genus endemic to the Western Ghats that thrive on heterogenous organic matter in the soil. In my father's eyes I was hallucinating alternative realities that threatened the monocrop fields of coffee so carefully nurtured under the adequate shade of thinned stands of *Grevillia robusta* native to southern Queensland and New South Wales in Australia (see figures 17.1 and 17.2). And in what my father cast as my fervid imagination of alternative plantations, he saw my refusal and rejection of his entire way of thinking about, and being on, the land.

I had become the feminist killjoy (Ahmed 2017) in recognizing and pointing out that plantation monocultures that emerged from coordinated efforts across time and space displaced, erased, and obliterated entire communities of persons and ecosystems, through inscribing landscapes of infertility solely to nurture the proliferation of one single plant: coffee.

My father and his kinfolks' management of plantations was a fantasy of control, of keeping in abeyance the anarchy that threatened their techno-pastoral imaginaries at the borders of their plantation properties. I define *techno-pastoral imaginaries* as the aspiration for orderly, hierarchical landscapes where land, beasts, and nature are managed through technical expertise to generate profits. Such technical expertise is perceived as an apolitical realm of decision making because rationality, science, and abstract technological considerations drive land-management practices (Rudrappa 2018). These techno-pastoral imaginations that govern South Indian plantation economies are akin to Donna Haraway's (1989) description of fiction as perceptions based on narratives in the making—active, contemporaneous acts of fashioning. These fictions, of techno-pastoral control of plantations, are necessary artifacts of individual and social life that make the everyday possible.

By the end of my five-month stay, toward summer 2019, I was bitten by mosquitoes and infected simultaneously with dengue and chikungunya. I returned to Texas and was hospitalized with severely high fevers and bone-breaking pain like I had never felt before. I have no memories of those three days I spent in the intensive care unit, but I emerged a new person. The viruses, I felt, had reconfigured the internal geographies of my body as they rapidly replicated. I was now wracked with neuralgia and had become a stranger in my own body. I occupied space and time in vastly different ways than I had before. I emerged from my five months in India feeling like an exile: I was exiled from the dreams I once had, the lands that I thought I could always go back to, and now, with these viral diseases, I was exiled from the body I once knew.

Disintegrations

Disintegration is foundational to sociology, from Durkheim's anxieties about theorizing widespread social change to Kelling and Wilson's (1982) "broken windows theory." In much of sociological literature, disintegration implies the falling apart of social order, where cohesive societies are broken up into individual constituents who feel no connection to each other or to a sense of tradition, order, stability, and tranquility. Displaced individuals, in Durkheim's famous formulations, are filled with anomie, figures of desolation, and, potentially, death. Disintegration is breakdown, erosion, waste, and decay.

Instead of these sociological meanings, I understand disintegrations here as individual epistemological crises that reorient people to other possibilities. Over these past few years, plagued with post-chikungunya and -dengue illnesses, I have ruminated on my disastrous return from South India in 2019. If tropical fevers are known to cause delirium and hallucinations, the opposite has happened to me. My fevers cured at least some of my many delusions. And it took a mosquito or two to teach me history.

I now understand that plantation economies and mosquitoes are intimate partners, the latter always loyally following where tropical monocultures are established. South Indian histories are filled with accounts of repeated widespread famines and irrigation projects designed to feed the frenzied grain and cotton markets fostered by laissez-faire colonial policies. With rampant land clearing, irrigation, and expanded agriculture has come another familiar colonial friend, that omnipresent being, the mosquito. The two viral diseases that I contracted are transmitted by two mosquitoes, the *Aedes aegypti* and the *Aedes albopictus. Aedes*

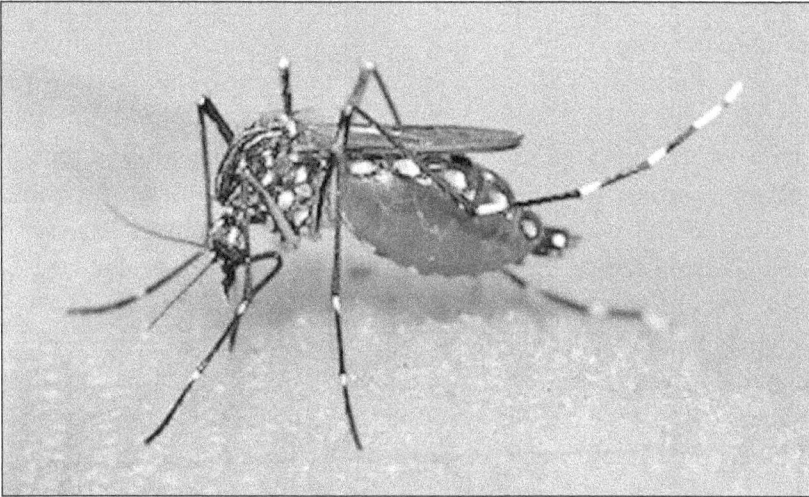

Figure 17.4. *Aedes aegypti*. Image from Ed Yong, *National Geographic*, August 24, 2011.
A. albopictus, or the Asian tiger mosquito, not shown here, has a striped underbelly.

aegypti originates on the African continent and is seen as the most successful invasive species in the world today (see figure 17.4). If you are in
South Asia, and you feel mosquitoes at your ankles in the morning and
not at the usual witching twilight hours, beware. You have made your
acquaintance with *A. aegypti*. Strikingly beautiful, with white markings
on black, this slender little mosquito moved out of Senegal and into Asia
and the Americas on ships that trafficked colonial commodities such as
sugar, cotton, silk, jute, indigo, and enslaved persons. As early as 1780,
the first epidemic of clinical dengue-like illness was recorded in Madras,
South India (Gupta et al. 2012).

The coffee plantations for which I felt such nostalgia, and problem-
atically do so even today, emerged from a colonial logic of cash crop
production in various parts of the world—sugar cane, cotton, tobacco,
tea, and coffee. Such expansions were possible only through the large-
scale dispossession of tribal and rural communities, and through the
conversion of men and women into property through the institution of
chattel slavery. Beginning in 1840, entire tropical evergreen forests on
the Western Ghats of Karnataka were cut down and replaced with coffee.
The colonial logics and practice of deforestation, plantation economies,

and slave and coolie labor of the 1700s and 1800s vastly expanded the practice of private property.

Those mosquitoes that bit me (or was it just one?) and those viruses they gave me opened my eyes. The Edenic gardens of my childhood, those coffee plantations where I experienced love, happiness, and belonging, emerged and were continually reproduced through violence. South Indian coffee plantation economies were established through large-scale ecological projects beginning in 1840 when Jenu Kuruba, Kaadu Kuruba, and Soliga peoples were driven out of their ancestral lands to make way for private property (see figure 17.5). They were converted to landless laborers who now worked on plantations carved on the lands to which they belonged. Or they were "illegal squatters" on state-owned forest land. To meet the labor demands of clearing the land and regularly weeding, spraying, and picking coffee beans, Mappila labor recruiters from Kerala brought in Tamil coolie laborers who, themselves, were late-nineteenth-century climate refugees, driven out of their own homes through decades of repeated famines. These Tamil laborers cleared bamboo off the land. Some trees were marked and enumerated as valuable teak or rosewood. Other trees deemed unnecessary were either cut down or thinned so that they would not shade the coffee that grew underneath. Tigers and Indian bison were hunted for sport. Wild elephants were trapped in large enclosures, or *keddah* operations, in order to domesticate them. Wild boar and spotted deer proliferated.

I have now come to recognize that the practice of private property in Malnad and the ownership of coffee-growing land is premised on erasures. My nostalgia for an idealized childhood, with aunts, grandmothers, and cousins, is built on the obliteration of people and communities, trees and forests that were homes to animals, annelids, arthropods, insects, and fungi. Yet, I would be lying if I denied that I continue to have a deep love for that land, a visceral sense of connection. Sometimes, when I close my eyes, I can smell it and become transported back, feet grounded among thinned silver oak trees, pepper vines, and coffee bushes. But my ability to act on my sense of belonging—of returning to what was once home—can only be realized through ownership. I can still visit my extended family on these lands, but I need to be a good guest. I cannot overstay, and I must temper my actions. I realize that through disinheritance, like the insurrecting populations of weeds, the

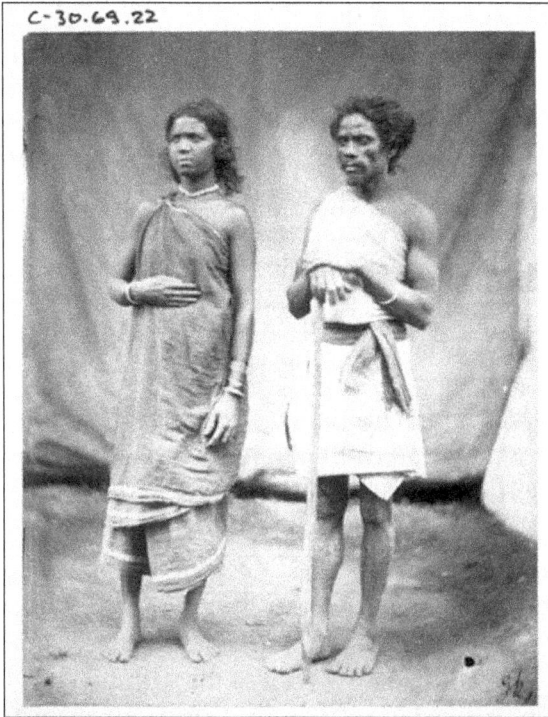

Figure 17.5. Jenu Kurubas, Kodagu Region (1859–1861). Basel Mission (subcollection), C-30.69.022 (reference number), International Mission Photography Archive, ca.1860–ca.1960 (collection), QC-30.001.0275.

mealy bugs and the faithful ants that nurture them, civets, pangolins, and elephants, I too have been exiled.

The ownership of coffee-growing land, and the practice of private property in Malnad, are premised on elisions. Elision is defined in Webster's dictionary as "the omission of an unstressed vowel or syllable in a verse to achieve a uniform metrical pattern." I use the term "elisions" to describe the processes of slippages, ways of overlooking, and omissions in plantation economies that go into reproducing monocultural crops, and their attendant monocultural cultivation practices that snuff out diversity and dissent.

But here I pause to raise three quick points regarding the practices of private property and the landscapes of infertility these practices tend to foster. First, emotional disentanglements from the idea of property seem impossible. How else to understand home other than as a place where there is a sense of ownership, a place that belongs to you, but also, to which you belong? Private property is the one tool that is available to migrants like me to inculcate a sense of belonging. In the worlds in which we live, to be exiled from the Nation of Property can potentially contribute to a feeling of rootlessness, a sense of always leaving but never arriving, and can be emotionally devastating. I am finally learning that the sense of belonging about which I still feel such nostalgia, is politically fraught. My belonging, a sense of familial love and care, was made possible through outright erasure and through its more subtle versions of elision and evasion.

Second, monocultural plantation economies are possible because of their socioeconomic and cultural underpinnings, organized through private property. Along with plants such as *Lantana camara* and *Parthenium hysterophorus*, both introduced from the American tropics, South Indian evergreen forest denizens are continuously trying to reestablish themselves. The suppression of such insurgent fertilities is made possible through the coordinated efforts of private property owners, each husbanding their lands with timely and judicious fertilizer and weedicide applications. Private property, then, entails not just ownership and the extraction of profits but also, within the context of plantation economies, individual caring responsibilities for the maintenance of coffee monocultures entailed in suppressing weeds and pests that proliferate. Coffee plantation owners, then, have a responsibility to themselves and to their neighbors to kill weeds and pests. What would it mean to work toward ecological restoration and increase biodiversity, while still holding onto the practices of private property in plantation economies?

Finally, my idealizations about restoration ecology in Malnad focused solely on reintroducing plant and animal species that are disappearing because of the death cultures of coffee. Yet, what did it mean to restore ecologies without Jenu Kuruba and Kadu Kuruba communities, who once called these lands home? In holding onto the notion of private property, by asking for what I believed to be mine and feeling devastated about the tragedy of my gendered exile, I was eliding histories of human dispossessions and exiles that preceded mine.

Disarticulations

First used by Samir Amin (1976), the term "disarticulation" explained the effects of uneven development brought about by colonialism. In his formulations, in the export-oriented economies under colonialism and neocolonialism, domestic working populations do not serve as the market for the goods they produce. Instead, the goods produced in the periphery by these Global South workers are destined for offshore consumer markets. Contrary to modernization theorists' postulations that economic growth in the peripheries would lead to greater social welfare, human development indices fell in export-oriented economies in the Global South.

The coffee plantations in South India are an exemplar of socioeconomic disarticulation, but my application here is different. I use disarticulations to explain the gaps and fissures between different modalities of reproduction across human worlds and nonhuman ecologies, which allow for the imagination of other possibilities than the ones we reproduce endlessly. I posit that disarticulations, these unintended cracks and fractures, can potentially open up possibilities for reworlding.

Overcome by disease and disinheritance, I returned to central Texas, which had not felt like home. However, like countless people during the global COVID-19 pandemic, I began gardening. Through digging soil and planting seeds, I have laid roots. But here too I live smack in the middle of a one-hundred-year flood plain, and on lands that have known other peoples (see figure 17.6). A dry creek bed lies behind the house; it flash-floods regularly and threatens to break its banks during torrential rainstorms. The part of the creek behind my home is not necessarily beautiful. The gushing rain waters in the creek wash in the detritus of Austin: plastic bags, T-shirts made in sweatshops, shopping carts. But the creek, too, reveals signs of other kinds of life. Amid water snakes, coyotes, barred owls, frogs, and anole lizards, the creek sometimes washes up arrowheads. The creek does not allow anyone to pretend otherwise. It reveals that other communities lived here and belonged to these lands. Tonkawa Indian communities were moved from these lands at the time of Austin's founding. The Comanches and Lipan Apaches, too, frequented these central Texas regions as they followed

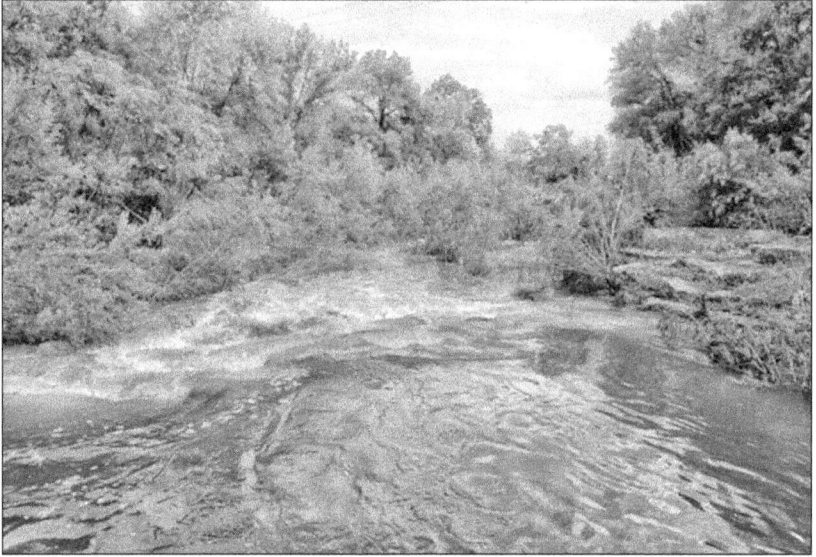

Figure 17.6. Shoal Creek, Austin Texas, after the Rains and with Pecan Trees in the Background. Credit: Texas Government Insider (2019)

routes of food supplies. They perhaps planted and nurtured the old pecan trees that dot my neighborhood up and down the creek.

Upon displacing indigenous communities, Anglo and Mexican settlers grew cotton on lands in central Texas, which in the early nineteenth century was part of Mexico. These labor-intensive cotton plantations could be sustained only through slavery, but by 1829 slavery was prohibited in most of Mexico, including Texas. Anglos and Mexicans worked together to secure the right to hold slaves against abolitionists in the Mexican government, which resulted in the Texas Revolution in 1836. Settlers sought independence from Mexico so that they could maintain the right to enslave people, and Texas joined the United States as a slave state (Torget 2018).

It is on these fraught, occupied territories that I have begun gardening every day. I am not very successful. Amidst the echinacea, paloverde, copper canyon daisies, and old pecan trees, my garden has a lush crop of different kinds of fungi—delicate little mushrooms, or bubbling masses that emit billowing clouds of black spores when disturbed (see figures 17.7 and 17.8). I do not know why the mushrooms reproduce so rapidly in my garden, what species they are, or why they appear in such abundance.

But I imagine the mycelia underneath, stretching in convoluted miles under and around the house, into the creek and beyond. I imagine the vast crisscrossing lines of communication, molecules of information transmitted to my garden from the family of coyotes that hides in the unoccupied plot of land three houses down, from the old pecan trees that grow all along the creek, and from the turkey buzzards that feed on what has died far beyond what I can see or hear.

Mushrooms live in parallel worlds to ours. Contrary to the kinds of forced fertilities and landscapes of infertility imposed through the practice of private property and the pursuit of profits, these fungi know no ownership and respect no boundaries. Through their mycelia they move molecules of information from one being to the other across vast spaces and

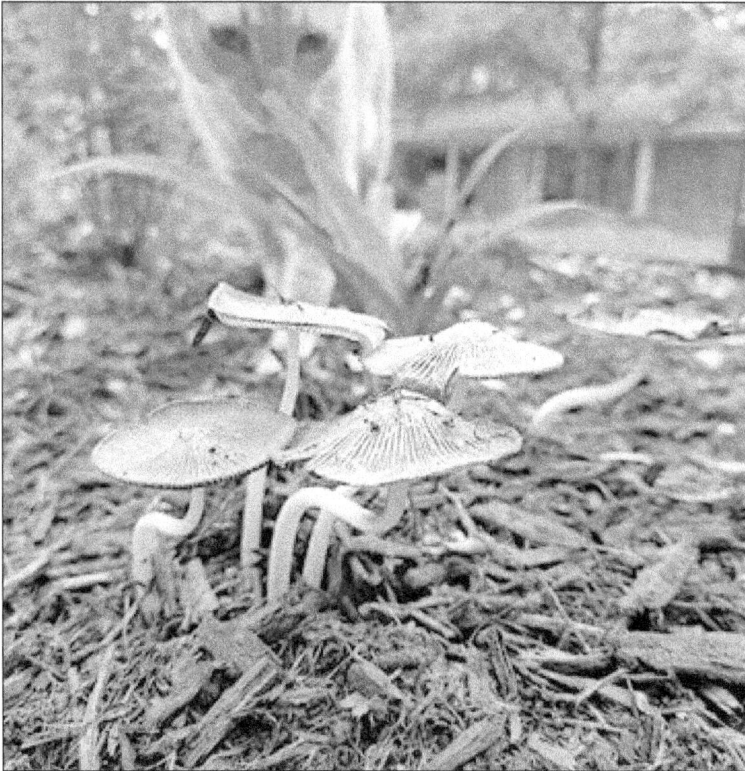

Figure 17.7. Chucklee the cat investigates the unidentified mushrooms in the garden I grow. Austin, Texas, March 2022. Credit: Picture by Author

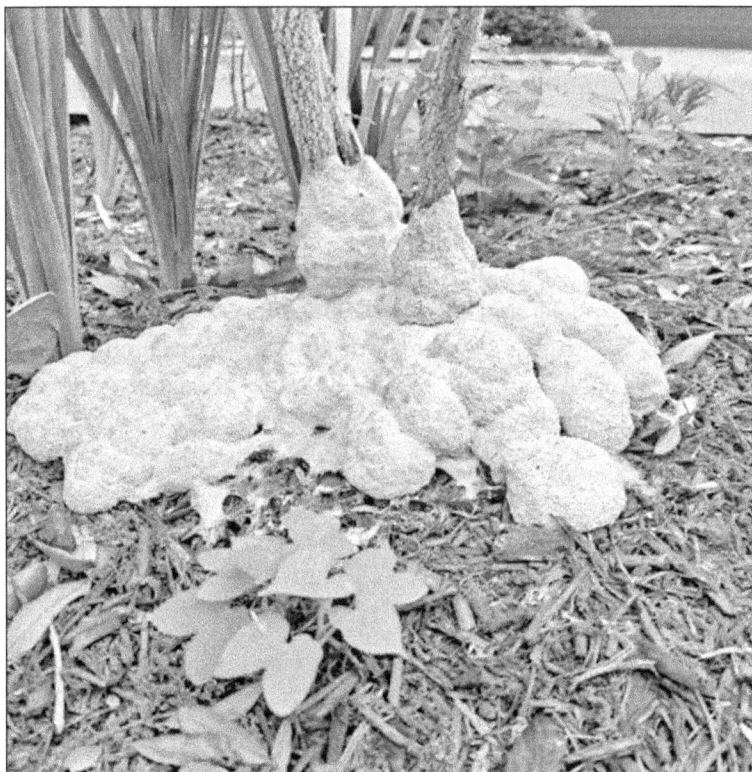

Figure 17.8. Unidentified Mushrooms in the Garden I Grow. Austin, Texas, March 2022. Credit: Picture by Author

time. I turn to the fruiting bodies of these mushrooms and their mycelia to defamiliarize myself from inherited notions of property and to disrupt habitual ways of knowing. They offer other configurations of reproduction and belonging outside of private property through inheritance.

Conclusion

Donna Haraway notes that we are deeply implicated in the conditions of our common inheritance. We are not simply passive observers or innocently located in particular places in the world. Instead, we are a part of the world and its ongoing activities in meaning making through eliding, effacing, and erasing. Haraway calls for a speculative fabulation, "a mode of attention, a theory of history and a practice of worlding" (Haraway 2016: 230). Speculative fashioning is rooted in everyday storytelling practices, but the stories we say matter. Worlding is the context in which concepts, things, people, and beings show up and take on significance to provide other perceptions of space, and other truths that remain hidden otherwise. Worlding is an engaged, active, ontological process.

Fungi provide metaphors for how to be and think about the world around us, rooted nowhere but with mycelia everywhere, deriving nurturance from decaying wood, animals long gone, and soil. These fungal mycelia transmit substance and information, connecting beings across vast spaces and time with little reverence for the borders of private property. Perhaps stories of human fertilities need to be like mushrooms, linking vastly disparate beings and nonbeings, revealing rhythms that are not easily apparent in stories that focus solely on people.

Yet, ethnographies of reproduction, given the nature of the work of ethnography itself, must necessarily recount individual stories of fertility and infertility. In retelling these highly individualized stories, ethnographers chronicle the gendered identities, familial values, and racialized institutions that are continually reimagined, reenacted, and, ultimately, reproduced. Ethnographic accounts reveal that deepened commodifications of human cells and bodily processes do not inevitably result in alienation but are life affirming and replete with the potential to create meaningful connections. But what does it mean when ethnographies simply affirm what we want to believe? Ethnographies, because they are steeped in showing how people understand their everyday lives, elide the fact that in order to make normative reproduction feasible, other human and nonhuman reproductions are repressed. Normative reproductions are made possible through the unequal distribution of life and death. Such asymmetry is partially made viable through the persistence of patriarchal families, gendered inheritance, and the practice of private property. These form a critical part of the scaffolding for normative reproduction.

On a surface level, the story of disinheritance and disease narrated here has nothing to do with reproduction. Yet, systems of beliefs, customs, primogeniture, inheritance, private property, and profits are the warp and weft that comprise reproduction. Who must die, and how many must die, in order for someone to live? What is a worthy life, and what are the social, political, and economic arrangements and costs of making that life happen? I suggest that there is something to learn by gazing intently just beyond the horizon of human in-fertilities, by bringing to focus what appears to be the blurred backdrop of human fertility. In such a consideration, I propose, the hidden registers of destruction and disintegration of other lives and people, so central to middle-class reproduction, might come into lines of vision. The stories of reproduction that are the preoccupation of demographers and reproductive sociologists must necessarily attend to the scaffolding that makes human reproduction possible. Like subterranean mycelia, narratives linking people, beings, and creatures may offer alternative ways of knowing, a reworlding, that open possibilities for considering reparative futures for damaged societies living on a damaged planet.

REFERENCES

Ahmed, Sara. 2017. *Living a Feminist Life*. Durham, NC: Duke University Press.

American Psychiatric Association. 2013. *Diagnostic and Statistical Manual of Mental Disorders*, 5th ed. Cambridge, MA: American Psychiatric Publishing.

Amin, Samir. 1976. *Uneven Development: An Essay on the Social Formations of Peripheral Capitalism*. New York: Monthly Review Press.

Bashford, Alison. 2014. *Global Population: History, Geopolitics, and Life on Earth*. New York: Columbia University Press.

Bourdieu, Pierre. 2013. *Outline of a Theory in Practice*. Cambridge: Cambridge University Press.

Castañeda, Claudia. 2002. *Figurations: Child, Bodies, World*. Durham, NC: Duke University Press.

Clark, Adele, and Donna Haraway, eds. 2018. *Making Kin, Not Population: Reconceiving Generations*. Chicago: Prickly Paradigm Press.

Collins, Jane L. 1988. *Unseasonal Migrations: The Effects of Rural Labor Scarcity in Peru*. Princeton, NJ: Princeton University Press.

Ehrlich, Paul, and Anne Ehrlich. 1968. *The Population Bomb*. San Francisco/New York: Sierra Club/Ballantine Books.

Gattuso, Reina. 2019. "Solved: The Mysterious Origins of Your Coffee's Worst Nightmare." *Atlas Obscura*, October 14. www.atlasobscura.com.

Gerrits, Trudie. 2018. "Reproductive Travel to Ghana: Testimonies, Transnational Relationships, and Stratified Reproduction." *Medical Anthropology* 37(2): 131–44.

Grandia, Liza. 2015. "Slow Ethnography: A Hut with a View." *Critique of Anthropology* 35(3): 301–17.

Gupta, Nivedita, Sakshi Srivastava, Amita Jain, and Umesh C. Chaturvedi. 2012. "Dengue in India." *Indian Journal of Medical Research* 136(3): 373–90.

Haraway, Donna. 1989. *Primate Visions: Gender, Race, and Nature in the World of Modern Science*. New York: Routledge.

———. 2016. *Staying with the Trouble: Making Kin in the Chthulucene*. Durham, NC: Duke University Press.

Inhorn, Marcia, and Pasquale Patrizio. 2015. "Infertility around the Globe: New Thinking on Gender, Reproductive Technologies, and Global Movements in the 21st Century." *Human Reproduction Update* 21(4): 411–26.

Kelling George L., and James Q. Wilson. 1982. "Broken Windows: The Police and Neighborhood Safety." *Atlantic*, March. www.theatlantic.com.

Malthus, Thomas Robert. 1798. *An Essay on the Principle of Population*. Chicago: J. Johnson.

Miyazono, Kengo, and Alessandra Salice. 2021. "Social Epistemological Conception of Delusion." *Synthese* 199: 1831–51.

Roberts, Dorothy. 1998. *Killing the Black Body: Race, Reproduction, and the Meaning of Liberty*. New York: Vintage Books.

Rudrappa, Sharmila. 2015. *Discounted Life: The Price of Global Surrogacy in India*. New York: New York University Press.

———. 2016. "What to Expect When You're Expecting: The Affective Economies of Consuming Surrogacy in India." *Positions: Asia Critique* 24(1): 281–302.

———. 2018. "Land, Women, and Techno-Pastoral Development in Southern Karnataka, India." *Reproductive BioMedicine and Society Online* 7(November).

Texas Government Insider. 2019. "Austin's Shoal Creek Erosion Control Project Estimated at $20M." *SPI Insights*, June 21. www.spartnerships.com.

Torget, Andrew J. 2018. *Seeds of Empire: Cotton, Slavery, and the Transformation of the Texas Borderlands, 1800–1850*. Chapel Hill: University of North Carolina Press.

Vinod Kumar, P. K., G. V. Manjunath Reddy, H. G. Seetharama, and M. M. Balakrishnan. 2016. "Coffee." In *Mealybugs and Their Management in Agricultural and Horticultural Crops*, eds. M. Mani and C. Shivaraju, 650–53. New Delhi: Springer.

Waldby, Catherine, and Melinda Cooper. 2014. *Clinical Labor: Tissue Donors and Research Subjects in the Global Bioeconomy*. Durham, NC: Duke University Press.

Whittaker, Andrea, Marcia C. Inhorn, and Francoise Shenfield. 2019. "Globalised Quests for Assisted Conception: Reproductive Travel for Infertility and Involuntary Childlessness." *Global Public Health* 14(12): 1669–88.

18

Heterotopian Ecologies of Abundance

Saving Seeds and (Bio)Diversity in London

KATHARINE DOW

What a waste, what a crime, to wreck a world so abundantly
full of different kinds of flowers.
—Olivia Laing, 2018

To respond to the climate crisis—a disaster on a more immense scale than anything our species has faced—we can
and must summon what people facing disasters have: a
sense of meaning, of deep connection and generosity, of being truly alive in the face of uncertainty. Of joy. This is the
kind of abundance we need to meet the climate crisis, to
make many, or even most, lives better. It is the opposite of
moral injury; it is moral beauty. A thing we needn't acquire,
because we already have it in us.
—Rebecca Solnit, 2023

This chapter explores the "quiet activism" (Pottinger 2016) of in situ seed
saving in London. Seed saving is the act of keeping and storing seeds
from the plants that one has grown. In this case, it refers specifically
to seeds from food plants. The seed savers I have encountered during
ethnographic fieldwork in London conceptualize seeds as encapsulat-
ing certain things: their genetic and environmental heritages (see Dow
2021), but also their relationships with, and the identities of, the people
who plant, grow, and save them. Saved seeds represent an alternative to
commercially bred hybrid seed, which proponents see as embodying
capitalist aims of profit maximization and enrichment of the few, but
also of the values of restriction, individualization, and limits, epitomized

by the plantation (Tsing 2004; Davis et al. 2019). London seed savers are enacting a more collective form of fertility and productivity, right in the belly of the capitalist beast.

I took my first steps into the world of seed saving in 2016. I had been reflecting on the parallels between the cryogenically enabled world of seed banking and assisted reproductive technologies (see Chacko 2022) and considering a new research project that would further develop my interest in the intersections between reproductive and environmental concerns. After several visits to seed swaps—small gatherings where people come together to swap saved and open-pollinated seeds[1]—and related events around England, I decided to home in on London, my home city, to investigate seed saving among small-scale, noncommercial food growers, focusing on their ideas about the relationship between human diversity and biodiversity, the conditions for growing food in a mega-city, and the ethical and political practice of non- and anticapitalist forms of exchange.[2]

I carried out patchwork ethnographic research between 2019 and 2021, switching to online interviews and meetings during the COVID-19 pandemic. The main point of contact throughout my research was the London Freedom Seed Bank, the first group of seed savers to emerge in the city about a decade ago (see Dow 2021; Dow and Doyle 2024). As well as interviewing the codirectors, steering group members, and growers in their network, I attended events, meetings, and informal gatherings. Some of these occurred in person and some online, depending on the COVID-19 lockdown restrictions in place at the time. In the summer of 2020 I accepted an invitation to join their steering group, which gave me the opportunity both to understand the values and practices that inform their work more deeply and to give something back to my research participants. Throughout the study I have been in contact with several other groups and community gardens who practice, or are interested in, seed saving, some of which I discuss in this chapter. In addition to representatives of these organizations, I interviewed individual seed savers throughout the course of this study. I conducted semistructured interviews with twenty seed savers in London (some, more than once). These data were supplemented by informal conversations, attendance at meetings, events, and workshops, and analysis of relevant textual, audio, and video content, from organizational websites to WhatsApp messages in seed savers' groups.

As I discuss in this chapter, seeds are "condensed nodes of fertility" (Sarah Franklin, personal communication). Almost all my participants have, in our conversations, referred to seeds as "life." This term refers to their status as reproductive units and their role in feeding other species, but also, and relatedly, to the profound and manifold meanings that they encapsulate. For my research participants, saved seeds encapsulate the collective values of sharing resources, nurturing environments and communities, and fostering diversity, which for many of them is also an explicit rejection of capitalist, neoliberal values.

The London seed savers I met during my research are interested not so much in saving seeds in the sense of preserving or rescuing them, but in nurturing the abundant diversity they offer when allowed to grow and pollinate openly, to adapt to their local conditions, and to travel between people and places through noncommercial exchanges. They aim toward *heterotopian ecologies*, in which all sorts of different creatures live alongside each other in conditions that foster plenty and diversity. This environment is "heterotopian" (Foucault 1967) not only because it celebrates difference and diversity but also because it is not utopian. While seeds and growing food give my research participants hope and joy, they also recognize that abundant diversity brings with it ambivalence. To use a horticultural metaphor, delicious tomatoes may attract bees, but might also entice slugs and succumb to blight. A heterotopian ecology does not necessarily embrace or welcome slugs or blight in and of themselves, but it does take them as part of a diverse world that is not predicated on controlling reproduction and fertility for commercial aims.

Encapsulation: "What Do Seeds Mean to You?"

Perhaps because they are generally very small, but encapsulate so much, seeds provide, for my research participants, an opening into bigger issues. Seed savers do not see seed saving as a single-issue form of activism but as a more manageable means to engage with other, perhaps weightier, issues, including biodiversity loss, climate change, the intensification of industrial agriculture, and the severing of ties among people, nature, and place. Several participants expressed a sense of being overwhelmed by the scale of the climate and biodiversity crisis and aware of the little they could do about it as individuals. Saving seeds offered participants a sense of agency, however small-scale, in the face of the enormous power and necropolitical behaviors of commercial seed companies.

On a sunny summer's day in August 2021, I visited the Seed Saving Network, which runs out of OmVed Gardens, a private garden and events space in Highgate, north London. Highgate is one of the most expensive areas of London. The garden was founded by the Leason family and funded through the philanthropic arm of their family's food business, Natco, which sells pulses, spices, and other South Asian foods in the United Kingdom and internationally. OmVed's mission is "to regenerate our relationship with the land, with food and with our human and non-human kin and to share what we are learning on [*sic*] the process, encouraging everyone to join our journey in different ways" (OmVed Gardens n.d.). In 2020, staff members, including Vicky Chown and Sonia Rego, established the Seed Saving Network with the aim of facilitating seed saving and sharing in London and beyond and building a database of information about seeds to have a better picture of how food growing and food growers are adapting to the changing climate (Seed Saving Network 2023).

Vicky, a White, working-class Londoner, is a very knowledgeable gardener and food grower. Sonia is a former academic who is now training to be a ranger in Scotland and is North American with South Asian heritage. Both are in their early thirties. I had spoken to them on the phone and in video calls before, but, due to the COVID-19 pandemic, this was the first time I met either in person. Following a delicious lunch of pasta with lion's mane mushrooms grown and cooked by Vicky, I interviewed her and Sonia about seed saving. At the end of the joint interview, I asked them both a question I have asked almost every interviewee to round up the interview: What do seeds mean to you? Vicky replied first, remarking that she had been on a train a few days previously, "dreaming out the window about seeds" and thinking about how they are "a promise of the future" and "a little secret thing that could go on forever and ever and ever." She explained that if you give someone a package of seeds, "you give this little dormant packet of things that can be stored for quite a while for when you're ready to plant them or when it's a good year for you to plant them, and then it can turn into a whole host of things that never stops."

Sonia continued in a pragmatic vein, "I guess seeds are food and we need food to live," going on to observe that this principle has been forgotten over the last few generations because of industrialization. Vicky picked up on this and mentioned the climate crisis, before quickly turning to thoughts of "a pretty huge apocalyptic-type event," concluding, "It'd be much more important for you to have a packet of seed in your pockets than a bottle of [crude] oil. You know what I mean? We don't realize just how important, like I said, it's the promise of it. If we lost 95 percent of our seeds now, we wouldn't probably survive as a species. Not that I know the stats for that, but it'd be very difficult to. Whereas, if we lost 99 percent of our fossil fuel, yes, things would change massively, but it's not [the end of the world]."

The following three quotations, in which each interviewee refers to seeds as "life" in one way or another, illustrate the richness of my research participants' feeling for seeds and their manifold meanings. The first is from Karen, a White woman in her fifties whom I met at a seed swap at a community garden near my home in east London. The second is from Simon, a Black man in his twenties who is involved in various community gardening projects in south London. The third is from Sophia, a German and Irish White woman in her twenties who was a codirector of the London Freedom Seed Bank at the time of our interview. The interview with Karen was in person and the other two were online. In each case, as with Vicky and Sonia, I asked, "What do seeds mean to you?"

> Without waxing too lyrical, I would say life. . . . I find it endlessly rewarding to take a seed from whatever source, be it from a packet or from a plant, and sow it, and watch those green shoots growing. . . . You don't garden for now; you garden for the future. And that to me is life affirming and creative and important and so, it's just the meaning of life stuff.
>
> And I think with the seeds, it's that not being in control. You never know if it's going to work. . . . Is there anything more rewarding than nurturing that seed? Suddenly you've given birth to it. For God's sake, don't let it die! And that is just brilliant, and I love that. (Karen)

> A phrase could sum it up, basically. The seeds of today are the flowers of tomorrow; the flowers of tomorrow are in the seeds of today. That's what seeds mean to me. There's so much power within a seed. Us as humans, I know it might not relate, but our mothers and fathers, there was a seed and an egg, similar principle, and out came life abundance. We have life, we

have so much to be appreciative for. It's just the same with a flower. Within that one seed, if that seed is put in the right conditions, soil, light, water, that seed is going to germinate. And depending on what species or genus that seed is, it's going to either create flowers for bees or fruits for insects, animals, and humans to eat. The power within a seed is exponential. The ramifications are too much. Seriously it's like, when I take seeds and I'm planting, it's just, I can't explain. (Simon)

I'm going to have a really cheesy answer. . . . I love seeds. I think they're beautiful, visually, and to touch them is amazing and the fact that they hold this whole potential. . . . It's something so humbling, and I think it's something so very, very real. Very material. Something that can be felt, and touched, and seen, and sensed, and experienced. Then that joy. Everyone experiences joy at something growing. That's, for me, the most essential part of being alive, because you can see life in seeds. [They're] kind of individuals, also—not individuals in the sense like humans are, but I really like seeing one seed grow and what it becomes and the relationship that goes along with that. Instead of just seeing it abstracted, or a species or kind of a whole. Something really personal, a very personal kind of thing. (Sophia)

Karen emphasized the life-giving properties of seeds, which encapsulate and animate the meaning of life. She also referred to the seed's capacity to bring forth life, or future generations, through time and the duty of growers to protect and care for plants ("For God's sake, don't let it die!"). Karen has worked with children throughout her career but does not have biogenetic children of her own. In this quotation, she makes a smooth analogy between sowing, growing, and protecting seeds and plants and giving birth. She thinks of growing plants as an act of nurture, creativity, and love. To watch the seed grow, she affirmed, is "endlessly rewarding"—and the fact that the seed is not entirely under her control, but literally has a life of its own, makes it all the more so. For Simon, seeds are at once present- and future-oriented. Like Karen, he directly analogized seed sowing to human fertility as well as to a parent's loving care and attention, but also talks about seeds' (immanent) power. He described "life abundance," but also gave a sense of abundance through his phrasing—"We have so much to be appreciative for" and "the power within a seed is exponential"—and linked this abundance with different species, from bees to humans.

Sophia was not alone in using romantic and emotional words like "love," "beauty," and "joy." Sophia, whom I have come to know well over the course of my research, is a sensitive and thoughtful person with left-wing anticolonial politics who thinks a lot about human diversity. So, when she makes a universalizing statement like, "Everyone experiences joy at something growing," it is worth paying attention. Along with other participants' sense of seeds' magic, power, and potentiality, she was expressing a shared sense that working with seeds is a way of getting (back) in touch with "nature," of (re)connecting with the other- or more-than human, of turning one's back on the political economic hegemony in favor of something less predictable, but altogether more delightful. Sophia's sense that this is something "everyone" finds joyful is normative, but also a reminder of Sonia's point about how seeds, and the plants that grow from them, are vital for human survival.

Abundant Diversity: "One for the Raven, One for the Crow, One to Rot, and One to Grow"

"Seed swapping is our way of resistance; it's our way of pushing back, not just for ourselves but also for future generations. It's about biodiversity." I heard these words on a bright but cold day in January 2017, at Seedy Saturday in Bristol in the southwest of England, when I was starting to plan my ethnographic study of seed saving. This event was one of several seed gatherings that take place, usually on weekends in January and February, across the United Kingdom, where amateur gardeners, allotment keepers, and smallholders gather to swap and acquire seeds they have saved from their own gardens.

The talk was attended by about thirty people, crammed into a side room in the venue. The speaker was Humphrey Lloyd, a member of the Landworkers' Alliance, a union for food producers in the United Kingdom that promotes agroecology and food sovereignty. A young White man dressed in jeans and a sweatshirt, he was an unassumingly persuasive rhetorician. Lloyd introduced his talk as a "potted history of the last eleven thousand years of seeds, from open pollination to GMOs" (genetically modified organisms). He smiled somewhat sheepishly at such an ambitious sweep of history, but his tone was serious and engaging. This is the history he told, based on my contemporaneous fieldnotes:

Before hybridization, all seeds were open pollinated. People saved their best seed, which led to incredible biodiversity. There were billions of slightly different landraces.[3] They never had huge yields, but they were stable and diverse. There's an old saying, "One for the raven, one for the crow, one to rot, and one to grow," which encapsulates the fact that with open-pollinated seed, you don't know how much has been pollinated, and usually around 75 percent isn't. So, open pollination is less reliable, but it is free of charge and so saved seed could be seen as a form of commons.

In the nineteenth century, Mendelian genetics led to the selective pollination of plants, the use of glasshouses, and plant hybridization. Traits could now be bred in, but the plants came to lose or lack diversity. Just think of a mule—inbreeding leads to sterility. Nowadays, farmers don't need to save seeds, but can buy them, but then they become no longer self-reliant. Hybridization improves yields, but only under certain conditions, and it relies on pesticides, fertilizers, and so on. The Plant Patent Act in the United States in the 1930s made saving F1 [first-generation] hybrid seeds illegal. Similar legislation came in in the United Kingdom in the 1960s.[4] The Green Revolution was essentially the exportation of the industrial agriculture model, including hybrid seeds, around the world. Foundations sent seed packages to developing countries to encourage capitalist development. In fact, this led to widening inequality and, although yields grew by 11 percent, hunger also grew by 11 percent because not all could afford food. Hunger is linked to food sovereignty. Genetic mutation seems like a continuation of this theme.

Petrochemical companies bought up seed companies, so they have an interest in farmers buying fertilizers and so on. One development was "terminator" genes, which breed in infertility so seeds can't be saved and reused. These have now become illegal, but the principle of preventing seed saving remains. A series of mergers and acquisitions mean that now ten biotech firms control 73 percent of seeds.

He concluded with his thoughts on seed swapping, which I quoted at the opening of this section.

In this densely woven potted history, it is possible to follow a thread of concern about reproduction and in-fertility through to sterility and finally endangerment, the ultimate inability to produce future generations. Lloyd described plant fertility becoming limited and controlled through human, rather than natural, selection. This human intervention, he said, has led to hunger and infertility—the opposite of the "life" that research participants described in response to my question about what seeds mean. So, the control of most of the world's plant seeds by large corporations that characterizes our current historical moment forces reliance on them for future fertility. As Lloyd implied, this is important for the survival of these plants, but also the survival of the humans and other species that rely on them and that produce future generations.

The saying, "One for the raven, one for the crow, one to rot, and one to grow," is diverse; various versions exist, featuring different creatures such as mice, cutworms, rats, and blackbirds. As Lloyd said, it expresses the fact that open-pollinated seed has a lower germination rate than hybrid seed. Yet he argued that, with the breeding practices that improve germination rates, much is lost along the way and that ultimately these practices may lead to sterility. The number "one," in this saying, expresses parts, shares, and systems—a way for biotic beings, many of them "pests," to rub along together in a somewhat ordered, knowable form. This phrase, with its roll call of different and notably humble beings, articulates a heterotopian ecology in which different creatures live alongside the plants that humans wish to grow—and have equal opportunities to reproduce future generations. So, the number one is also a way of expressing plenty, abundance, and diversity, rather than individualism. Notably, the word "rot" indicates that along with growth comes decay and prompts us to think of the regenerative possibilities of compost that are so often at the forefront of gardeners' minds (Haraway 2016).

Lloyd told a story in which technological innovation and commercial investment led to hunger, inequality, biodiversity loss, and the consolidation of power in the hands of an increasingly small few. Saved and open-pollinated seeds represent both an alternative and the precursor to commercially bred seed. Lloyd contrasted the anthropogenic fertility of industrialized agriculture, characterized by the biotechnological model of fertility control, with the more "natural" forms of fertility, characterized by cycles, loops, and ecologies. Lloyd and my research participants see commercially bred seed as embodying capitalist aims of profit maxi-mization and enrichment of the few, with an inclination toward values of restriction, individualization, and limits. We can see this in the way Lloyd used numbers—his declensionist history starts with "billions of slightly different landraces" and arrives at a world in which "ten biotech firms control 73 percent of seeds." Since 2017, this figure has become even starker: now, just four corporations own 60 percent of commercial seeds (Barber 2019; see also MacDonald 2019).[5] As the saying "One for the raven . . ." indicates, open-pollinated seeds only have a 25 percent germi-nation rate, so they are not hyperfertile, but they are "stable and diverse." So, with commercialized breeding, it is not that plants have gone from a state of hyperfertility to infertility but that they have gone from abun-dant diversity to uniformity in the service of stable commodification.[6]

In my conversations with London seed savers, biodiversity relates to greater food security and greater natural abundance:

> JULIE: Diversity means a better resistance; whether it's a virus, or a disease, or anything like that, or a better resistance to the way weather can be very changing here. So, if you'd had only, let's say, one type of tomato in your garden, and then you had a really cold, wet summer—if this tomato is not adapted to it, it will die.
>
> HELENE: I'm actually a writer in food and agriculture and just had no idea about how serious our plant biodiversity situation is in terms of climate change resilience and things like that. And the fact that I think we get 90 percent of our calorific intake globally from ten crop varieties, that is crazy, and we are really playing with fire in quite a big way. And I think we've lost something like 94 percent of our vegetable varieties. That we don't know about that and we don't talk about that every day is astonishing to me and that I had no idea about that. . . . We're just really putting ourselves quite seriously at risk of mass food insecurity in the quite near future.

Both Julie and Helene, who are young White women, both involved with London Freedom Seed Bank, used numbers and quantification to explain why seed saving is vital. Julie discussed how relying on one variety of tomato may well lead to food insecurity when humanity is faced with an unpredictable climate, implying that the more varieties one grows, the more likely it is that one will have a good crop. Helene cited percentages to get across the scale and urgency of both biodiversity loss and people's reliance on corporations for food. Other seed savers have talked about how one plant can contain hundreds of seeds, giving a sense of natural abundance. For example, Janie, who runs a community growing group in south London and is a White woman in her sixties, remarked,

> I love new growth, and seeing that coming through is the most excit-
> ing thing. I love it when the trees, I love the spring flowers, as a kind of
> early beginning. And then when you sow the seeds, it's just magical. That
> that tiny, tiny thing could grow into something so huge. And produce so
> many thousands of seeds itself. And that is the miracle. . . . All of that, in
> that tiny thing. I love that. . . . That there's so much in one seed. So much
> information and so much capacity. And how few seeds we actually need
> to grow our own food.

In these examples, quantity is associated with life, fecundity, and growth. The contrast to this natural plenty is the insecurity of the mono-crop. Seed saving recognizes that the reproduction of a *variety* of plants is vital to survival, which suggests both a sense of humans' interdependence with other species and an understanding that, without reproduction or fertility, whether in soil, plants, or people, there is no future.

Heterotopian Ecologies

Seed-saving practice and activism offer a vision of a different world—a heterotopia (Foucault 1967) that accommodates, rather than eliminates, difference. Heterotopian ecologies are filled with different ideas, values, species, and varieties—worlds in which diversity is abundant and fostering diversity is a critical responsibility for humans. In ecology, "population abundance" is a term that expresses how common particular species are in a selected area—so, effectively, it is another term for population size. The way I am using "abundance" instead picks up on the more colloquial meaning of abundance as plenty. I suggest we think about an abundance of interrelated and interdependent kinds rather than an abundance of individuals. "Abundant diversity" celebrates the wondrous excesses and messy bounties of life. It exhorts us to think about how to rearrange our worlds to foster multiple ways of living rather than limiting the reproduction of particular kinds.

In proposing heterotopian ecologies, I am building on Rosemary-Claire Collard, Jessica Dempsey, and Juanita Sundberg's (2015: 323) "Manifesto for Abundant Futures." They draw attention to the losses in biological variety and abundance that extractive capitalism, fueled by colonialism, has brought about and argue that we should, in response, be striving for "a world filled literally to the brim with different creatures." They conjure a world in which reproduction is not controlled and managed as it has been by colonial regimes or for commercial ends, but instead for a more equal and more diverse world in which fertility can flourish for as many species as possible. This manifesto echoes the aims of reproductive justice (Ross and Solinger 2017), with its attention to the infrastructures that make life possible and impossible for different "kinds," and which urges us to think about reproduction beyond fertility and conception and consider the environments in which people raise and care for kin.

Eva Giraud et al. (2019) consider abundance a "constitutive element of the Anthropocene." They discuss pests, parasites, and pathogens, complicating the hopefulness of some accounts of multispecies kinship in the face of climate change, while pointing out that such "undesirable" life forms are themselves reflective of and entwined with "failed 'technofixes,' colonial legacies, and contemporary inequalities" (Giraud et al. 2019: 357). Thinking about the different abundant life forms that inhabit the earth and their competing needs, rights, and means of survival confronts us with ethical and political questions about what and who is supported to live, reproduce, and thrive. As the saying "One for the raven . . ." suggests, abundance incorporates the positive and negative valences of bounty—the rot alongside the growth. This is why I suggest thinking of these practices as heterotopian rather than utopian. Abundant diversity is a serious muddling along together, an experiment in plenty. Thinking through in-fertility with abundance can allow room for those who do not, cannot, or will not reproduce (biogenetically) (Davis 2015), as well as avoiding easy associations between fertility, growth, productivity, and success.

As stated in the introduction to this book, "The idea that fertility can no longer be taken for granted, and is instead in dire need of help, is one of the reversals that most defines the new reproductive order and its accompanying fertility logics, orientations, and industries" (Franklin and Inhorn, Introduction). Fertility, infertility, and in-fertility all speak to the ideas of "life," "power," and "abundance" that my research participants discussed with me. All of these ideas also relate to temporality. In the twentieth century, fertility was often associated with the future and, in particular, with ideas of scientific progress, rational planning, and economic growth; these ideas were borne out in quite literal ways in the development of industrialized agriculture and seed breeding. The temporality of this way of thinking is linear; it is an ideology in which inputs are tightly controlled and outputs are maximized in number and limited in kind. Seed savers are pushing back against this thinking and the practices that support it through a counterideology of abundant diversity. Simon talked about the similarities between seeds and human gametes, discussing how, with the "right conditions," "out comes life abundance." His reference to conditions is astute—seed savers are striving for abundant diversity, a set of conditions in which multiple species can reproduce alongside each other. He described the "exponential" power encapsulated within a seed—this power is both its inherent fecundity and its ability to support heterotopian ecologies by creating flowers and fruits that other species can eat, reminding us of seed savers' belief that seeds should not only be abundant in their diversity but should be shared with others.

Conclusion

Although open-pollinated seeds have a germination rate of approximately one-quarter, seed savers think of seeds as full of immanent potential. The small, quiet practice of saving seeds may not make much of a dent in the monopolies of the agribusinesses that legally own most seeds or to shift the plantation thinking that sustains them, but it speaks to a vision of a different world and a different future, which I call a heterotopian ecology. Seed saving and its goal of abundant diversity is about resisting a worldview of ever-diminishing possibilities that is epitomized by monocrops.

Reflecting on the myth of Persephone, the ancient Greek queen of the underworld and goddess of spring and nature, who personifies the life cycle of crops grown from seed through her own abduction to the underworld and reemergence with spring, Tracey Hetherington (2021) reminds us not only of the tight relationship between fertility and agriculture, but that fostering not only fertility but biodiversity is crucial to survival in a changing climate in which previously reliable crops may fail. In heterotopian ecologies, fertility and the future are tightly bound, but this is a fertility unfettered by capitalist values like uniformity, hyperproductivity, or individuality. It is, instead, open, shared, and unpredictable. And, as Persephone and "One for the raven . . ." remind us, death is, still, part of the cycle—those seeds that do not grow may still feed birds or rot and enrich the soil.

Many of my research participants described seeds as "life," in an attempt to express the multitude of meanings and the potential encapsulated by these tiny objects. This sense of immanent magic is at once reproductive and earthy; it is an attempt to describe the unknowable process that happens when a small object being planted in soil becomes a full-grown plant, with its own further seeds, emerging (or not). It is also a way of expressing the unfinished nature of seeds, the ways in which they are porous to their environments and conditions. Many made analogies between human children and seeds (and with some interesting temporal slippage between seeds, seedlings, and plants) and spoke of seeds as containing the means to perpetuate the future. But there was also a sense that, while seeds might contain all this miraculous potential within them, this could not be fully controlled by humans, and for many this was part of a seed's magic, or power. Saved and open-pollinated seeds grow out through the generations in a way that eludes total control. But, as Karen said, this sense that humans are not completely in control is part of the magic and the joy: "Is there anything more rewarding than nurturing that seed?"

NOTES

1   Most commercially available seeds are hybrids bred in controlled settings, while open-pollinated seeds are left to pollinate freely. Open-pollinated seeds have more genetic variety and are more suitable for saving than seeds from hybrids.

2   Given the location of this research, I use British terms throughout. For those not familiar with these, British people refer to what Americans call "yards" as "gardens." In London, gardens are often quite small, due to population density and the expense of owning a property large enough to have significant outdoor space. Allotments are areas of land, usually in towns or cities, which are set aside

for growing food crops on a noncommercial basis. They can be found across the United Kingdom (and in other countries, such as Germany, France, and Denmark). They are subdivided into plots that are rented for a small annual fee and tended by individuals, families, or friends. The land is usually owned by local councils, but some are owned and managed by charities. In London, the waiting list for allotments is often several years long. "Community gardens" in the United Kingdom tends to refer to gardens that are communally managed as nonprofit initiatives and that offer space for (food-)growing, but also function as a leisure space for members, local residents, and visitors, though there is sometimes blurring between these and allotments.

3 "Landrace" refers to plants that have been saved and grown out across several generations in a particular location and are considered to be adapted to that location.

4 For more on this, see Müller-Wille and Brandt (2016) and Van Dooren (2007).

5 Despite my last name of Dow, I have no relation to Dow Inc.

6 Notably, "uniformity"—along with "distinctness" and "stability"—is one of the key characteristics that helps determine a seed producer's property rights over a newly bred variety.

REFERENCES

Barber, Dan. 2019. "Save Our Food: Free the Seed." *New York Times*, June 7. www.nytimes.com.

Chacko, Xan Sarah. 2022. "Stringing, Reconnecting, and Breaking the Colonial 'Daisy Chain': From Botanic Garden to Seed Bank." *Catalyst* 8(1): 1–30.

Collard, Rosemary-Claire, Jessica Dempsey, and Juanita Sundberg. 2015. "A Manifesto for Abundant Futures." *Annals of the Association of American Geographers* 105(2): 322–30.

Davis, Heather. 2015. "Toxic Progeny: The Plastisphere and Other Queer Futures." *PhiloSOPHIA* 5(2): 231–50.

Davis, Janae, Alex A. Moulton, Levi Van Sant, and Brian Williams. 2019. "Anthropocene, Capitalocene, . . . Plantationocene? A Manifesto for Ecological Justice in an Age of Global Crises." *Geography Compass* 13(5): 12438.

Dow, Katharine. 2021. "Bloody Marvels: In Situ Seed Saving and Intergenerational Malleability." *Medical Anthropology Quarterly* 35(4): 493–510.

Dow, Katharine, and Sophia Doyle. 2024. "'Saving the Knowledge Helps to Save the Seed': Generating a Collaborative Seed Data Project in London." In *Digital Ecologies: Mediating More-Than-Human Worlds*, eds. Jonathan Turnbull, Adam Searle, Eva Giraud, and Henry Anderson-Eliott. Manchester, UK: Manchester University Press.

Foucault, Michel. 1967. "Of Other Spaces, Heterotopias." *Architecture, Mouvement, Continuité* 5: 46–9.

Giraud, Eva, Eleanor Hadley Kershaw, Richard Helliwell, and Gregory Hollin. 2019. "Abundance in the Anthropocene." *Sociological Review Monographs* 67(2): 357–73.

Haraway, Donna J. 2016. *Staying with the Trouble: Making Kin in the Chthulucene*. Durham, NC: Duke University Press.

Hetherington, Tracey. 2021. "Fertility's Fate: Agrarian Anxieties and the Social Life of Seed." In *Seedways: The Circulation, Control, and Care of Plants in a Warming World*, eds. Bengt G. Karlsson and Annika Rabo, 207–26. Stockholm: KVHAA.

Laing, Olivia. 2018. *Crudo*. New York: Picador.

MacDonald, James M. 2019. "Mergers in Seeds and Agricultural Chemicals: What Happened?" Economic Research Service, U.S. Department of Agriculture, February 15. www.ers.usda.gov.

Müller-Wille, Staffan, and Christina Brandt. 2016. "From Heredity to Genetics: Political, Medical, and Agro-Industrial Contexts." In *Heredity Explored: Between Public Domain and Experimental Science, 1850–1930*, eds. Staffan Müller-Wille and Christina Brandt, 3–25. Cambridge, MA: MIT Press.

OmVed Gardens. N.d. www.omvedgardens.com. Accessed on January 25, 2024.

Pottinger, Laura. 2016. "Planting the Seeds of a Quiet Activism." *Area* 49(2): 215–22.

Ross, Loretta, and Rickie Solinger. 2017. *Reproductive Justice: An Introduction*. Berkeley: University of California Press.

The Seed Saving Network. N.d. https://seedsaving.network/. Accessed on February 5, 2024.

Solnit, Rebecca. 2023. "What If Climate Change Meant Not Doom—but Abundance?" *Washington Post*, March 15.

Tsing, Anna L. 2004. *Friction: An Ethnography of Global Connection*. Princeton, NJ: Princeton University Press.

Van Dooren, Thom. 2007. "Terminated Seed: Death, Proprietary Kinship, and the Production of (Bio)Wealth." *Science as Culture* 16(1): 71–94.

19

Fruitility Activism

Restoring Roots, Branches, and Rot Holes in the
English Orchard Revival

SARAH FRANKLIN

One of the most prominent and powerful examples of the new role
for fertility as a sign of "quality of life"—not just its quantity—is the
increasing overlap between environmental and reproductive activism.
In this chapter, I explore the roots of British orchard activism to offer a
brief case study of how in-fertility idioms and causal reproductive logics are being used to mobilize community activism to protect what are
perceived to be collective social and environmental goods. One of my
objectives is to suggest that the perception of both human and nonhuman fertilities as communal, shared resources with diffuse and enduring
benefits for society is not only, or even primarily, a pre-industrial or
indigenous perspective but an enduring tradition that can be traced
to the very epicenter of industrialization, in the British home counties
from the sixteenth century onward. This is an important way to further
explore the suggestion also made in other chapters of this section that
the new in-fertility politics emerging in the context of rapidly declining
birth rates in the first quarter of the twenty-first century have important
and widespread historical precedents. Indeed, some of these in-fertility
activisms and social-environmental justice movements are quintes-
sentially industrial and modern, with strong roots in local resistance
movements dating back centuries.

English orchards are a particularly useful example of grassroots fertility activism, both because they play such a prominent role in the history of rural communities and because they have become the subject of
a newly explicit fertility-protection campaign in contemporary Britain,

which I would characterize as *fruitility activism*. A nationwide movement to establish, document, revive, and celebrate the unique fertility
of traditional orchards has grown rapidly since the 1990s, supported by
charities and organizations such as the UK Orchard Network, in an attempt to "reverse the decline of orchard crop and biodiversity," as well
as to "promote a wider understanding of the value of orchards . . . to
benefit wildlife, humans and our heritage" (UK Orchard Network n.d.).
Through such networks, local community orchard projects across the
British Isles connect to share resources and establish a focal point for
policy, in particular by planting and restoring community orchards, including increasingly in urban areas such as London. The prominence of
community orchard projects is now evident at a variety of institutional
levels—from schools, churches, universities, and city parks to television
shows, food festivals, and local government.

The County Council of South Cambridgeshire where I live, for example, formally incorporated the preservation of traditional orchards
into its Biodiversity Action Plan in 2009, specifically noting the unique
"biodiversity value" of "old orchards" (South Cambridgeshire County
Council 2009; see also Robertson and Wedge 2008). To aid efforts not
only to restore but revive old orchards, other community- and volunteer-
led charities, such as the East of England Apples and Orchard Project
(EEAOP), have begun to repropagate 250 rare, regional, and endangered
apple varieties by grafting them onto new rootstock, which they now
sell online. Available from early November for seventeen pounds each,
many of these varieties sell out within a month due to their increasing popularity for large and small local orchard projects. I have planted
twenty of these trees in the disused agricultural plot beside our house
and thus have become something of a fruitility activist myself. This has
also enabled me to appreciate the ways in which the new interest in protecting traditional orchards articulates many key elements of emerging
fertility vernaculars. These include the broad links among food, environment, and agriculture described in several chapters of this section, as
well as the connections between these overarching macro-themes and
more personal choices about consumer products, lifestyle, parenting,
diet, and education that constitute the new in-fertility politics we argue
characterize the new reproductive order.

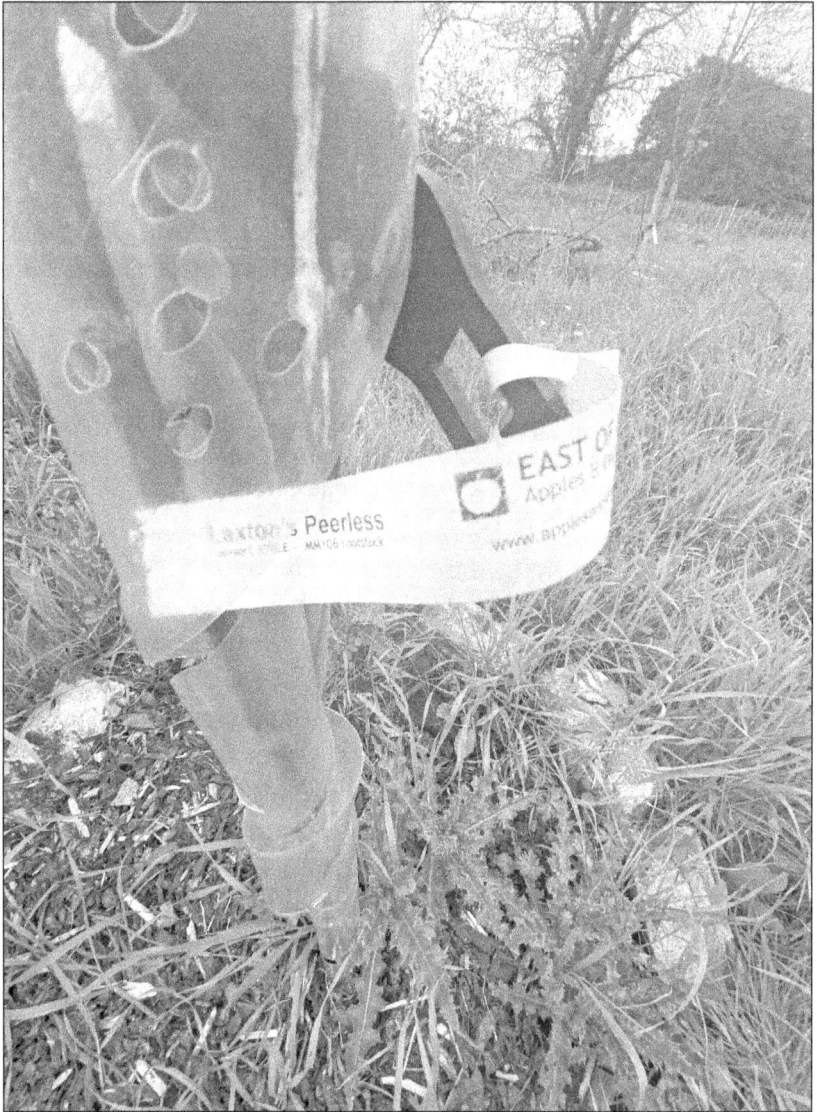

Figure 19.1. Image from Author's Home Orchard. Credit: Picture by Author

It may seem a large leap from the problem of Britain's current fertility woes to the future of the traditional English apple orchard, but as several chapters in this volume suggest, these links are more intuitive than they seem. Indeed, the connections between the history of the English apple tree and the future of UK demography arguably belong to a new form of common sense that is increasingly legible and logical—as well as pervasive. The new fertility vernaculars of species loss, birth strikes, and organic produce join together concerns about reproductive health, environmental justice, and social inequality. In the new in-fertility logics connecting plastic bags to falling birth rates, an explicit calculus of reproductive cause and effect links consumer waste to low sperm counts and premature reproductive aging. These new in-fertility vernaculars—or "grammars," to use Chaparro-Buitrago's term (chapter 15)—not only link economic, political, and social activities and values to reproductive outcomes but also help to articulate alternative reproductive options and hopes as well as activisms. Tracing these changing perceptions of reproductive causality, and demonstrating how very broadly encompassing this analytic perspective quickly becomes, is one of the main objectives of this volume.

By adopting this approach, we are not only "dragging reproduction to the center" by arguing that neither fertility nor reproduction is a narrow topic. We further propose that a new reproductive order is in the process of emerging in which "fertility figures," "fertility grammars," and "fertility symbols" are becoming increasingly dense and sticky, as well as powerful, signifiers in social, cultural, and political life. In the new reproductive order, fertility is no longer a simple metric, or demographic concern—or even any particular number or rate associated with national or economic concerns, such as supplying the labor market, supporting the elderly, or populating rural areas. Increasingly, fertility has become, to use Donna Haraway's (2016) words, a means of "worlding"—meaning that it represents a question mark about what kind of world people want to live in in the future, and how to get there. In this chapter, I explore one kind of world—full of delicious apples and fruitility activism—as it plays out in the English countryside.

Orchard Activism: An Apple a Day?

Apple Days are a good place to start to appreciate the ways in which the movement to restore community orchards articulates a range of connections between a specific activity and a wider set of social and cultural values, and also how these connections are politicized through a form of collective in-fertility consciousness raising. The increasingly popular Apple Days that now take place across the United Kingdom in October combine practical, economic, and educational purposes with recreational, cultural, and celebratory activities in much the same way that orchards have been home to a mix of community and social functions for centuries (Williamson 2020). The popular option of bringing apples to be identified at an Apple Day by expert fruit breeders in places like the Cambridge Botanical Garden simultaneously acts as a means of preserving and enhancing horticultural heritage and diversity, and sharing the rich apple lore that has been cultivated on Cambridgeshire soil to yield varieties such as Histon Favourite, Cockett's Red, Barnack Beauty, and the Perfection apple bred in Bluntisham in 1960. Apple Days are promoted by local schools and horticultural societies, as well as by the County Council and the University of Cambridge, to increase awareness about the environment and local history, and thus promote environmentally friendly food production, the recognition and protection of local biodiversity, an appreciation of soil structure, and an awareness of decarbonization and its connection to these issues.

All of these topics have a particular significance in the English home counties, such as Bedfordshire, Hertfordshire, Essex, Kent, and Cambridgeshire, which are famous for their prolific orchards (Masset 2012). The rich legacy of orchard cultivation for which these regions are known combines commercial fruit growing with domestic gardening and the integration of many fruit-related activities into the seasonal calendar, year-round. Considered neither strictly agricultural nor woodland, orchards have for centuries occupied a special status in the minds, villages, hearts, and homes of the residents of the British countryside. They are both agricultural and domestic, cultivated and wild, and often physically located in between residential buildings and arable fields. Often enclosed, orchards were places of merriment, celebration, leisure, and ritual activity, as well as of productive horticultural cultivation—in both village small-holdings and large estates. Year round, the care and tending of orchards is intimately interwoven with all aspects of domestic life—from eating and drinking orchard products to heating the home with firewood collected from pruning and feeding domestic livestock with leftover fruit, leaves, and mash. Birds, bees, butterflies, and iconic British mammals such as hedgehogs, dormice, and badgers thrive in the orchard environment, while also churning and fertilizing its uniquely rich soil. Orchard activities such as cider making help shape the annual farming cycle and are enmeshed with folklore and tradition, as well as seasonal rituals, such as the autumn decoration of Green Men, the Corn Queen for the harvest, and the Flower Festivals in May. Many of these festivals are explicitly, and one might even say abundantly, concerned with fruitility.

Fruitility Value

Biologically and culturally, as well as economically, orchards are perceived as uniquely fertile in several senses. Home to a huge variety of flora and fauna, orchards are increasingly heralded for their exceptionally biodiverse environments, which regularly support more than double the average number of species of woodlands, rivers, fields, bogs, heath, or even ponds. The fertility of orchards is, moreover, multidimensional in terms not only of time and space but of kind and type, linking the reproductive lives of insects, birds, mammals, trees, and humans with those of micro-organisms, including fungi—all feeding into the constant cyclical churn of digestion, decomposition, and metabolic exchange that stokes the fertility of the all-important orchard soil. On its website, the People's Trust for Endangered Species (PTES), a UK organization founded in 1977, showcases the diversity of old orchards on a special page dedicated to "Orchard Habitat." "Traditional orchards," it notes, "contain a mosaic of habitats important to wildlife and provide food, shelter and breeding sites for many different species" (People's Trust for Endangered Species n.d.).

The unique fertility value of the orchard as a "mosaic habitat" is built up not only through the accumulated activities and deposits from a variety of flora and fauna (nesting birds, pollinating insects, bat poo, rotting wood, and worm holes), or even their accumulated and often symbiotic interactions (all linked to the mycorhizomal web connecting all the trees), or the physics of seasonal adjustments (frost, circadian cycles, high winds). A key element in the fertility value of the mosaic orchard habitat is the interconnectedness of the multiple regenerative

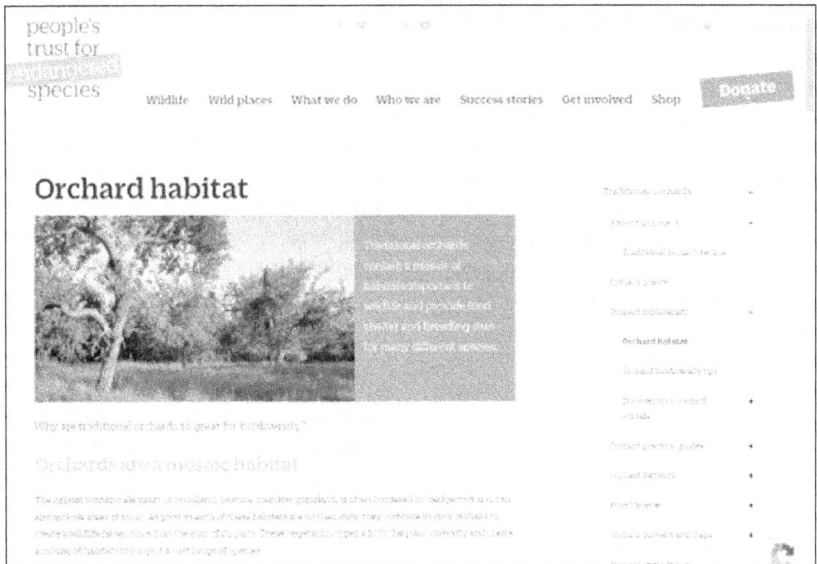

Figure 19.2. The People's Trust for Endangered Species, one of Britain's oldest country-side protection charities, dedicates an entire section of its website to traditional orchard preservation. Credit: People's Trust for Endangered Species (n.d.)

feedback loops that work on short-, medium-, and long-term cycles: the flash-in-the-pan mating cycles of moths that are embedded in the seasonal flowering cycle of wild meadows that are in turn supported by the centuries-long life cycles of trees, hedges, and orchards themselves—each cycle as interdependent on the others as the birds and the bees are on the nectar whose sweet exchanges yield the thumping rain of fat apples that fall to the ground by the thousands every autumn.

In addition to being ecological "mosaics," orchards are valued as a kind of fertility combinatorium, mixing together woodland, pasture, meadow, grassland, hedgerow, and scrub habitats on a single site. The richness of the orchard ecosystem is amplified by the bio-engine of standing dead wood in old orchards, where trees as much as a century old "veteranize" and senesce, hollowing out into roomy, cavernous rot houses that shelter a vast array of busy inhabitants (Grüebler et al. 2013). Formerly perceived as useless relics of once-productive orchards, ancient decaying fruit trees have emerged as fertility heroes, acquiring a newly exalted status in the age of mass extinctions. Covered with nooks and crannies on their rough exterior bark, these trees are riven with cozy rot holes that boost microbial activity while providing nutrients and support for rare species of lichen, mold, and moss that crave their humid microclimates. Old apple trees offer "an incredible habitat for all manner of invertebrates, fungi, birds, bats and other small mammals" that in turn interact with the surrounding plants, shrubs, trees, and soil (People's Trust for Endangered Species n.d.). Their appeal to so many coresidents further benefits the orchard ecology through the generative waste the visitors leave behind; the insect, animal, and bird deposits, feathers, bones, shells, carcasses, and other detritus that litter the ground and gradually feed into the rich regenerative soil cycles, which are especially biophilic because the orchard detritus, clutter, and decay are not "tidied up," as the wheatfields or coppiced woodlands are, instead being left to rot. Indeed, it is the extensive copresence of death and decay with regenerative processes of germination and sustenance that creates the unique multispecies fertility cycles for which old orchards are so highly prized. According to the PTES website, "Aging trees naturally die-back (senesce) and begin to hollow out, helping them to remain standing, recycling nutrients and ultimately thriving for longer. Dead and decaying wood, therefore, does not necessarily mean that a tree is in poor health. It will still be able to survive and produce fruit for many years to come whilst providing valuable habitat" (People's Trust for Endangered Species n.d.).

At once an embodiment and a symbol of biodiversity, the traditional apple orchard has come to be seen as a new "fertility figure," in Wahlberg's terms (chapter 6), celebrated as a new horticultural superpower in the era of both climate change and cost-of-living increases. Orchards have reemerged from their sleepy rural state of neglect as new community projects helping to energize a social contract linking local food production, increased environmental protection, and ecological awareness in new, ethical fertility chains of both logic and practice.

Rural Rides

The formation of bio-conscious community groups such as the PTES in the 1970s corresponded to a significant shift in British public perceptions of land management and the rural landscape more generally, as the alleged benefits of industrial agriculture began to give way to concerns about the

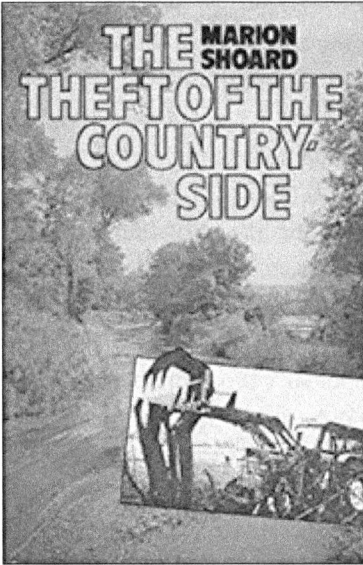

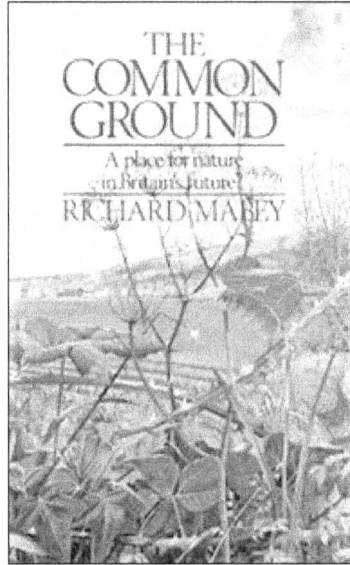

Figures 19.3 and 19.4. Two Best-Selling Books Published in 1980 by Marion Shoard and Richard Mabey That Helped to Catalyze the Countryside Protection Movement in the United Kingdom to Protest against the "Sterile Landscapes" Associated with Industrial Agriculture

ecological damage caused by the heavy use of pesticides, herbicides, and fertilizers. Marion Shoard's (1980) *Theft of the Countryside* was one of the leading publications to expose the hidden costs of the agricultural subsidies that allowed farmers to profit from turning the countryside into food factories at the expense of wildlife, meadows, rivers, and open land.

Shoard's best-selling book alleged that British taxpayers were unwittingly funding the destruction of one of their most valuable economic assets; she proposed a number of specific remedies, such as the establishment of countryside planning authorities. Without better protection of rural landscapes, she warned, the unique character of the English countryside would be destroyed by a runaway agricultural obsession with efficiency and profit that would transform rural England into a featureless and sterile landscape.

In the same year that Shoard's book cover prominently featured a tractor savagely destroying a hedgerow, nature writer Richard Mabey

(1980) published his now-iconic plea for British rural landscape preservation, *The Common Ground: A Place for Nature in Britain's Future?* This searing account of the destruction of vast swathes of British countryside in the name of economic progress ran to twelve editions between 1980 and 1993 and catalyzed the formation of the first rural protection organizations such as the PTES. Documenting the relentless destruction of the British countryside in the postwar period, the book offered a forensic and excoriating account of the terminal and cumulative losses of wildlife, birds, meadows, plants, ancient ecosystems, and other irreplaceable natural assets caused by industrial farming. At every level, from the economic and environmental to the aesthetic and historical, Mabey (1980) catalogued the damage and tallied up the costs. His book helped establish the principle of connecting communities to nature conservation and landscape preservation that has since become an entrenched feature of British law, governance, and policy.

Orchards do not feature in either Shoard's or Mabey's books, and they largely escaped the notice of conservationists during the 1980s and the 1990s, in part because they are so closely linked to agricultural production. Indeed, the expansion of orchard cultivation from the middle of the nineteenth century onward was a form of industrialization that had much in common with other branches of modern agriculture and the birth of "factory farming," including new techniques of plant breeding and orchard design to maximize the yield from smaller, more productive dwarf trees that could be more easily harvested to produce higher profits.

It was during the twentieth century that the creation, cultivation, and refinement of English orchards peaked in areas of the country, such as Cambridgeshire, that became known for their vast orchards and associated industries (Barnes and Williamson 2022). The new "orchard counties" both supported extensive local fruit preservation industries and supplied both large cities and overseas distributors with freshly picked produce by rail. With support from the British government and investment in more intensive cultivation practices, including heavy use of insecticides and pesticides and the use of dwarfing rootstalk to create smaller trees, UK production of orchard fruit increased to nearly 275,000 acres by 1950. Fewer types of apples were grown on more and faster-growing trees in tightly packed commercial orchards that became, in effect, Taylorized fruit factories supplying world-famous companies such as Tiptree, Robertson's, Coopers, Wilkins & Sons, and Chivers.

Older, unmodernized, and "worn out" traditional orchards came to be seen both as increasingly unproductive and even as commercially wasteful while the increase in international trade reduced demand overall for British soft fruit from the 1960s onward. By the 1970s the government was firmly advocating the use of only seven varieties of apple and the grubbing out of unproductive orchards to make way for more profitable and efficient food production. By 1990, more than 90 percent of British orchards—old and new—had been destroyed in the name of national economic progress (Macdonald and Gates 2020).

An Apple a Day . . .

Already by the late 1980s, however, the fragments of remaining old orchards were beginning to acquire an important new set of functions. The first Apple Day, commemorating the rebirth of the orchard as an aesthetic, communal, and environmental asset, was held in 1990. By the early twenty-first century, the restoration of old orchards had begun to gain additional favor through a host of new links to key government priorities, such as improving public health and nutrition, greening urban areas by creating city farms, growing food more locally and with fewer energy costs, protecting biodiversity, and preserving local traditions and landscapes. Apple advocates began to emerge as not only social, economic, and environmental heroes but cutting-edge problem solvers for everything from reducing antisocial activity to stimulating economic growth. By 2020, the UK-wide Orchard Project had declared its goal "for every household in the UK's towns and cities to be within walking distance of a productive, well-cared for, community run orchard" (Orchard Project n.d.).

This new fruitility activism is not only future oriented, however. With increased attention to the iconic role of the apple tree in literature, folklore, and rural tradition comes a renewed appreciation of the ancient role of orchards as places to celebrate seasonal changes and the harvest. Rural rituals such as "wassailing" in January, when village processions celebrate the vital contribution apples make to good health (as well as hard cider), are being revived in urban centers such as London as well

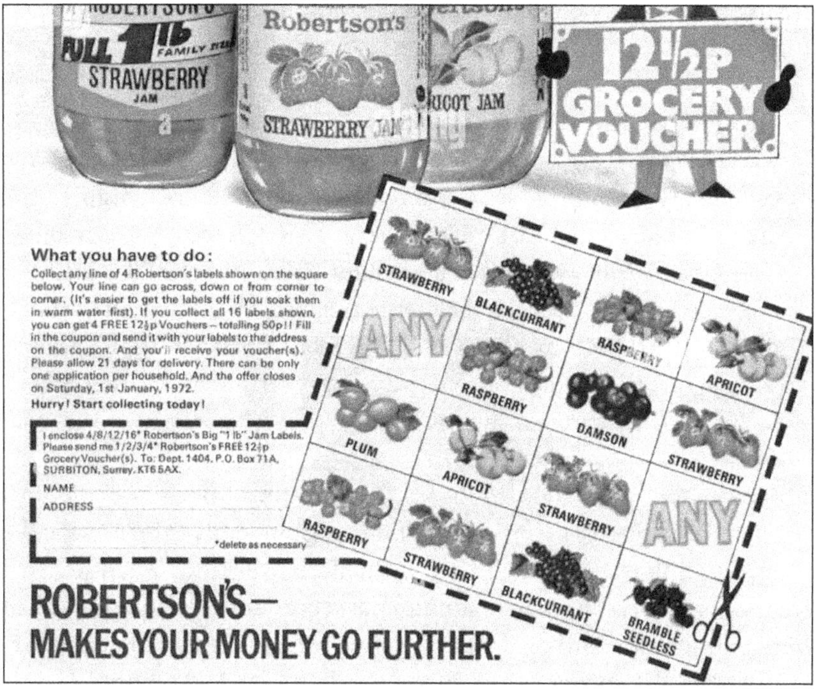

Figure 19.5. A 1972 Magazine Ad for Robertson's Food Products. Large fruit-processing companies such as Tiptree and Robinson were still harvesting from thousands of acres of orchards in the 1970s, but by the end of the 1980s, 90 percent of British orchards had been deemed agriculturally useless and "grubbed out"—i.e., destroyed.

as in the countryside. Media coverage of such events has become an autumn staple, with online sites such as tradfolk.com and cideruk.com, as well as national television news stations and mainstream newspapers, extolling the lost arts of apple orchard cultivation and merriment.

Although traditionally associated with the countryside, the revival of traditional orchards and the planting of new community gardens and fruit trees now plays an equally important role in cities across the United Kingdom, where they not only provide spaces for outdoor activity and supply fresh food to inner cities but also serve as symbols of community care, environmental awareness, economic "leveling up," post-COVID "building back better," and social justice (Clifford and King 2011). As the Orchard Project explains on its website in a blog on racial justice from director Kath Rosen, the value of the urban orchard is important not only to the nation's health and recovery but to its rich multicultural past, its unique horticultural traditions, and its ongoing struggle to overcome racial injustice:

> We work primarily in cities—the most racially diverse parts of the UK—where we aim for every household to be within walking distance of a community orchard. . . . It's worth noting that the UK's rich history of orchards stems from racially diverse beginnings. It is only thanks to the work of indigenous farming communities across the world that traditional orchards exist: apples themselves originate from Kazakhstan and the skill of grafting came from China. Our modern and heritage UK fruit varieties are the product of generations of observations, tending, and stewardship from growers in the UK and beyond. (Rosen n.d.)

From this point of view, orchards are not only "mosaic" ecological habitats but both emblems and literal embodiments of the productive intermingling of diverse cultural influences over time. Each orchard tree not only preserves and continues but reproduces a unique history of human migration and diversity, as well as skill and accumulated expertise, within the communities surrounding them. The orchard is thus more than a simile, or even synecdoche; it is instead a living testament to all these influences, which are carried forward through its own fruit and fertility. In this way, orchards and their communities are imagined to cultivate one another. As the Orchard Project director's blog goes on to emphasize, orchard planting regenerates this same relation for the future: "We are passionate about celebrating local distinctiveness and diversity. Every orchard is as unique as the community it supports. When we design a new orchard with a local group, we choose varieties and species of fruit that both reflect local history (like the Hounslow Wonder that was developed in that area) and the people who live there now" (Rosen n.d.). This analogy between communities of trees, communities of people, legacies of cultural diaspora, and contemporary cosmopolitan multiculturalism is extended to biodiverse ecosystems: "There is huge strength in diversity, both for people and for wildlife. It is curious how many of the ecological benefits we talk about in regards to community orchards are often mirrored in the communities who benefit from them. The underground network of mycorrhizal fungi that connect all the trees above them, sharing nutrients and providing mutual protection, are, like the network of people connecting around the trees, stronger by working and being together" (Rosen n.d.). The Orchard Project's ambitious goal mentioned above, of every UK household being within walking distance of a community orchard, is about more than health and well-being, or even environmental safeguarding and biodiversity preservation. It is not only about wildlife, trees, and birds—or rare lichens, saproxylic insects, and the booster-effect of tree hollows. The community vision connected to the orchard community has become one that is not only diverse, inclusive, sustainable, and resilient but serves as a model of and for the "societies we desperately need" and that better reflects the needs of the communities of which orchards are a part.

> We still have a lot of work to do and are still learning. At the moment we are completing feasibility work with new partners, who are black or global majority led, to develop orchard programmes that better reflect need in these communities. We know we have a long way to go in terms of truly addressing racial injustice through our work and also that we may not always get things right. But we are led by a vision that as a biodiverse orchard system teaming with wildlife is much more resilient, so are diverse organisations. We need everyone's voices, strengths and solutions to help create the equitable, resilient, sustainable societies we desperately need. (Rosen n.d.)

Crucially, then, the orchard is at once a model of community and a community project—a model of interactive, codependent, reciprocal care, productivity, and survival. This new emphasis on fruitility ethics was recently proposed as a possible basis for new legislation empowering communities to register lot communal assets, such as old orchards, for protection (Walker 2023). The frutility ethos has at the same time, and unsurprisingly, also become a significant market trend (Keech 2017; Sharpies 2003). New products, such as cider made from community contributions of apples that would otherwise go to waste, further embody the emphasis on cocreating new solutions.

In the same way that fruitility consciousness has mobilized community activism to save old orchards, where newly planted saplings from rare older varieties of apple come to literally embody the mosaic

Figure 19.6 and Figure 19.7. Screenshots of Hawkes London Website. The UK Orchard Project works in partnership with craft cideries such as Hawkes to combine food waste reduction and carbon-negative production in the manufacture and marketing of ethical products such as "Urban Orchard" cider.

histories of the communities around them, so too it is now possible to imbibe these histories as newly branded orchard products packaged to provide urban apple cider in a can.

Conclusion

The codependence of the birds and the bees, the pollinating insects and the flowering apple buds, the decomposing wood and the nesting bats, whose poop energizes the soil micro-flora and algae communities, as well as earthworms burrowing beneath the surface of the wildflower meadows decorating the old apple orchard offer not only a mosaic model for community, resilience, or biodiversity—but also of fertility, or what I have described here as fruitility. The carefully cultivated fertility of fruit orchards, which, like maize or wheat, cannot retain their most highly productive form without near-continuous human tending, is itself a product, something that must be made as well as maintained. In turn, and unsurprisingly, the cultivation of orchards, as well as orchards themselves, become symbols of human fertility—both individual and collective, as well as cultural and horticultural.

The use of orchards for weddings is another growing trend, echoing the long-standing association of mistletoe—an orchard flower—with romance and fertility, but now with fruitility as well. This transfer of the orchard idiom to marriage and conjugal fertility, as well as communal, collective, and ecological regeneration, is a helpful and timely reminder that fertility is not always imagined as individual, biological, or medical—even in its most familiar human form. An important aspect of the new eco-cultural turn toward old orchards is the way in which changing perceptions of their reproductive complexity not only attribute greater value to their intersectional fruitilities but engender new practices, behaviors, and possibilities. Community orchards represent a collectivized investment in regeneration that in turn articulates a wide range of intersecting social, ethical, and cultural values. New definitions of economic cost and benefit are branches of the same apple tree that yields a model of future social justice, urban renewal, and community diversity. The celebration of old orchards as symbols of an altered awareness of the causes of human economic, environmental, and social precarity—and prosperity—reverses the previous perception of them as useless and uneconomical. It reconstitutes standing dead veteranized apple trees as consciousness-raising tools in the battle against climate change, overconsumption, and eco-blindness. Here, in the old—and renewed—orchard, a vision of a fertility multiverse, and of the regenerative bio-churn of old, dead wood into new life, provides an antidote to the heavy headlines about rising sea levels and extinction rates. Here, among the out-of-date apples, the neglected varieties, the parasitic fungi, and the nesting beetles is nothing short of a fertility paradise—bursting into bloom beneath the bright blue sky.

REFERENCES

Barnes, Gerry, and Tom Williamson. 2022. *English Orchards: A Landscape History*. Oxford: Oxbow Books.

Clifford, Susan, and Angela King. 2011. *Community Orchards Handbook*. New York: Bloomsbury.

Grüebler, Martin U., Sabrina Schaller, Herbert Keil, and Beat Naef-Daenzer. 2013. "The Occurrence of Cavities in Fruit Trees: Effects of Tree Age and Management on Biodiversity in Traditional European Orchards." *Biodiversity and Conservation* 22: 3233–46.

Haraway, Donna J. 2016. *Staying with the Trouble: Making Kin in the Chthulucene*. Durham, NC: Duke University Press.

Keech, Daniel. 2017. "Social Enterprises with Environmental Objectives: Saving Traditional Orchards in England and Germany." *Geographical Journal* 183(2): 164–74.

Mabey, Richard. 1980. *The Common Ground: A Place for Nature in Britain's Future?* London: Hutchinson.

Macdonald, Benedict, and Nicholas Gates. 2020. *Orchard: A Year in England's Eden*. London: William Collins.

Masset, Claire. 2012. *Orchards*. London: Bloomsbury Publishing.

Orchard Network. N.d. www.orchardnetwork.org.uk. Accessed on February 5, 2024.

People's Trust for Endangered Species. N.d. https://ptes.org. Accessed on February 5, 2024.

Robertson, Heather, and Chris Wedge. 2008. "Traditional Orchards and the UK Biodiversity Action Plan." In *Orchards and Groves: Their History, Ecology, Culture, and Archaeology*, ed. Ian D. Rotherham, 109–18. Devon, UK: Wildtrack Publishing.

Rosen, Kath. N.d. "Racial Justice and Community Orchards." The Orchard Project. www.theorchardproject.org.uk. Accessed on February 5, 2024.

Sharpies, Ann Elizabeth. 2003. "Cider and the Marketing of the Tourism Experience in Somerset, England: Three Case Studies." *Journal of Travel & Tourism Marketing* 14(3–4): 49–60.

Shoard, Marion. 1980. *The Theft of the Countryside*. London: Temple Smith.

South Cambridgeshire County Council. 2009. *Biodiversity Action Plan*. www.scambs. gov.uk.

Walker, Fergus. 2023. "Community Orchards: Tragedy or Victory of the Commons." The Orchard Project. www.theorchardproject.org.uk.

Williamson, Tom. 2020. "English Orchards in History: Production, Aesthetics, and Myth." *Studies in the History of Gardens & Designed Landscapes* 40(3–4): 197–215.

Afterword

In-Fertilities in the New Reproductive Order

ADITYA BHARADWAJ

The notion of "in-fertilities" reverberates with potential, teeming with conceivability that is lively in its seeming stillness. In-fertilities alter imaginaries, practices, and experiences of the human in-capacity to reproduce selves and others. The notion of in-fertilities—explicitly plural—also instantiates an interplay of presences and absences awaiting reproduction, thus exposing the fuzzy boundary between an imagination of a fertile presence and an infertile absence. In-fertilities are profoundly phenomenological. The experience of each—absence (infertility/fertility) and presence (fertility/infertility)—typifies the other. It is in the presence of one that we confront the absence of the other, thus rendering the absent present, locatable, tangible, and impactful. In-fertilities as a conceptual arc shape the extensive research featured in this epic volume. This majestic book heralds the dawn of a new era in which human reproduction and its experience transcend crass biopolitical enumeration, ideological prescription, and banal measurement. The new reproductive order straddles both a willful expression and an ethical assertion—for instance, a simultaneous celebration of child-free living and proactive "quest for conception"; devastating critiques of egregious medicalization as well as a determined embrace of a dazzling array of technological mediations; political resistance and critique and socio-political mobilization.

The idea of in-fertilities structuring the new reproductive order must also be read as an invitation to examine the kinds of structures, ideas, and norms we consider reproducing. For instance, how might we conceive and embrace "new" kinds of motherhoods? That is, how might the recreated sense of maternal connection appear in the absence of the notion of motherhood, a concept seemingly (irreversibly) tainted by structural patriarchy? Under what conditions could configurations of queer kinship, for instance as exemplified by gay fatherhood, assert their independence from ideologically prescriptive terminology, such as "dad" and "father"? As Michel Foucault may have averred, What new can emerge in its place, take its place? This quest may stimulate other provocations: instead of creating something new, can we approach the idea of reproduction in a different manner and resist the allure of novelty altogether? That is, can we envision the new reproductive order as a quintessential supplement, one that replaces and also adds? But, how do we make sense of this absent newness in the face of a time-tested anthropological truism—that reproduced difference births newness?

This question gains salience as we pause to consider in-fertilities in contexts and formations, variously conceived as Third World, developing world, resource-poor settings, or "other cultures." Here, too, as in the Euro-American formations, fertility is valorized and sacralized in equal measure. In these settings, the biopolitical overreach often stigmatizes certain kinds of fertilities as a premodern pathology and family planning as a modernist panacea. The imagined traditions become ever more deeply embedded in local communities, only to ostracize infertility as a fertile failure. Once we begin outlining the cultural contours of marginalized lives infected with infertile stigma, coproduced by health policy neglect and socially entrenched prejudice, we begin to better appreciate the complex ways in which reproductive precarity becomes stratified in-fertility. Perhaps it is worth asking, What kind of new reproductive futures will become further stratified and despised in the new reproductive order? In the meantime, the in-fertilities of the dispossessed and the marginal, especially those enduring violent cycles of climatic change, wars, displacement, and extreme levels of socioeconomic peril, will routinely appear and disappear, announcing their presence with deafening clarity.

The new reproductive order demands a new ethicality, one that unremittingly interrogates the conditions under which persons, communities, and international orders enact, reject, and/or embrace infertilities. In this, we must remain attentive to the new conditions that are fomented into existence. Most importantly, this new ethicality also means enacting and embracing a different (new) kind of politics and asking, How can we then liberate ourselves from ideological demands imposed on us by the very notion of reproduction, without giving up on reproducing? How might we clasp onto in-fertilities as the only potent act of resistance in the face of a crass pro- and antinatalist bio-politicization?

This book is a giant leap in this new direction. It remains fully attentive to the irony implicit in heralding the "new" and acknowledging the new demands it imposes on us. It is a spectacular distillation of decades spent at the forefront of reproductive scholarship, as well as the front line of reproductive politics. The editors of this landmark volume have transformed the field of anthropology of reproductive in-fertilities. Thanks to this unwavering commitment—and the conceptual bravura and ethnographic splendor inscribed in the chapters of this opus—we now see much more clearly how to begin the process of extricating infertility and fertility—"in-fertilities"—from an unproductive binary entrapment sunk in an oppositional quicksand. This shift also behooves us to explore how we might better decipher and reconceive the absent presences and present absences that undergird the structural foundations of human reproduction. The book convincingly shows how the late liberal separation between infertility and fertility has now truly departed. This movement will likely herald monumental shifts as the world slips into a new reproductive order, one in which the interplay of biology and ecology birth unprecedented scientific and social challenges for the discipline of biomedicalized "gyn-ecology." The scientific texture and structure of reproductive knowledge must now converse with environmental and food sciences just as the structures underlying the discipline of demography must confront its cooptation as a scribe to the biopolitical logics of neoliberal governance.

More fundamentally, the notion of the new reproductive order brilliantly captures the emerging resistance toward, and appraisal of, a well-established neoliberal perichoresis: state, capital, science. Similarly, a critical alignment among desire, choice, and consumption typifies the new reproductive order. While this configuration is producing unprecedented opportunities for action and expression, the triumvirate of state, capital, and science is also proffering staggering opportunities to profit from child desire and instrumentalize (and monetize) choice as a culturally mediated imperative.

The dazzling array of scholars in this volume who together announce the new reproductive order through their committed scholarship have truly ignited this heartfelt endeavor. This masterful, erudite tome, bunting together a spectacular range of offerings, pushes us to also receive what the editors eruditely unpack and explain as "reproductive cause and effect," or the alterations in perceptions, pursuits, and experiences of reproductivity, both individually and collectively.

In this respect this book is so much more than a harbinger of a new reproductive order. It firmly establishes in-fertilities as forever emerging from global disorders; cooked in a cauldron of unprecedented sociopolitical heat; altered, perhaps irreversibly, in a climate of rapid change; swept up in a wave of emerging queer configurations and relationalities; and ensconced in new bio-political configurations as yet unknowable. In other words, new in-fertilities in a new world order.

ACKNOWLEDGMENTS

All anthologies require special teams, and this one has had the support of an international cast of supporters for over a decade. Each chapter of this book was authored by a member of the Changing In-Fertilities Project (CIFP), codirected from 2014 to 2024 by Sarah Franklin in the Department of Sociology at the University of Cambridge and Marcia C. Inhorn in the Department of Anthropology at Yale University. We are grateful to the Wellcome Trust [Grant 209839/Z/17/Z], which generously funded our ambitious global research program from 2018 to 2022, as well as our public outreach program during this same period [Grant 209839/Z/17/Z]. A further Open Access publication grant was funded by the Trust in 2024.

We are especially grateful to the Reproductive Sociology (ReproSoc) Research Group, located in the Department of Sociology at the University of Cambridge and directed by Professor Franklin, for hosting and supporting the CIFP during its initial development, the research activities it funded, and the preparation of this volume. Formative international CIFP conferences were held at Yale in 2015, at Yale-NUS College (YNC) in Singapore in 2019, and at Cambridge in 2018 and 2022. We are grateful to all three universities for their support, and in particular to ReproSoc administrators Lois Gibbs and Chantal Novak of Cambridge for their logistical genius. At Yale, Jennifer DeChello, Marleen Cullen, Cristin Siebert, and Marwa Khaboor provided invaluable conference support, as did numerous staff members at YNC, where President Joanne Roberts deserves special thanks for her generous financial support of our spectacular Singapore CIFP conference.

We also want to thank the remarkable team of forty international scholars from sixteen different countries who contributed to the work of the CIFP—many of whom were part of this project from its inception, and roughly half of whom are included in this volume. The work represented in the nineteen brilliant chapters that make up this volume is based not only on pathbreaking field research across the globe but on a uniquely collegial, collaborative, creative, and caring team effort. Thanks must go to all the study participants and collaborators on almost every continent who made this research possible. Without their willingness to participate, this comparative in-fertility research project would never have been possible.

Within months of having held our highly successful in-person conference in Singapore in the autumn of 2019, we found ourselves in the midst of an unprecedented global epidemic, with all its draconian restrictions and pervasive uncertainties. It was a great relief to discover that online research collaboration was not only possible but could be even more inclusive, accessible, and rewarding than face-to-face meetings. For many of us, our CIFP Zoom room became one of the key places where we could reboot, refresh, and take stock at our monthly meetings hosted by Professor Franklin between 2019 and 2023.

The process of producing this book has been a source of great joy. We thank Jennifer Hammer, senior editor at New York University Press, who spurred us on with her initial interest, an advanced contract, careful reading of our manuscript, and always constructive editorial comments. We also thank the anonymous reviewers—plus one nonanonymous reviewer, Professor Rayna Rapp, a true icon in the world of feminist reproductive anthropology—for incredibly helpful and constructive suggestions for revision. Bonnie Rose Schulman did a heroic job of compiling and copyediting this volume twice, both before and after the book was revised and submitted. Without her expert guidance, submission of the final manuscript would not have been as seamless. Larry Sweazy did a masterful job of indexing this large book, with all of its chapters. We also thank Emily Wright for her superb copyediting, and the entire production staff at NYU Press, particularly Alexia Traganas, for bringing this book to fruition. The NYU Press design team created the striking cover featuring the celestially beautiful work of Gina Glover, an artist focusing on the new reproductive order.

ABOUT THE CONTRIBUTORS

ADITYA BHARADWAJ is Professor and Chair of Anthropology and Sociology at the Graduate Institute of International and Development Studies, Geneva. His principal research interest is in the area of assisted reproductive, genetic, and stem cell biotechnologies and their rapid spread in diverse global locales. He is the author or coauthor of four books, including *Conceptions: Infertility and Procreative Technologies in India* (2016) and *Global Perspectives on Stem Cell Technologies* (2017).

DAPHNA BIRENBAUM-CARMELI is Professor at the Faculty of Social Welfare and Health Sciences in the Department of Nursing at the University of Haifa. Her interests focus on the political and social implications of medical technologies, especially gender, health, and the politics of reproductive medicine. Her research concentrates on reproduction-related issues and the interface of health care and state politics. She is the author of *Tel Aviv North: The Making of a New Israeli Middle Class* (2000).

MWENZA BLELL is a Senior Lecturer in the School of Geography, Politics, and Sociology at Newcastle University. Her interest in biosocial medical anthropology focuses on data-driven health research and technological development, particularly the sociopolitical contexts in which new health data technologies and ethical and governance infrastructures are situated.

JULIETA CHAPARRO-BUITRAGO is a Wellcome Trust early career fellow in Reproductive Sociology at the University of Cambridge. Her work builds on the interdisciplinary fields of fertility studies, decolonial feminisms, reproductive justice, and Latin American studies. Her research probes long-standing colonial structures, whether through fertility control or exposure to contaminants, that shape indigenous and peasant women's reproductive lives.

KATHARINE DOW is an independent researcher and writer. She was previously Senior Research Associate in Sociology and Deputy Director of the Reproductive Sociology Research Group (ReproSoc) at the University of Cambridge. Her main research interests are the ethical questions provoked by reproduction and assisted reproductive technologies and the interconnections between concerns about the environment and reproduction. She is the author of *Making a Good Life: An Ethnography of Nature, Ethics, and Reproduction* (2016).

NANA OKURA GAGNÉ is a cultural anthropologist at the Graduate School of Asia-Pacific Studies, Waseda University, Tokyo, Japan. She formerly taught in the Department of Japanese Studies at the Chinese University of Hong Kong. Her research explores how global capitalism impinges upon local ideologies and existing sociocultural relations, including gender relations, family relations, and socioeconomic relations. She is the author of *Reworking Japan: Changing Men at Work and Play under Neoliberalism*, and she has published in *American Ethnologist, Anthropological Theory, Ethnography*, and the *Journal of Contemporary Asia*.

TRUDIE GERRITS is Emeritus Associate Professor in the Anthropology Department at the University of Amsterdam. Her research focuses on reproduction, and particularly infertility and assisted reproductive technologies in sub-Saharan Africa and the Netherlands. She is the author of *Patient-Centred IVF: Bioethics and Care in a Dutch Clinic* (2016).

SANDRA P. GONZÁLEZ-SANTOS is an independent researcher, coordinator of transdisciplinary research groups in the National Art Center, and Lecturer at the Universidad Iberoamericana and at the National Autonomous University of Mexico in the Bioethics program. She is the author of *A Portrait of Assisted Reproduction in Mexico: Scientific, Political, and Cultural Interactions* (2020).

RIIKKA HOMANEN is Academy Research Fellow in Gender Studies at Tampere University, Finland. Her research explores ethics and social relations, such as kin, class, gender, sexuality, and race/ethnicity, in reproduction. More recently her interests have particularly focused on reproductive outsourcing in the multi-billion-dollar transnational fertility industry and markets.

TSIPY IVRY is Professor of Anthropology and Chair of the Graduate Program in Medical and Psychological Anthropology at the University of Haifa. She conducts ethnographic research in Japan and Israel. Her research interests include local formations of reproductive responsibilities and reproductive decision making, rabbinically mediated assisted conception and postdiagnostic termination decisions in Israel, pregnancy and obstetrical care in the aftermath of earthquakes in Japan, the implementation of NIPT, and the Japanese style of genetic counseling. She is the author of a comparative double ethnography, *Embodying Culture: Pregnancy in Japan and Israel* (2010).

VENETIA KANTSA is Professor of Anthropology, Director of the Laboratory of Family and Kinship, and Chair in the Department of Social Anthropology and History, University of the Aegean, Greece. Her research focuses on lesbian (in)visibility, same-sex families, new forms of parenthood, kinship in the context of assisted reproduction, interrelations among kin, medical technology, law and religion, and relations between human and nonhuman entities. She is author or coauthor of two books, including *Out of Body, Out of Home: Assisted Reproduction, Gender, and Family in Greece* (2015) and editor or coeditor of six books, including *(In)Fertile Citizens: Anthropological and Legal Challenges of Assisted Reproduction Technologies* (2015).

NITZAN PERI-ROTEM is Senior Lecturer in the Department of Social and Political Sciences, Philosophy, and Anthropology, University of Exeter. Her research involves the ways in which fertility patterns are shaped by social and cultural factors, as well as inequalities in accessing assisted reproductive treatment and other aspects of reproductive health. Her recent projects include examination of the role of health and lifestyle factors in explaining fertility differences by education.

ROBERT PRALAT is Research Associate at THIS Institute in the Department of Public Health and Primary Care at the University of Cambridge. His research focuses on how people respond to cultural changes and advances in medicine that enable them to become parents, with a particular focus on sexual minorities and men living with HIV.

SHARMILA RUDRAPPA is Professor and Chair of Sociology at the University of Illinois, Chicago. Her research focuses on race and migration, markets in assisted reproductive services, and medical sociology. She is author of two award-winning books, *Ethnic Routes to Becoming American: Indian Immigrants and the Cultures of Citizenship* (2004) and *Discounted Life: The Price of Global Surrogacy in India* (New York University Press, 2015).

MARCIN SMIETANA is an Affiliated Lecturer in the Reproductive Sociology Research Group (ReproSoc) at the University of Cambridge, where he was previously a Senior Research Associate. He holds the post of Research Fellow at Ca' Foscari University of Venice within the European Research Council project "PregDaT." Currently he also holds the post of Postdoctoral Researcher at Queen Mary University of London and is an Affiliated Researcher with the AFIN-Barcelona research group at the Autonomous University of Barcelona. His research focuses on gay men who create families through surrogacy and adoption in the United Kingdom, the United States, and Spain. He adopts perspectives from the sociology of reproduction, queer kinships, queer reproductive justice, as well as race and whiteness studies.

SORAYA TREMAYNE is Founding Director of the Fertility and Reproduction Studies Group (FRSG) and Research Affiliate at the Institute of Social and Cultural Anthropology (ISCA), University of Oxford, and the former Director of International Gender Studies at the University of Oxford. Her research focuses on the politics of reproduction in Iran with a focus on religion, population policies, and assisted reproductive technologies. She is the author, editor, or coauthor of five books, including *Inconceivable Iran: To Reproduce or Not to Reproduce?* (2022).

LUCY VAN DE WIEL is a Lecturer and Postgraduate Research Director in Global Health and Social Medicine at King's College London. Her research focuses on the introduction of new reproductive technologies such as egg freezing, IVF, and embryo selection. She explores how these technologies give insight into broader developments within the sector, including the datafication of reproduction and the financialization of fertility. She also researches telemedical abortion in the post-*Roe* landscape. She has published an Open Access book on egg freezing called *Freezing Fertility: Oocyte Cryopreservation and the Gender Politics of Aging* (New York University Press, 2020).

SIGRID VERTOMMEN is Assistant Professor of Gender and Health Studies in the Sociology Department at the University of Amsterdam and a postdoctoral researcher at the Centre for Research on Culture and Gender at Ghent University. She conducts feminist research on the global politics of (assisted) reproductive technologies, including transnational surrogacy, egg donation, adoption, and other forms of "motherwork," in Israel/Palestine, Georgia, and Belgium. She is currently writing her book manuscript, *Fertility Frontiers: Israel/Palestine through the Lens of Assisted Reproduction* (forthcoming).

AYO WAHLBERG is Professor and Chair in the Department of Anthropology, University of Copenhagen. His research focuses broadly on the field of social studies of biomedicine, including work on traditional herbal medicine (in Vietnam and the United Kingdom), selective reproductive technologies (in China and Denmark), and health metrics (in clinical trials and global health). He is the author of the award-winning *Good Quality: The Routinization of Sperm Banking in China* (2018) and coeditor of *Selective Reproduction in the 21ˢᵗ Century* (2017).

ANDREA WHITTAKER is Professor of Anthropology in the School of Social Sciences, Monash University. Her research focuses on the study of global medical trade and mobility, oocyte mobilities in southern Africa, and reproductive travel and biotechnologies in the Asia Pacific, including issues of gender, religion, bioethics, and global regulation of the trade. She is the author and editor of six books, including *Thai in Vitro: Gender, Culture, and Assisted Reproduction* (2015) and *International Surrogacy as Disruptive Industry in Southeast Asia* (2018).

ABOUT THE EDITORS

SARAH FRANKLIN is Emeritus Professor of Sociology at the University of Cambridge, and the founding Director of the Reproductive Sociology Research Group (ReproSoc). Over four decades, her research has explored the social aspects of new reproductive and genetic technologies, as well as the history and culture of IVF. She has written and coauthored nine books and coedited five volumes, including *Biological Relatives: IVF, Stem Cells, and the Future of Kinship* (2013) and the 25th anniversary edition of *Embodied Progress: A Cultural Account of Assisted Conception* (2022).

MARCIA C. INHORN is the William K. Lanman Jr. Professor of Anthropology and International Affairs in the Department of Anthropology and the Whitney and Betty MacMillan Center for International and Area Studies at Yale University, where she has also served as Chair of the Council on Middle East Studies. Her research focuses on Middle Eastern gender, religion, and reproductive health issues, particularly the social impact of infertility and assisted reproductive technologies in Egypt, Lebanon, the United Arab Emirates, and Arab America. She is the author of six award-winning books on these subjects, including *The New Arab Man: Emergent Masculinities, Technologies, and Islam in the Middle East* (2012), and coeditor of fourteen additional volumes. Her newest book, *Motherhood on Ice: The Mating Gap and Why Women Freeze Their Eggs* (New York University Press, 2023), is based on a US National Science Foundation study of 150 American women who froze their eggs, primarily due to the absence of male partners.

INDEX

NOTE: Page references noted with an *f* are figures; Page references noted with a *t* are tables

abortion: access to, 207; Arab families, 38; in China, 126; laws, 38; Middle East, 42; selective, 30

abundance, natural, 357

abundant diversity, 354–358

access: to abortion, 207; to ARTs in sub-Saharan Africa, 240–241; to citizenship, 78; to fertility clinics, 98

acquisition of children *(apoktisi pedion)*, 67

active pursuit of pregnancy *(ninkatsu)*, 28, 48, 49, 62; birth of, 52–57; in practice, 58–61

activism: orchard revivals in (Great Britain), 364–369 *(see also* orchard revivals in [Great Britain]); quiet, 348; reproductive justice (RJ) movement, 5

adoption, 77, 78

affordability, 225. *See also* costs; of in vitro fertilization (IVF), 8

Africa: batching (clinical work for mobility), 245–250; clinicians and mobile knowledge, 242–243; fly-in fly-out (FIFO) clinical staff, 243–245; HIV+ status in, 247; interviews, 241–242; mobile reproductive labor, 238–240; sub-Saharan, 238; in vitro fertilization (IVF) in, 238

agroecology, 354

Ahemmed, Baiju P., 246

Ahmadinejad, Mahmoud, 189

Ahmed, Sara, 20, 78

AIDS, 112, 113

Aitken, Robert John, 210

Algeria, 31, 32

Alibaba, 136

altruistic surrogacy, 106, 111*f,* 254, 266–268. *See also* surrogacy

Amin, Samir, 341

Amini, Mahsa, 195

Anthropocene, 282, 359

antisemitism, 157. *See also* Israel

anxieties of fertility (Finland), 280–281

anxiety, fertility, 2. *See also* fertility

apoktisi pedion (acquisition of children), 67

Apple Days (UK), 367–369, 374

apples, 365, 366*f,* 367, 377; cider, 377; flowering cycles of, 370; varieties of, 368. *See also* orchard revivals in (Great Britain)

Application of Methods of Medically Assisted Reproduction, 71

apps, fertility, 3

Apricity, 228

Arab families: abortion and, 38; assisted reproductive technologies (ARTs), 36*t;* balancing families, 43; contraception, 33–35; demographics, 33; fertility and, 29, 31*t,* 32*t;* fertility decline, 31–33; reproductive changes in, 144; selective technologies and, 37–41; technological convergence, 29–31, 41–43 *(see also* technological convergence); in vitro fertilization (IVF), 35–37

Aristotle University of Thessaloniki, 70
armed conflict, 14
Arthrosphaera genus, 335
artificial intelligence (AI), 229, 232.
   See also automation
Asia, 42; pursuit of pregnancy in Japan,
   47–49. *See also* Japan
assisted reproduction (Israel), 145–153
assisted reproductive technologies
   (ARTs), 1, 3, 27, 30; access to in sub-
   Saharan Africa, 240–241; in Africa,
   240 (*see also* Africa); Arab families
   and, 29, 36*t* (*see also* Arab families);
   boom of in Greece, 73–74; changing
   Greek families, 74–76; in China, 126
   (*see also* China); context of in Japan,
   57–61; development of in Japan,
   52–57; in Greece, 67–68, 70–73
   (*see also* Greece); in Iran, 192
   (*see also* Iran); in Israel, 142 (*see also*
   Israel); in Japan, 47, 309 (*See also*
   Japan); laws (Greece), 71; in Mexico,
   163–164, 170 (*see also* Mexico); post-
   ART labor in Georgia, 259–261; proximate determinants of fertility, 200,
   206–207; regulations, 173; welfare of
   children, 80
asylum, Iranians in United Kingdom
   (UK), 184
Australia, 223; mobile reproductive labor
   in, 239
automated cryopreservation technology,
   230
automation: automated efficiency,
   228–232; embryo incubation, 230; in
   vitro fertilization (IVF), 221, 228–232
autonomy, patient, 233
awareness, fertility, 18
Azarashvili, Zurab, 266

backwardness, trope of, 125, 126, 128
balancing families, 43
barbasco (wild yam), 166

bare branches (*guang gun;* 光棍), 127,
   134–135
batching (clinical work for mobility),
   245–250
behaviors: fertility, 17; in-fertilities, 17;
   sexual, 11
best interests of the child, 79–80
Billari, Francesco, 10
bio-conscious community groups, 371–374
biodiversity (in London, England),
   348–350; abundant diversity, 354–358;
   COVID-19, 351; meaning of seeds,
   350–354
Biodiversity Action Plan (2009), 365
bioethics, 72
biological parenthood, queer families, 95
biology, fertility in the natural world, 5
biomedical factors and fertility, 209
biotechnological developments, 68
birthing bee (*synnytystalkoot),* 281
birth rates, 10, 11; decline in births (Israel),
   145; in Japan, 50; pledging to boost
   (China), 129
bisexual: clinically assisted reproduction,
   93; identifying as, 87
Blake, Judith, 199, 200, 201, 202, 203, 204,
   205, 210, 213
bodily constitution *(taishitsu),* 49
Boivin, Jacky, 205
Bongaarts, John, 202, 210, 211, 215
Bongaarts's model, 203, 204, 205, 210.
   See also proximate determinants of
   fertility
Bourdieu, Pierre, 334
Braidotti, Rosi, 130
breadwinning housewives (Georgia), 260.
   See also surrogacy
Briggs, Laura, 4, 274
broken windows theory (Kelling and
   Wilson), 336
brokers, fertility, 2
Brown, Louise, 35, 36, 70
business decisions, 227, 228, 231

Cambridge Botanical Garden, 368
Cameroon, 242; fly-in fly-out (FIFO)
    clinical staff, 244. *See also* Africa
Campaign for the Regulation of the
    Family (Iran), 187
Canaka, Vasso, 77
capitalism, 142, 359
carbon emission, 15
career women, egg freezing technologies,
    129
Carlos, Monica, 75
Catholicism, 163, 177
Caucasus Barometer, 259
Cerro Corona mine (Peru), 293
Chalkidou-Chalkidis, Aspa-Pako, 78
Changing In-Fertilities Project (CIFP),
    15–19, 210
Chernobyl accident (Russia), 319, 320
childbirth in Japan, 310, 311–313. *See also*
    Japan
child is a gift *(sazukarimono),* 49
childlessness, 147; involuntary
    childlessness in Iran, 192–194
children: Arab families, 32 (*see also*
    Arab families); best interests of
    the child, 79–80; decline in births
    (Israel), 145; desire for parenthood,
    94, 95; health, 42; involuntary
    childlessness in Iran, 192–194; queer
    families, 86, 87, 88, 90–93 (*see also*
    queer families)
"Children Are Joy, Children Are Bless-
    ing," 147
China, 4; bare branches *(guang gun;* 光
    棍), 127, 134–135; Communist Party,
    129; COVID-19 in, 128; DINKs *(dīngke
    yizú;* 丁克一族), 127, 136–137; elderly
    populations in, 129, 130; lack of births,
    126; leftover women *(sheng nu;* 剩
    女), 127, 131–133; mating gaps in, 131,
    135; one child policy, 125, 211 (*see also*
    one child policy [China]); overview of
    fertility figures, 128–130; populations

in, 136; three-child policy, 127, 130–137;
    two-child policy, 126
Chown, Vicky, 351, 352
chuño (dehydrated potato), 303
cider, 377. *See also* orchard revivals in
    (Great Britain)
cideruk.com, 375
circle of care (Kimberly Theidon), 302
citizenship, reproductive, 69
clean mining, 297, 298. *See also* mining
    in Peru
climate change, 350. *See also* biodiversity
    (in London, England)
clinicians and mobile knowledge, 242–243
Cobble, Dorothy Sue, 267, 269
coffee, 330f, 332f, 333f; disarticulations,
    341–344; disintegration, 336–340; in
    India, 329–336 (*see also* India)
coffee berry borer *(Hypothenemus ham-
    pei),* 333f
Cold War, 166
collaboration, 225
collapse of demographics, 128
Collard, Rosemary-Claire, 359
colonialism, 14, 337. *See also* India
commercial surrogacy, 254, 266–268.
    See also surrogacy
commodification, stable, 357
*The Common Ground: A Place for Nature
    in Britain's Future?* (Mabey), 372,
    372f, 373
Communist Party (China), 129
conception, 16; in Japan via IVF, 52; quest
    for, 383
condoms, 169. *See also* contraception
congenital anomalies, fetuses with, 29
Constantini, Naama, 151
consumerism, 168, 171
contamination, *chuño* (dehydrated
    potato), 303
contraception, 27; Arab Families, 33–35;
    in China, 126; methods, 34; in Mexico,
    167

costs: altruistic surrogacy, 111f; rising costs of surrogacy, 112–116; of surrogacy, 105, 106, 107, 108, 108f, , 109–112; in vitro fertilization (IVF), 8, 110f, 225, 241

County Council of South Cambridgeshire, 365

COVID-19, 5, 9, 10; biodiversity (in London, England), 349, 351; in China, 128; fertility and, 9; in India, 341; in Israel, 156; in Peru, 296

Croll, Elisabeth, 42

crows, 356

cryopreservation, 70

C-sections, 57; surrogacy, 265. *See also* pregnancy

cycles, birth, 11

databases, 273–275. *See also* population databases (Finland)

data-driven digital economy issues, 275. *See also* Finland

data economies (Finland), 286. *See also* Finland

Davis, Kingsley, 199, 200, 201, 202, 203, 204, 205, 210, 213

decision making, 231

decline in fertility: of Arab families, 31–33, 31t, 32t; in Iran, 183

de-commodifying reproductive transactions, 227

Deda, Kartlis, 254, 255f

deforestation (in India), 337

de Gortari, Carlos Salinas, 177

dehydrated potato *(chuño),* 303

Demographic Center (Israel), 143

demographics, 10, 11–15; Arab families and, 33; collapse of, 128; Finland, 274; Greece, 73, 75; Iran, 185–190; Japan, 52; Jews as demographic threat, 143; proximate determinants of fertility, 199–200 (*see also* proximate determinants of fertility); statistical modeling, 207–292

Dempsey, Jessica, 359

DEMUS–Women's Rights Advocacy Group, 293

Deng Xiaoping, 125

Department of Social Anthropology and History at the University of the Aegean, 69

designer babies, 57, 128

determinants of fertility, 199–200. *See also* proximate determinants of fertility

DINKs (*dīngke yizú;* 丁克一族), 127, 136–137

disarticulations (India), 341–344

disasters, 309. *See also* Japan; vulnerabilities (in Japan)

Discounted Life: The Price of Global Surrogacy in India (Rudrappa), 327

discrimination, 74

disintegration of coffee, 336–340

disorientation, feeling of, 94, 95

diversity, 368. *See also* biodiversity (in London, England)

divorce, 49, 75. *See also* families; marriage

Dobbs v. Jackson Women's Health Organization (2022), 5

documentation of destruction of Great Britain countryside, 373

Dow, Katherine, 301

earthquakes: ecosystem model of maternity, 313–316; in Japan, 309 (*see also* Japan); moral panic after, 316–321; Oomachi's birth story (Japan), 311–313

East of England Apples and Orchard Project (EEAOP), 365

Echeverría, Luis, 165

economics: downturns, 9

economies: coffee (*see* coffee); in India, 327–329; in-fertile, 219–220

ecosystem model of maternity, 313–316

education: and fertility, 212f; in Finland, 277

educational attainment (Jewish women), 150, 150*f*

efficiency: automated, 228–232; fertility, 18 (*see* fertility efficiency); scalar, 222–228, 235

egg donors, 3, 58, 70; queer families and, 90

egg freezing, 7, 133, 230, 233; LGBTQ+, 233, 234; technologies, 129; in United Kingdom (UK), 230; in United States, 230

Egypt, 32, 35

elderly populations (China), 129, 130

Elson, Diane, 257

embryologists, 227

embryos: incubation, 230; models, 16; transferring, 246; in vitro fertilization (IVF), 29

Endangered Daughters: Discrimination and Development in Asia (Croll), 42

England, 87; orchard revivals in (Great Britain), 364–367 (*see also* orchard revivals in [Great Britain]). *See also* United Kingdom (UK)

environmentalism, 56

environments: in-fertile, 291–292; maternal, 312

epistemic defects, 334

Erlich, Anne, 328

Erlich, Paul, 328

Essay on the Principle of Population (Malthus), 328

ethics (Finland), 277

Ethiopia, 242. *See also* Africa

ethnonationalism, 14

eugenics (Finland), 278–280

Europe, 10; automated cryopreservation technology, 230; IVF Surveillance Consortium (IEC), 71; reprohubs, 68; as a world force, 155

European IVF Surveillance Consortium (IEC), 71

European Social Fund, 69

European Society of Human Reproduction and Embryology (ESHRE), 70

European Union (EU), divorces in, 75

Europe Rainbow Map and Index (ILGA-Europe 2023), 76

Even, Geula, 153, 154*f*

exports (Peru), 297. *See also* Peru

extractivism. *See* reproductive extractivism (Peru)

families: Arab (*see* Arab families); best interests of the child, 79–80; changing Greek, 74–76; fertility treatments in Japan, 49–52; formations in Japan, 49–52 (*see also* Japan); gay couple and straight surrogacy, 105–109; *gran familia Mexicana* (great Mexican family), 165, 176; heterosexual, 27; in-fertile, 27; models in Finland, 285; non-normative, 57; nuclear heterosexual family model, 81; process of creating, 87, 88; queer families in Great Britain, 86, 87–88 (*see also* queer families); traditional family models (Greece), 75, 76

family balancing, 41

Family Federation of Finland, 278, 280

family planning, 33. *See also* contraception; in China, 125, 126, 128 (*see also* China); investments, 171; in Iran, 191; methods, 34; Mexico, 166–168

fatherhood: Lebanese men and, 35; queer families, 87, 88 (*see also* queer families)

*fatwa*s, 39

feedback, 224

female empowerment (Iran), 189

feminism, 1; in India, 328, 329; in Iran, 184; Marxist feminists, 258, 261; science and technology studies (STS), 256

feminist anthropologists, 13

feminization of reproductive politics, 184

FemTech, 18

(In)Fertile Citizens study (2012-15), 69

fertility, 1, 2; accessing clinics, 98; anxieties of fertility (Finland), 280–281; anxiety, 2; in apple orchards, 369 (*see also* orchard revivals in [Great Britain]); apps, 3; Arab decline, 31–33, 31*t*, 32*t*; Arab families and, 29 (*see also* Arab families); awareness, 18; behaviors, 17; biodiversity (in London, England), 350 (*see also* biodiversity [in London, England]); biomedical factors and, 209; brokers, 2; control, 1; COVID-19 and, 9; decline, 1; decline in fertility in Iran, 183, 194–195; demographics, 11–15; destinations, 73; drivers of change, 6; education and, 212*f*; efficiency, 18; fertility-protection campaigns (Great Britain), 364, 365; free fertility treatments, 192; goals, 103; internetization, effect on, 10; investments, 223; in Iran, 182–184 (*see also* Iran); in Israel, 153–159; Jewish women in Israel, 148*f*; labor, 18; lack of births in China, 126; marketing, 8; marketization of, 3, 221; in Mexico, 163–164 (*see also* Mexico); in the natural world, 5; planning, 7, 18; preservation, 233 (*see also* egg freezing); presumed-to-be-fertile women, 8; private equity–funded groups, 226; proximate determinants of, 199–200 (*see also* proximate determinants of fertility); rates in Greece, 76; rates in Japan, 51*f*; remodeling, 6–11; replacement, 30; situated, 200; situating, 17; social changes and, 48; socioeconomic factors and, 209; spreadsheet, 103–105 (*see also* spreadsheet fertility); transitions, 255 (*see also* surrogacy); treatments, 47, 133; treatments in Japan, 49–52; ultra-low, 28; valor of, 384; value, 3, 18

fertility efficiency, 221–222; automated efficiency, 228–232; scalar efficiency, 222–228, 235; treatment, 232–235

fertility figures (China), 125; overview of, 128–130; three-child policy (China), 130–137

fertility rates: of Arab families, 29 (*see also* Arab families); in Finland, 273; in Israel, 149, 151*t*, 158

fertility regimes, 182, 185. *See also* Iran

fertility-trap, 211

fertilizers (India), 331

fertinomics, 3, 17, 103, 219

fetal reduction, 29, 30, 37

fetuses with congenital anomalies, 29

Final Solution (Hitler), 152

Finland: anxieties of fertility, 280–281; demographics, 274; education in, 277; eugenics, 278–280; fertility rates in, 273; homogeneity, data, and politics, 281–283; marketing, 276; population databases, 273–275 (*see also* population databases [Finland]); reproductive injustice in, 283–285; repropolitical anxieties, 280–281

Finnish data landscape, 275–278. *See also* population databases (Finland)

Finnish Sámi populations, 282, 283

Finns Party, 281

f-kyū (female leave), 56

flowering cycles (apples), 370. *See also* orchard revivals in (Great Britain)

fly-in fly-out (FIFO) clinical staff, 239, 242, 243–245

food: food chain, 15; security, 357; sovereignty, 354

Ford Foundation, 166

Former Soviet Union (FSU), 147, 148, 148*f*

Foucault, Michel, 383

Franklin, Sarah, 103, 118, 350

free fertility treatments, 192

free trade agreements, 168

freezing eggs. *See* egg freezing

frozen-thawed embryo transfer (FET), 51*f*

fruitility activism, 365. *See also* orchard revivals in (Great Britain) fruitility value, 369–371

Fujimoru, Alberto, 297

Fukushima accident (Japan), 319

funin treatments, 54

future families, envisioning, 89

Gambino, Evelina, 259

gametes (bioscapes), 240

Gammeltoft, Tine, 30

gay: clinically assisted reproduction, 93; identifying as, 87; queer families (*see* queer families); rights, 76, 77

gay-father families: gay couple and straight surrogacy, 105–109; infertility, 107; researching, 103–105; spreadsheet fertility (*see* spreadsheet fertility); surrogacy costs, 109–112; in vitro fertilization (IVF), 104

gay men, 3, 87; study of gay fatherhood, 89. *See also* queer families

Gaza, 4; October Hamas attack, 160

General Secretariat of Research and Technology, 69

genetic disorders, 29, 37, 43; prevention of, 39 (*see also* preimplantation genetic diagnosis [PGD])

genetic isolation, 276

genetic testing, preimplantation, 223

genocide, 4

George, Babu P., 73

Georgia: global fertility chains, 258; housewifization of surrogates, 260, 261–265; post-ART labor in, 259–261; privatization of healthcare in, 259; prohibition of commercial surrogacy, 266–268; reproductive worker's inquiry of surrogacy, 257–259; surrogacy in, 254–257

Georgian Public Service Development Agency, 255

Ghana, 242. *See also* Africa

Gietel-Basten, Stuart, 138, 207

Gillis, John, 89

Ginsburg, Faye, 12, 14, 17

Giraud, Eva, 359

global fertility chains, 256; Georgia, 258; Israel, 258; Palestine, 258

globalization, 168–171

Global North, 243

Global South, 341

Glyphosate, 331

goals, fertility, 103

gold mining, 298. *See also* mining in Peru

Gold Ore Processing (Kappes/Manning), 298

Goldscheider, Calvin, 207

Google Babies, 2

Gordon, Avery, 274, 275

governance of women's reproductive choices, 56

grammars, in-fertility, 367

gran familia Mexicana (great Mexican family), 165, 176

Great Britain: gay-father families, 103 (*see also* gay-father families); orchard revivals in, 364–367; queer families in, 86, 87–88 (*see also* queer families). *See also* United Kingdom (UK)

"Great Replacement" theory, 4

Greece: ART laws, 71, 72; assisted reproduction in, 67–68; assisted reproductive technologies (ARTs), 70–73; best interests of the child, 79–80; boom of ART, 73–74; changing Greek families, 74–76; demographics, 73, 75; (In) Fertile Citizens study (2012-15), 69; fertility rates in, 76; nuclear heterosexual family model, 81; parenthood in, 78; reproductive heterosexism, 68, 76–79; repronational familialism, 68; traditional family models, 75, 76

Greek Family Law (1983), 74

Greenhalgh, Susan, 6, 12, 17, 19, 130, 200, 207

Green Revolution, 6, 355

greying Finland, 281. *See also* Finland
groups, private equity–funded fertility,
     226

Haaretz, 155
habitats, orchard revivals in (Great
     Britain), 371
The Handmaid's Tale (Atwood), 191
Haraway, Donna, 128
haunted records, 275. *See also* population
     databases (Finland)
health campaigns, 56
Hebrew University, 152
hereditary traits, 278
heroine mothers, 143
heteronormative families, 57, 58
heterosexual families, 27
heterosexual intercourse, unprotected,
     204
heterotopian ecologies, 350, 358–360.
     See also biodiversity (in London,
     England)
Higashio, Riko, 54, 55*f*
high fertility (Israel), 157
high-order multiple pregnancies
     (HOMPs), 29, 37
Hitler, Adolf, 152
HIV+ status, 112, 114, 169; in Africa, 247
Holocaust, 143, 155. *See also* Israel
home insemination, 110
homogeneity, data, and politics (Finland),
     281–283, 284
homosexuality, 86, 87, 88. *See also* gay;
     queer families
hope technology, 16
housewifization of surrogates (Georgia),
     260, 261–265
housing prices (Israel), 156
Huamanlozo, Rosa, 302
Hu Jiye, 137
Human Fertilization and Embryology
     Authority (HFEA), 112
human rights, 76, 274

hybrid seeds, 348, 355. *See also* seeds,
     saving
Hypothenemus hampei (coffee berry
     borer), 333*f*

iFertility, 103
incubation, embryos, 230
Independence Day (Israel), 153
independent clinics, 223
India: COVID-19 in, 341; disarticulations,
     341–344; disintegration, 336–340;
     economies in, 327–329; feminism in,
     328, 329; modernization in, 341; sur-
     rogacy, 257, 327; women workers in,
     329–336
Indian lace makers, 261
individualism, 356
in-fertilities, 2, 5, 7, 14; behaviors, 17;
     economies, 219–220; environments,
     291–292; families, 27; nations, 123–124;
     new reproductive order of, 383–386;
     situating, 17; uncertainty of, 11;
     vernaculars, 367
infertility, 1, 2; in the Arab Middle East,
     193; demographics, 11–15; in India,
     327–329 (*see also* India); LGBTQ+
     parents, 107; marketing, 8; measure-
     ments, 205–206; men, 37; in Mexico,
     164; social, 50; social changes and, 48;
     treating, 29
*Infertility around the Globe: New Thinking
     on Childlessness, Gender, and Repro-
     ductive Technologies* (Inhorn/van
     Balen), 13
infertility trap, 14
The Infertility Trap (Aitken), 210
inheritance, 71
Inhorn, Marcia C., 13, 129, 131, 193, 240, 256
insemination, 77, 110
intermediate variables, proximate
     determinants of fertility, 200–202
International Federation of Fertility
     Societies (IFFS), 70, 240

International Monetary Fund (IMF), 8
internetization, effect on fertility, 10
intracytoplasmic sperm injection (ICSI),
  37, 71; in Israel, 142 (*see also* Israel);
  numbers of neonate births, 51*f*
intrauterine device (IUD), 167
intrauterine insemination (IUI), 58, 233,
  234; queer families, 93
investments: family planning, 171; fertility, 223; return on investment (ROI),
  223, 225, 226, 235; in vitro fertilization
  (IVF), 224
investors (United Kingdom [UK]), 227
in vitro fertilization (IVF): add-on
  technologies, 221; affordability of, 8;
  in Africa, 238 (*see also* Africa); Arab
  families, 35–37; Arab families and, 29
  (*see also* Arab families); automation,
  221, 228–232; costs, 110*f*, 225, 241;
  embryos, 29; gay-father families, 104
  (*see also* gay-father families); growth
  of, 29; inception of, 1; investments,
  224; in Iran, 192 (*see also* Iran);
  Islamic support of, 36; in Israel,
  142 (*see also* Israel); marketing, 8;
  Middle East, 35; numbers of neonate
  births, 51*f*; queer families, 93; risks,
  234; scaling, 223; surrogacy, 256
  (*see also* surrogacy); United Kingdom (UK), 112
involuntary childlessness in Iran, 192–194
Iran: decline in fertility in, 183, 194–195;
  demographics, 185–190; family planning in, 191; feminism in, 184; fertility in, 182–184; involuntary childlessness in, 192–194; laws, 190; new
  antinatalist policies (1990–2011), 187;
  Pahlavi Dynasty (1925–1979), 186, 187;
  population according to censuses,
  188*t*; population policies of, 184–185;
  Qajar Dynasty (1785–1925), 185, 196;
  Theocratic Pronatalist Approach
  (1980), 186–187; total fertility rates

(TFRs) in, 183; ultraconservative pro-
  natalist policies (Iran; 2011–Present),
  189
Iranian Bureau of Women's Affairs, 189
Iran-Iraq War (1980-88), 187
Iran Open Data, 191
Iraq, 32
Islam, 29; support of IVF, 36. *See also*
  Arab families
Islamic Fiqh Council, 39
Islamic Organization for Medical Sciences, 39
Islamic Republic of Iran. *See* Iran
Islamic Revolution (1979), 186
Israel, 4; assisted reproduction, 145–153;
  childlessness in, 147; COVID-19 in,
  156; educational attainment (women),
  150*f*; fertility in, 153–159; fertility rates
  in, 149, 151*t*, 158; founding of, 142;
  global fertility chains, 258; high fertility in, 157; Holocaust, 155; October
  Hamas attack, 160; populations in,
  145; present and future, 153–159;
  reproduction in early years, 143–145;
  reproductive politics among Jews in,
  142–143; resilient pronatalism, 145–153;
  test-tube babies in, 145; total fertility
  rates (TFRs) in, 144*f*
IVF platform, 16
Ivry, Tsipy, 56

James, Selma, 258
Japan: active pursuit of pregnancy
  (*ninkatsu*), 48, 49; birth rates in, 50;
  context of ARTs in, 57–61; demographics, 52; development of ARTs in, 52–57;
  earthquakes in, 309; ecosystem model
  of maternity, 313–316; fertility rates in,
  51*f*; fertility treatments, 49–52; moral
  panic (after earthquakes), 316–321;
  Oomachi's birth story, 311–313, 321;
  pursuit of pregnancy in, 47–49;
  vulnerabilities in, 309–311

Japanese Ministry of Health, Labour, and Welfare, 318
Japan Society of Obstetrics and Gynecology (JSOG), 57, 58
Japaridze, Sopo, 259, 267
Jews in Israel, reproductive politics among, 142–143. *See also* Israel
Jing Song, 131
Jones, Howard, 70
Jones Institute Foundation in Reproductive Medicine, 70
Jordan, 32, 35
Juarez, Benito, 177
justice, reproductive justice (RJ) movement, 4, 5

Kappes, D. W., 298
Karanadze, Revaz Telia, 267
Kashani-Sabet, Firoozeh, 184
Katan, Hanna, 151, 152
keddah operations, 338
Khamenei, Ayatollah, 182
Khazali, Ensieh, 191
Khomeini, Ayatollah, 186, 187
Kindbody, 228
kinship, 71
Kuwait, 31
Kvernflaten, Birgit, 129

Lab of Family and Kinship Studies, 69
labor, fertility, 18
lack of births (in China), 126
land management (in India), 333
landscapes of infertility, 329
Landworkers' Alliance, 354
Lantana camara, 340
large-scale global industry (finances-capes), 240
Law 3089 (Greece - 2002), 77
laws: abortion, 38; in China, 126; commercial surrogacy (Georgia), 266–268; in Finland, 277; Iran, 190;

Reform Laws (Mexico), 177; surrogacy, 254 (*see also* surrogacy)
laws (Greece), 72; Application of Methods of Medically Assisted Reproduction, 71; assisted reproductive technologies (ARTs), 71; Greek Family Law (1983), 74; Law 3089 (Greece - 2002), 77
Lebanese men and fatherhood, 35
Lebanon, 30
leftover women (*sheng nu;* 剩女), 127, 131–133
legislation: in Finland, 277; surrogacy, 254 (*see also* surrogacy)
lesbians, 87, 88; clinically assisted reproduction, 93; identifying as, 87. *See also* queer families
LGBTQ+: egg freezing, 233, 234; in Mexico, 174; parents, 107
LGBTQI+, 18, 27, 28
Libya, 31, 32
Lloyd, Humphrey, 354, 356
London, England: abundant diversity, 354–358; biodiversity in, 348–350; heterotopian ecologies, 358–360
London Freedom Seed Bank, 349, 352, 357
loss of biodiversity, 350. *See also* biodiversity (in London, England)

Malthus, Thomas Robert, 328
Mammo, Laura, 119
"Manifesto for Abundant Futures" (Collard/Dempsey/Sundberg), 359
Manning, T. J., 298
Mantzavinos, Themis, 70
manufacturing maybe-babies, 229
Mao Zedong, 125
Maratou-Alibranti, Laura, 75
marketing: Finland, 276; in vitro fertilization (IVF), 8
marketization of fertility, 3, 221, 255, 256. *See also* commercial surrogacy

marriage: decline in marriage rates (Greece), 76; planning, 47; single men/women in Japan, 50

Marriage Market Takeover (2016), 132, 133*f*

Martin, Emily, 299

Marxism, 258, 261. *See also* feminism

maternal environments, 312

mating gaps in China, 131, 135

Mattingly, Cheryl, 310, 312, 321

maybe-babies, 229

measurements, infertility, 205–206

Medical Birth Register (Finland), 281

Meiji period (1868–1912), 49

men: birth of one son, 40; gay (*see* gay men); gay-father families (*see* gay-father families); infertility, 37; infertility treatments, 48; Lebanese men and fatherhood, 35; single men/women in Japan, 50; support of Arab women use of contraception, 34

Merrill-Crowe, 299

metals, mining, 299. *See also* mining in Peru

methods, contraception, 34

Mexican Constitution, 175

Mexican Council of Gynecologists and Obstetricians, 172

Mexican Medical Association of Reproductive Medicine (AMMR), 172

Mexican Revolution (1910–1917), 164

Mexican Social Security Institute, 165

Mexican World Trade Center, 170

Mexico, 342; assisted reproductive technologies (ARTs) in, 170; Catholicism, 163 (*see also* Catholicism); contraception in, 167; current reproductive agenda, 168–174; family planning, 166–168; fertility in, 163–164; globalization, 168–171; individual liberty in, 169; infertility in, 164; LGBTQ+ in, 174; neoliberalism, 168–171; *Puericultura* and *Esterilología* (1930s–1970s), 164–166; Reform Laws, 177; reproductive agenda reflections, 175–177; reproductive rights in, 175; social media in, 177; sterilization in, 166

Middle East: abortion, 42; assisted reproductive technologies (ARTs), 36*t*; infertility in, 193; in vitro fertilization (IVF), 35

Mies, Maria, 260, 267

mining in Peru, 296–298; reproductive metaphors in processes, 298–300. *See also* Peru

Ministry of Education (Japan), 319

Mitsotakis, Kyriakos, 67

mobile knowledge, clinicians and, 242–243

mobile reproductive labor, 238–240; in Australia, 239; batching (clinical work for mobility), 245–250; fly-in fly-out (FIFO) clinical staff, 239. *See also* Africa

models, embryo, 16

modernization (India), 341

moral panic (after earthquakes), 316–321

moral vulnerability (Cheryl Mattingly), 310, 312

mosaic habitats, 370

mosquitoes (India), 336, 337*f*

Mother Georgia (statue), 254, 255*f*

motherhood: new types of, 383; queer families, 86, 87, 88

Motherhood on Ice: The Mating Gap and Why Women Freeze Their Eggs (Inhorn), 131

Mothers (Xu 2013), 125

motherworkers, 267, 268. *See also* surrogacy

Mozambique, 242. *See also* Africa

multifetal pregnancy reduction (MFPR), 29, 37, 41. *See also* fetal reduction

multispecies reproductive justice framework, 282

Muña, Estanislao, 300, 301

mushrooms, 343*f*, 344*f*

Muslims, 36; in Iran, 186; women, 189.
See also Islam
Muslim World League, 39

Nagasaki atomic bomb (Japan), 319, 320
Nahman, Michal, 256
Namibia, 242; fly-in fly-out (FIFO) clinical staff, 244. See also Africa
Natality Committee (Israel), 143
National Authority for Medically Assisted Reproduction, 72
National Authority of Assisted Reproduction, 72
National Census (Iran), 187
National Health Service (NHS), 107, 112
National Sanitary Risk Commission (COFEPRIS), 172
National Water Agency (Peru), 301
natural abundance, 357
neoliberalism, 168–171, 176
new antinatalist policies (Iran; 1990–2011), 187
new Arab family, 33–35. See also Arab families
new reproductive order, 2, 19
new reproductive order of in-fertilities, 383–386
new reproductive technologies (NRTs), 13. See also assisted reproductive technologies (ARTs)
new world order, 240
ninkatsu (active pursuit of pregnancy), 28, 48, 49, 62; birth of, 52–57; in practice, 58–61
nonheterosexual forms of reproduction, 79
non-normative families, 57
Nordic welfare state citizenship, 275–278. See also Finland
North American Free Trade Agreement (NAFTA), 168, 170, 178
Not Infertility, but TGP Trying to Get Pregnant (Higashio), 54, 55f

nuclear heterosexual family model, 81
numbers of neonate births, 51f

October Hamas attack (Israel), 160
Office of the United Nations High Commission for Human Rights (OHCHR), 191
Oman, 31, 32
OmVed Gardens (London, England), 351
one-child (China), 125, 211
Oomachi's birth story (Japan), 311–313, 321
Orban, Viktor, 4
orchard revivals in (Great Britain), 364–367; activism, 367–369; bioconscious community groups, 371–374; fruitility value, 369–371; function of orchards, 374–379; habitats, 371
Organization for Economic Cooperation and Development (OECD), 142, 150
Orihuela Quequezana, Roberth, 300, 302, 303
ovarian hyperstimulation syndrome (OHSS), 246, 247

Pahlavi Dynasty (1925–1979), 186, 187
Palestine, 4, 134; global fertility chains, 258
Pande, Amrita, 257
pandemics, 9. See also COVID-19
Panhellenic Association of Doctors of Assisted Reproduction, 70
Papataxiarchis, Evthymios, 75
Paraquat-di-chloride, 331
Paraskou, Anastasia, 73
parenthood: in Greece, 78; queer families, 88–90 (see also queer families); questioning, 96–99
parenting rights, 87
Parthenium hysterophorus, 340
Pasivos Ambientales: Los Residuos de la Minería que Nadie Quiere Asumir

(Environmental Liabilities: The Mining Waste That No One Wants to Take Responsibility For [Queque-zana]), 300

paternity: legitimacy of gay, 98; queer families, 90

pathways to parenthood, 87

patient autonomy, 233

Patrizio, Pasquale, 223

Pavone, Vincenzo, 256

peasants (Peru), 297, 298, 301. *See also* Peru

Pediatric Neurosurgery (Tel Aviv Medical Center), 151

People's Trust for Endangered Species (PTES), 369, 370, 370*f*, 371–374

Peru: COVID-19 in, 296; mining in, 296–298; National Water Agency, 301; reproduction in a multispe-cies register, 300–304; reproductive grammar (Peru), 293–296; reproduc-tive metaphors in mining processes, 298–300

pesticides (India), 332. *See also* India

planning fertility, 7, 18

plantation economies, 337. *See also* India

policies, Iran population, 184–185. *See also* regulations

politics: among Jews in Israel, 142–143 (*see also* Israel); feminization of re-productive, 184; population databases (Finland), 273–275 (*see also* population databases [Finland])

Population Bomb (Erlich and Erlich), 328

Population Council (Mexico), 166

population databases (Finland), 273–275; anxieties of fertility (Finland), 280–281; eugenics, 278–280; Finnish data landscape and, 275–278; reproductive injustice in Finland, 283–285

Population Fund, United Nations (UN), 129

populations: assessing changes in, 9; in China, 136; increasing, 4; Israel, 142; in Israel, 145; lack of births in China, 126; population policies of Iran, 184–185

Porcon, Granja, 294

pregnancy, 3. *See also* fertility; infertility; active pursuit of pregnancy *(ninkatsu)*, 48, 49; conception in Japan via IVF, 52; ecosystem model of maternity, 313–316; pursuit of, 28; pursuit of in Japan, 47–49; surrogacy, 261–265 (*see also* surrogacy); teenage, 171

preimplantation genetic diagnosis (PGD), 29, 30, 37, 38, 39, 41, 42, 43

preimplantation genetic testing, 223

Prelude, 231

preservation, fertility, 233. *See also* egg freezing

presumed-to-be-fertile women, 8

Princeton European Fertility Project, 6

private equity–funded fertility groups, 226

processes, 224; *chuño* (dehydrated potato), 303; mining in Peru, 299 (*see* mining in Peru)

process of creating families, 87, 88. *See also* queer families

Progyny, 228

prohibition of commercial surrogacy, 266–268

pronatalism, 145–153, 158, 160

proximate determinants of fertil-ity, 199–200; assisted reproductive technologies (ARTs), 200, 206–207; beyond statistical modeling, 207–212; criticisms of, 202–207; intermediate variables, 200–202

Puericultura and *Esterilología* (Mexico; 1930s–1970s), 164–166

pursuit of pregnancy, 28, 47–49

Qajar Dynasty (1785–1925), 185, 196

Qatar, 32

quality of life, 364
queer families: biological parenthood, 95; children, 90–93; egg donors, 90; gay-father families, 103–105 (*see also* gay-father families); in Great Britain, 86, 87–88; navigating disorienting reproductive imaginations, 93–96; outcome and processes, 90–93; paternity, 90; questioning parenthood, 96–99; researching reproductive imaginations, 88–90; spreadsheet fertility, 103–105
questioning parenthood, 96–99
quiet activism, 348

racial hygiene, 278. *See also* eugenics
radioactivity, effects of, 319
Raisi, Ebrahim, 190
Rapp, Rayna, 12, 14, 17
Reagan, Ronald, 13, 221
Reform Laws (Mexico), 177
Register of Congenital Malformations (Finland), 279
Register on Induced Abortions and Sterilizations (Finland), 280
Register on Infectious Disease (Finland), 280
Rego, Sonia, 351, 352
regulations: assisted reproductive technologies (ARTs), 173; Iran population policies, 184–185
Reinis, Kia, 203
remodeling fertility, 6–11
replacement fertility, 30
repro-activity, 28, 47, 48
reproduction: feminist perception of, 1; independence of, 296; nonheterosexual forms of, 79
reproductive actors (ethnoscapes), 240
reproductive cause and effect, 2
reproductive citizenship, 69
reproductive extractivism (Peru), 295, 300–304. *See also* Peru

reproductive grammar (Peru), 293–296. *See also* Peru
reproductive heterosexism, 67–68, 76–79; assisted reproductive technologies (ARTs), 70–73; best interests of the child, 79–80; boom of ART, 73–74; changing Greek families, 74–76; (In)Fertile Citizens study (2012-15), 69
reproductive imaginations, 28, 86, 87–88; navigating disorienting, 93–96; outcome and processes, 90–93; questioning parenthood, 96–99; researching, 88–90
reproductive injustice in Finland, 283–285
reproductive justice (RJ) movement, 4, 5
reproductive politics: feminization of, 184; population databases (Finland), 273–275 (*see also* population databases [Finland])
reproductive rebellion, 184, 195–196
reproductive rights (Mexico), 175
reproflows, 256
reprohubs, 68
repronational familism, 68
repronationalism, 123
repropolitical anxieties, 274, 280–281
reproscapes, 219, 256
researching: gay-father families, 103–105; reproductive imaginations, 88–90
resilient pronatalism (Israel), 142, 145–153
restricted access to abortion, 207
return on investment (ROI), 223, 225, 226, 235
rhythm methods, 58
Rights of the Child (UN), 79
Rinne, Antti, 281
rising costs of surrogacy, 112–116
risks in vitro fertilization (IVF), 234
Rivera, Flora, 301
Robertson's Food Products, 375*f*
Rockefeller Foundation, 166
Roe v. Wade (1973), 5
Roma populations (Finland), 282

Rosen, Kath, 375
Roseneil, Sasha, 97
Rose Revolution (1991), 259
Rotkirch, Anna, 207
Rudrappa, Sharmila, 327
Ruppin, Arthur, 143
rural rituals (UK), 374. *See also* orchard revivals in (Great Britain)
Russia, 4
Rwanda, fly-in fly-out (FIFO) clinical staff, 244

Saakashvili, Mikheil, 259
Safe Lunch Box Movement, 320
same-sex rights, 76. *See also* queer families
Sámi populations (Finland), 282, 283
Sasser, Jake, 128
Saudi Arabia, 31, 32, 35
sazukarimono (child is a gift), 49
scalar efficiency, 222–228, 235
scaling up in vitro fertilization (IVF), 223
science and technology studies (STS), 256
seasonality, 11
security, food, 357
seeds, saving, 348–350. *See also* biodiversity (in London, England); heterotopian ecologies, 358–360; hybrid seeds, 355; London Freedom Seed Bank, 349; meaning of seeds, 350–354; swaps, 349, 355
Seed Saving Network, 351, 352
seeking surrogacy overseas, 114
selective abortion, 30
selective reproduction, 30
selective reproductive technologies (SRTs), 30, 126. *See also* China
selective technologies (Arab families), 37–41
sex, frequency of, 205
sex selection, 39, 40, 42
sexual activity, 204–205
sexual behavior, 11

sexually transmitted diseases (STDs), 171
sexual orientation, 87; identifying, 87; in Israel, 147
sharing best practices, 225
shifting reproductive agendas, 163, 164. *See also* Mexico
Shoal Creek, Austin Texas, 342*f*
Shoard, Marion, 372, 372*f*, 373
short-term trends, 10
Simeonidou, Charis, 75
Simpson, Bob, 241
Single Man (2010), 134
situated fertility, 200
situating fertility, 17
Smart, Carol, 89
Sobotka, Tomáš, 10, 207
social good (of body politic), 74
social infertility, 50
socialism, 142
social media (Mexico), 177
social policy, 153
social science research, 88–90
socioeconomic factors: and fertility, 209; Finland, 276
soil depletion, 15
Solidarity Network, 258, 259, 267
son selection, 40
sorting maybe-babies, 229
South Africa, 242; fly-in fly-out (FIFO) clinical staff, 244. *See also* Africa
South African Society for Reproductive Medicine and Gynaecological Endoscopy (SASREG), 242
South America, Peru, 296. *See also* Peru
Spain, 73
sperm donors, 112, 113
spousal equality (in Greece), 74
spreadsheet fertility, 103–105; gay couple and straight surrogacy, 105–109; overseas surrogacy, 115*f*; rising costs, 112–116; surrogacy costs, 109–112
Sri Lanka, 241
stable commodification, 357

stakeholders, 13

standardization, 235

statistical modeling, 207–212

Steptoe, Patrick, 70

Stergiou, Katerina, 78

sterility, 205

sterilization, 278–280; in China, 126; in Mexico, 166. *See also* eugenics

straight surrogacy, 106. *See also* surrogacy

Strathern, Marilyn, 13, 80

sub-Saharan Africa, 238; access to ARTs in, 240–241; batching (clinical work for mobility), 245–250; fly-in fly-out (FIFO) clinical staff, 243–245; HIV+ status in, 247; interviews, 241–242. *See also* Africa

Sudan, 32

Sundberg, Juanita, 359

Sunni Muslims, 36, 37. *See also* Islam

surrogacy, 58; altruistic, 254; costs of, 105, 106, 107, 108, 108*f*, 109–112; gay couple and straight, 105–109; in Georgia, 254–257 (*see also* Georgia); house-wifization of surrogates (Georgia), 260, 261–265; India, 257, 327; prohibition of commercial, 266–268; reproductive worker's inquiry of, 257–259; rising costs, 112–116; seeking overseas, 114; traditional, 106

survivors, Holocaust, 155

synnytystalkoot (birthing bee), 281

Syria, 31, 32

Tadashiku Kowagaru (Yamashita), 319

taishitsu (bodily constitution), 49

Tal, Alon, 153

Tamil laborers, 338

Tanzania, 242, 244. *See also* Africa

Tarlatzis, Vassilis, 70

Tatar populations (Finland), 282

technological convergence, 29–31; Arab families, 41–43 (*see also* Arab families); Arab fertility decline, 31–33

teenage pregnancy, 171

testing, preimplantation genetic, 223

test-tube babies, 35; in Israel, 145. *See also* in vitro fertilization (IVF)

Texas (United States), 342, 343, 343*f*

Thatcher, Margaret, 13, 221

Theft of the Countryside (Shoard), 372, 372*f*

Theidon, Kimberly, 302

Theocratic Pronatalist Approach (1980), 186–187

Third International Population Conference (1974), 186

Thompson, Charis, 1

three-child policy (China), 127, 130–137

Tianhan Gui, 133

timing (on birth totals), 11

TMRW automated cryopreservation technology, 230

Tonkawa Indian communities, 341

total fertility rates (TFRs), 31, 32, 202; in Iran, 183; in Israel, 144*f*

trade agreements, 168, 170, 178

tradfolk.com, 375

traditional Chinese medicines, 54

traditional family models (Greece), 75, 76

traditional surrogacy, 106, 111*f*. *See also* surrogacy

traits, hereditary, 278

transatlantic surrogacy arrangements, 114

transitions, fertility, 255. *See also* surrogacy

treatments: assisted reproductive technologies (ARTs), 50 (*see also* assisted reproductive technologies [ART]); fertility, 47, 133; fertility efficiency, 232–235; free fertility, 192; *funin*, 54; in vitro fertilization (IVF) (*see* in vitro fertilization [IVF])

trends, short-term, 10

Tronti, Mario, 258

two-child policy (China), 126, 127*f*. *See also* China

Uganda, 242. *See also* Africa

UK Orchard Network, 365

UK Orchard Project, 374, 375, 376, 377, 378*f*

ultraconservative pronatalist policies (Iran; 2011–Present), 189

ultra-low fertility, 28

United Arab Emirates (UAE), 30, 32, 40

United Kingdom (UK), 28; biodiversity in, 348–350 (*see also* biodiversity [in London, England]); costs of surrogacy, 105, 106; egg freezing, 230; gay couple and straight surrogacy, 105–109; gay-father families, 103 (*see also* gay-father families); investors, 227; Iranian asylum in, 184; National Health Service (NHS), 107, 112; navigating disorienting reproductive imaginations, 93–96; orchard revivals in, 365–367 (*see also* orchard revivals in [Great Britain]); private equity–funded fertility groups, 226; queer families, 86, 87, 88; queer family outcome and processes, 90–93; questioning parenthood, 96–99; researching reproductive imaginations, 88–90; rising costs of surrogacy, 112–116; spreadsheet fertility, 103–105

United Nations (UN), 8; Population Award (Iran), 187; Population Fund, 129; Rights of the Child, 79; World Fertility Survey, 200; *World Population Prospects,* 9

United States, 5; automated efficiency, 229; egg freezing technologies, 129, 230; Former Soviet Union (FSU) immigrants in, 147; Jewish community fertility rates, 151*t*; surrogacy in, 114; Texas, 342, 343, 343*f*

University of Athens, 70

UN Population Division Report (2021), 9

value, fertility, 3, 18

van Balen, Frank, 13

Varghese, Alex C., 246

vasectomies, 169. *See also* contraception

vernaculars, in-fertility, 367

Vienna Institute of Demography, 10

vulnerabilities (in Japan), 309–311; earthquakes, 309; ecosystem model of maternity, 313–316; moral panic (after earthquakes), 316–321; moral vulnerability (Cheryl Mattingly); Oomachi's birth story (Japan), 311–313, 321

Wahlberg, Ayo, 30

Wales, 87. *See also* United Kingdom (UK)

wars: Cold War, 166; Iran-Iraq War (1980-88), 187; in Israel, 145; Mexican Revolution (1910–1917), 164; October Hamas attack (Israel), 160; war crimes, 4

wassailing, 374. *See also* orchard revivals in (Great Britain)

weedicides, 331

welfare states (Finland), 275–278. *See also* Finland

Wellcome Trust, 15

Western Ghats of Karnataka (India), 337

Weston, Kath, 80

wild yam *(barbasco),* 166

withdrawal (contraception method), 34

Wojcicki, Anne, 231

Wojcicki, Susan, 231

Woman in the Body: A Cultural Analysis of Reproduction (Martin), 299

wombs, 327. *See also* pregnancy; surrogacy; women

women: agency (in Iran), 184; Arab, contraception, 33–35; Arab families, 32 (*see also* Arab families); in China, 126 (*see also* China); educational attainment, 150*f*; egg freezing technologies, 129; fetal reduction, 37; in India, 327 (*see also* India); infertility in Japan, 52; infertility treatments, 48; Jewish women reproductive practices, 150; men's control over bodies, 31; Muslims, 189; presumed-to-be-fertile, 8;

women (*cont.*)
    single men/women in Japan, 50; surrogacy (*see* surrogacy); workers in India, 329–336
worker-mothers (Georgia), 260
World Bank, 8
World Fertility Survey (UN), 200
World Health Organization (WHO), 8, 129
worldmaking, 128
World Population Prospects (UN), 9
World War II, 280
Wu Cangping, 125

Xi Jinping, 129
Xu Huijing, 125
Xu Zaozao, 133

Yamashita, Shunichi, 319
Yanacocha mine (Peru), 293
Yanagisako, Sylvia, 74
Yemen, 31, 32
Yingchun Ji, 131
Yoriko, Katsuma, 320

Zacharaki, Sofia, 67
Zambia, 242. *See also* Africa
Zionism, 143

www.ingramcontent.com/pod-product-compliance
Lightning Source LLC
Chambersburg PA
CBHW031137020426
42333CB00013B/414